The
Acupressure
Atlas

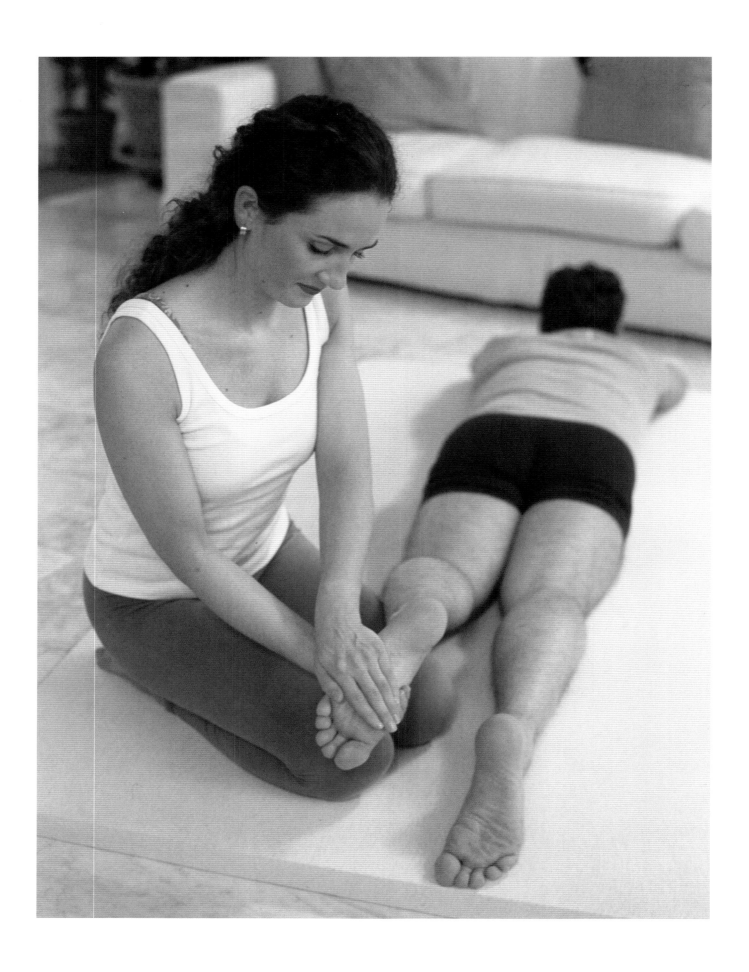

The Acupressure Atlas

Bernard C. Kolster, M.D., and
Astrid Waskowiak, M.D.

Translated from the German by Nikolas Win Myint

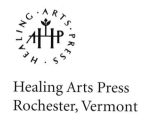

Healing Arts Press
Rochester, Vermont

Healing Arts Press
One Park Street
Rochester, Vermont 05767
www.HealingArtsPress.com

Healing Arts Press is a division of Inner Traditions International

Originally published in German under the title *Knaurs Atlas der Akupressur* by Verlagsgruppe Weltbild GmbH, Steinerne Furt 67, 86167 Augsburg
Sonderausgabe für Droemersche Verlagsanstalt Th. Knaur Nachf., München

First U.S. Edition published in 2007 by Healing Arts Press

Note to the reader: This book is intended as an informational guide. The remedies, approaches, and techniques described herein are meant to supplement, and not to be a substitute for, professional medical care or treatment. They should not be used to treat a serious ailment without prior consultation with a qualified health care professional.

Library of Congress Cataloging-in-Publication Data
Kolster, Bernard C.
 [Knaurs Atlas der Akupressur. English]
 The acupressure atlas / Bernard C. Kolster and Astrid Waskowiak ; translated from the German by Nikolas Win Myint.—1st U.S. ed.
   p. cm.
 "Originally published in German under the title Knaurs Atlas der Akupressur by Verlagsgruppe Weltbild GmbH."
 Includes bibliographical references and index.
 ISBN-13: 978-1-59477-207-8 (pbk.)
 ISBN-10: 1-59477-207-X (pbk.)
 ISBN-13: 978-1-59477-175-0 (hardcover)
 ISBN-10: 1-59477-175-8 (hardcover)
 1. Acupressure—Atlases. 2. Reflexology (Therapy)—Atlases. I. Waskowiak, Astrid. II. Title.
 RM723.A27K6513 2007
 615.8'222—dc22
                                                              2007018419

Printed and bound in India by Replika Press Pvt. Ltd.

10 9 8 7 6 5 4

Text layout by Priscilla Baker
This book was typeset in Minion, with Agenda used as a display typeface

Contents

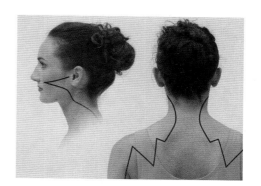

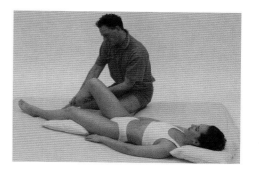

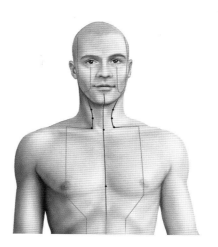

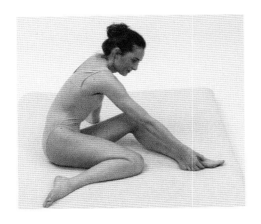

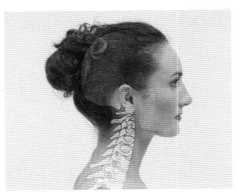

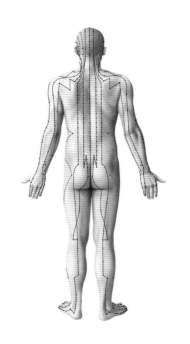

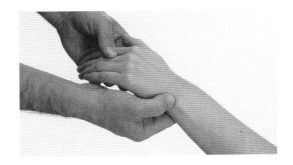

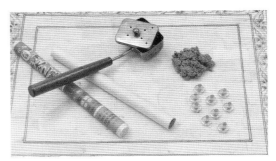

Preface

Do you frequently have trouble falling asleep? Do you suffer from a sensitive stomach, or is your neck frequently tense? The incidence of sensory ailments like these has been on the rise in Western countries over the years. However, despite the fact that many people suffer from them, these ailments are often accepted as facts of life. People who are chronically stressed do not find the time or the strength to look after their health and address the risks to it. The many medications that are widely available today seem to work reliably and without risks, but they are replacing our own responsibility for our health. For those who are not content to accept ailments as facts of life or to take medication on a regular basis, acupressure may offer a solution.

A component of traditional Chinese medicine, acupressure has the goal of regulating life energy and creating a harmonious balance in the body, which in turn will lead to stable health. Acupressure offers the possibility of taking our well-being into our own hands and looking after our own health. The effectiveness of acupressure is not limited to the prevention of illness. When our body's defensive systems fail, acupressure helps alleviate ailments and accelerates the healing process. Give your body the gift of correctly applied acupressure therapy, and you are giving it the attention and care that will keep you healthy. In fact, you will find that minor ailments like repeated colds or chronic pain will no longer leave you helpless.

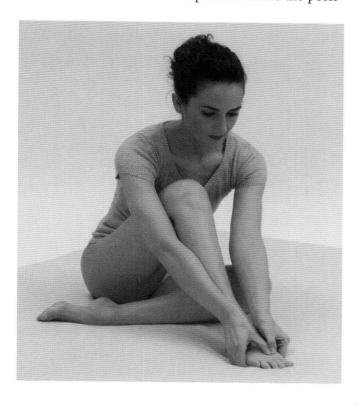

In this comprehensive guide you will find acupressure applications that have been specially compiled to help you address common ailments and illnesses or support an existing medical therapy. To optimize the utility of this book, look for useful information about the historical background, applications, and limitations of acupressure, as well as its proper application, in the first part of the book. It is important to read this part first to get a solid grounding in the principles and workings of acupressure. You are then ready to turn to the second part of the book, which offers individual applications to address illnesses. After this section, you will find information about wellness massages that you can use to quickly and effectively relax the entire body.

Wishing you good health,
Dr. Bernard Kolster

Introduction

Acupressure is a massage technique that originated in China; it is used to harmonize the body and to prevent or alleviate ailments and physiological disturbances.

Activating Body and Life Energies Naturally

Holistic is more than a slogan in today's society. When applied to our entire lifestyle, it means living in harmony with the environment and oneself. Only a well-balanced person can give his or her best in relationships and jobs. In today's Western medicine, holistic approaches aim to treat the individual, rather than the symptoms. People are feeling increasingly uncomfortable with technocratic medicine and treatment that is measured in minutes. For example, digestive problems are frequently subjected to extensive examinations that lead to nothing more than a diagnosis of a "sensitive stomach" or chronic gastritis. Often, no concrete cause for the symptoms is found, even though the suffering of the patient is real. What often follows is a therapy comprising medication to address the symptoms, and perhaps a few basic diet instructions. For patients, this is frequently an unsatisfactory situation, because the root cause is not identified or addressed.

A holistic health approach attempts instead to view the patient as a whole, rather than focusing on the specific symptoms. In this way the therapist can develop a comprehensive picture of the illness process. Very often a number of psychological factors cause the ailment at hand. Recognizing and treating these factors is an important precondition for a successful healing process. In addition, it is important to recognize that health and well-being are very much linked to personal responsibility. Those who rely on medication to relieve symptoms often experience rapid improvement at the onset of treatment, only to find that many of the symptoms soon return.

Acupressure is part of a fundamental healing system. *Acu* comes from Latin and means "point"; *pressure* is self-explanatory. In acupressure, certain points or zones of the body are pressed or massaged with the fingers. These pressure techniques are a component of a Chinese therapeutic massage called *tui na* (see page 11). This massage has ancient origins; it was even described in the *Huang Di Nei Jing*, a classic text of Chinese medicine that, remarkably, was written more than two thousand years ago by the legendary Yellow Emperor. It is likely that healing massages with acu-

In acupressure you locate precisely defined points on your body and massage or press them.

8

pressure were a predecessor to acupuncture, in which certain points are treated with very thin needles.

Equally surprising is the subtle knowledge that existed in this ancient time about the human body. The body in this tradition was described not only as a collection of organic functions but as an individual that formed part of the cosmos.

Preventive Approaches of Chinese Medicine

Chinese massage encompasses a lot more than simple massage techniques. Embedded in a philosophical holistic concept, it sees the individual as part of a larger whole. According to this thought, illnesses are the result of energy imbalances in the body. These energies can be brought out of balance through external factors such as cold, heat, wind, diet, and many other factors. Internal emotions can also cause energy imbalances in the individual and thus lead to illness. Most people are familiar with the consequences of greed, depression, pain, and fear on physical well-being. Such internal factors can have very negative consequences for our health. In a holistic health approach, the goal is to find the cause that led to the illness. Only when the cause is known can the actual illness be treated.

Indeed, Chinese medicine goes a step further: it aims to prevent illnesses by giving people the necessary tips for staying healthy. In the Western health concept, this equates to preventive medicine. Preventive medicine is gaining increasing attention in Western culture, in part for a series of very obvious reasons: health creates well-being and reduces costs to the health system for the provision of medical services, to name but two. Prevention is in the power of individuals: everyone is responsible for themselves and their well-being. And everyone today can inform themselves about any number of healing methods. For example, universities, community colleges, and community centers offer a range of health-related classes.

It is noteworthy that the preventive approach forms the basis of the Chinese understanding of health, which has developed over thousands of years. The job of Chinese healers in ancient times was to develop instructions for health, for which they were paid. In contrast, should a patient fall ill, treatment was free of charge. The effectiveness of a physician was judged in this sense: a good physician prevents illnesses from occurring, while a bad physician treats illnesses.

But the maintenance of good health, as indicated above, is also an individual responsibility. The ways and means by which individuals apply the instructions and tips offered by a healer are the deciding factor. Health is an active process that assumes that individuals will work for themselves. Acupressure offers a good, proactive means for taking our health into our own hands and maintaining our well-being. In addition, it is a good way to alleviate a wide range of minor ailments.

The following pages offer the basic information you will need to effectively and appropriately use acupressure.

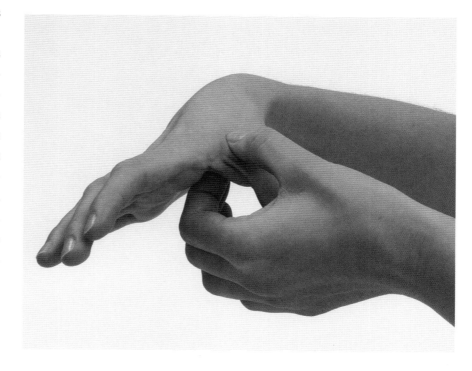

A range of pressure techniques are used for the different points.

The Basics of Acupressure

The Origins and Principles of Acupressure

The knowledge behind acupressure comes from China and is embedded in the overall structure of traditional Chinese medicine, which is one of the oldest medical systems in the world. The first comprehensive written text from traditional Chinese medicine dates to 2600 BC and incorporates the discussions of the legendary Yellow Emperor with his personal physicians about the causes of and treatment possibilities for illnesses. Since the late nineteenth century, traditional Chinese medicine has been practiced in Europe.

Traditional Chinese Medicine

When people talk about Chinese medicine today, the first thing that comes to mind is often acupuncture. In reality, traditional Chinese medicine is an interplay between a number of therapy forms that complement each other: acupuncture, movement therapy, massage, herbal medicine, and dietary principles are all embedded in a complex holistic system that sees the individual as part of a large, comprehensive system. The system of traditional Chinese medicine can be divided into external and internal therapy.

External Therapy

External therapy includes acupuncture, physical applications, and massage, as well as health-inducing exercises.

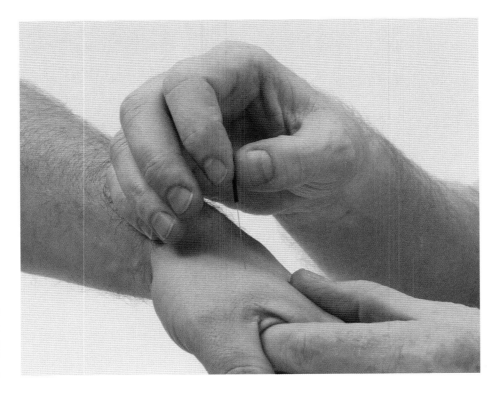

Acupuncture is based on the ancient knowledge of acupressure.

Acupuncture

Acupuncture is the component of traditional Chinese medicine that is best known in the West. Acupuncture is based on the concept that the human body contains a number of energy pathways, called meridians or channels (see page 32). Within these meridians circulates life energy, called *qi* (see page 20). At certain points around the body, this energy can be influenced by the insertion of thin needles. The insertion of the needles aims to direct qi in such a way that it is distributed optimally throughout the body.

Moxibustion

Moxibustion complements acupuncture. Here, the patient receives warmth, either directly through the heating of the acupuncture needles or indirectly through the warming of certain points or areas of the skin. The combination of acupuncture and moxibustion is called *zhen jiu,* which translates as "poking and burning." The application of warmth across an area is accomplished through the burning of mugwort. Before each application, the therapist has to decide whether warmth should be introduced via points or areas.

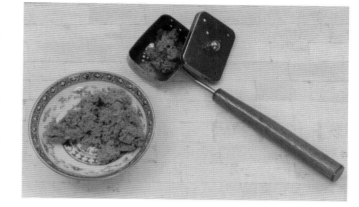

Mugwort is used for moxibustion. It is sometimes kept in a special moxa box during treatment.

Massage

Another external therapy is healing massage, called *tui na. Tui* means "to push" or "to stroke," and *na* means "to grasp" or "to knead." Tui na comprises a complex array of different massage grips that are chosen and applied based on the sensitivities and presented symptoms of the patient.

Like acupuncture, tui na has harmonizing effects on the circulation of qi. Although tui na is a complicated system with a number of different techniques, many grips and their effects can be compared to those of classic Western massage.

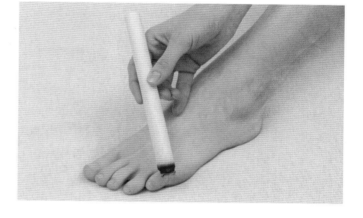

One variant of moxibustion is the use of a moxa cigar.

Breathing and Movement Therapy

The prevention of illnesses plays an important role in traditional Chinese medicine. The goal is to live in harmony with the energy of the seasons and the requirements of body and mind. Prevention is achieved through a conscious diet that includes high-value nutrients and active gymnastic exercises that include breathing practices.

The forms of this therapy best known in the West are *qigong* and *tai chi,* systems of movement and breathing exercises that stimulate flexibility and smooth functioning of the body to actively contribute to the maintenance of health. In addition, relatively complicated movement sequences stimulate the ability to concentrate.

Qigong and tai chi have long been popular exercises in China, where people regularly meet outdoors early in the morning to practice together.

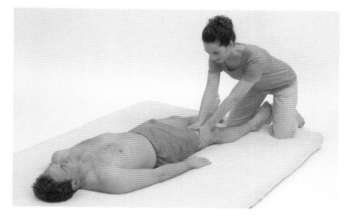

An important component of Chinese healing massage is the moving and stroking of certain parts of the body.

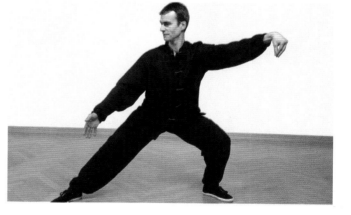

Tai chi and qigong are breathing and movement exercises common throughout China.

Internal Therapy

The second pillar of traditional Chinese medicine is prevention of illness through healthy diet and the application of herbs.

Herbalism: The Healing Powers of Plants

Many herbs and plant-based formulas can be effectively used to treat a wide variety of ailments. In China, systematic research and the development of herbal medicine over thousands of years led to a unique system in which healing herbs that complement and strengthen each other are used in mixtures. Chinese herbal formulas are made up of several herbs, including a main active ingredient, called the "emperor"; a number of additional ingredients that strengthen the effectiveness of the emperor, called "ministers"; and ingredients to improve the taste of the formula, as may be required in the case of very bitter ingredients, called "assistants."

The common goal of both external and internal therapies is the prevention of illness. This goal supports the mission of a healer in traditional Chinese medicine, which is to advise his or her patients in such a way as to prevent the onset of illness. This is a fundamental difference between traditional Chinese and Western medicine. Western medicine, in contrast to traditional Chinese medicine, focuses on the treatment of illness and has as its primary goal the removal of illness symptoms.

Summary

- Like acupuncture, acupressure is part of traditional Chinese medicine.
- Traditional Chinese medicine differentiates between internal and external treatments.
- External treatments include exercises that promote health (such as qigong), acupuncture, acupressure, and massage.
- Internal treatments include the use of traditional herbs, dietary therapies, and the use of medicine (animal- and mineral-based components).
- Traditional Chinese medicine uses these different measures to prevent and treat illnesses and to restore health after illness.

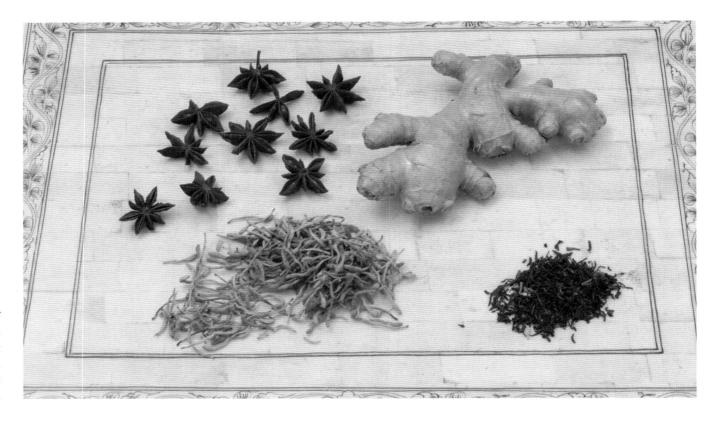

The use of healing herbs is very important in traditional Chinese medicine.

The History of Traditional Chinese Medicine

Like acupuncture, acupressure is grounded in the understanding of meridians, or body pathways in which life energy circulates (see page 32). This understanding developed in prehistoric times in China and was refined over thousands of years. However, we have indications that knowledge of energy pathways in the human body was also present in Europe in prehistoric times. For example, Oetzi, a Stone Age hunter whose mummy was unearthed in the Alps in 1991, bears tattoos that we know to outline points of the Urinary Bladder meridian (see page 39).

The first written record of traditional Chinese medicine is the classic work *Huang Di Nei Jing* (The Yellow Emperor's Book of Teachings about Internal Medicine). According to legend, this book is based on the investigations of Emperor Huang Di (circa 260 BC), who was interested not only in the political affairs of his country but also in medicine. He regularly questioned his personal physicians about the causes of and treatments for illnesses. *Huang Di Nei Jing* records these discussions, which to this day form the foundation of medical training in China.

The introduction of book printing in China in the tenth century led to the dissemination of other works that contained teachings about the meridians. Among these is *Explanations of the Fourteen Main Pathways*, published in 1341. From one of the most influential Chinese physicians, Li Shizhen, who lived between 1518 and 1593, we have *Investigations of Eight Unpaired Pathways*. And one of the most important books of Chinese medicine is *Ben Cao Gang Mu*, published in 1596 and consisting of fifty-two volumes describing nearly two thousand medications. Two generations of Chinese physicians worked on its completion.

Contact with Europe

Starting in the seventeenth and eighteenth centuries, Portuguese and Dutch sailors brought the knowledge of traditional Chinese medicine to Europe. Because of the similarities between the arrangement of the energy pathways on the human body and the arrangement of longitudes on their maps, they coined the term *meridians*, which is in use in the West to this day. Meridians are the lines along which lie the acupressure and acupuncture points.

Beginning in the late nineteenth century, with contact between China and Europe becoming increasingly frequent, Western medicine was introduced in China. With the founding of the republic in 1911, China became increasingly oriented toward the West. In medicine, scientific views and methods were introduced, and traditional Chinese medicine was no longer supported by the state.

In contrast, in Europe there was increasing interest in Chinese medical teachings beginning around 1930. European researchers, primarily in Austria, France, and Germany, began to systematically investigate the foundations of Chinese medicine. And back in China, starting in 1949, traditional Chinese medicine began once again to be supported by the state, now under Mao Tse-tung, since it represented a relatively cheap way of providing health care for China's large population.

Since the 1950s, certain aspects of traditional Chinese medicine have once again been taught in Chinese universities, and research on their effectiveness is being conducted. Today, three medical systems exist side by side in China: traditional Chinese medicine, Western medicine, and a combination of the two systems.

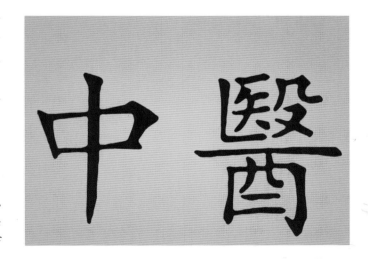

This illustration shows the Chinese characters for the term *traditional Chinese medicine*.

The Five Phases of Transformation

The concept of the five phases of transformation originates in Chinese philosophy. Since this system is designed to explain the world, it is used in traditional Chinese medicine as well. According to the philosophy of Chinese Taoism (see page 18), the world and every living thing exist in a steady, fluid cycle. The transformation phases symbolize the different stages of this cycle, which is known as the creation cycle.

Each transformation phase is accorded a specific element that gives it its name:

- Wood
- Fire
- Earth
- Metal
- Water

In the fluid creation cycle, each element leads to another, or transforms itself into another (hence the term *transformation phases*). For example, if one applies the model

to the seasons, the wood phase corresponds to spring, the season of growth. This growth leads to the fire phase, which is linked to great heat and represents the summer. From the fire in turn comes the earth phase (or ash), which corresponds to late summer, the time of harvest. The fall, a time of cooling down, is represented by the metal phase. In winter nature rests and landscapes are at times covered under snow, as represented by the water phase. Water is also the precondition for new life arising, for example, in the form of a growing plant in the spring.

As long as the elements influence each other in the appropriate direction (as indicated in the diagram), there is harmony in the organism. However, if the direction is reversed, meaning one transformation phase exhausts the previous one or one transformation phase cannot sufficiently nourish the one to come, disharmony results. In this case we speak of a disturbed creation cycle.

The individual transformation phases control and regulate one another. This results in the control cycle:

- Water extinguishes (controls) fire.
- Fire melts (controls) metal.
- Metal cuts (controls) wood.
- Wood, in the form of trees with their root networks, consumes (controls) the nutrients of the earth.
- Earth controls water in the shape of the shores. (See page 15 for illustration.)

Disharmonies in the control cycle occur when, for example, fire is overwhelmed by metal or earth is covered by water. A disturbed control cycle is called an "overwhelming" or *wu* cycle.

The system of the transformation phases can also be applied to bodily functions. Indeed, this model can help describe the relationships between individual organs. For example, the wood transformation phase is associated with the liver and gallbladder. Fire is associated with the heart and small intestine as well as blood vessels and

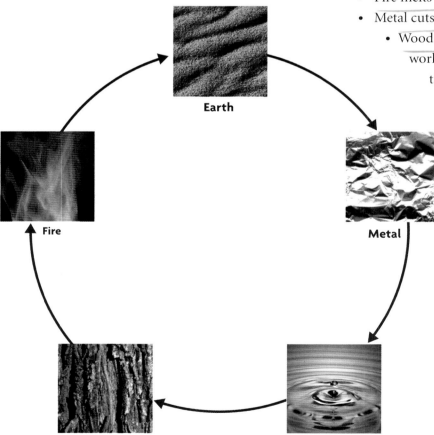

Earth

Fire

Metal

Wood

Water

In a healthy organism, the transformation phases influence each other in a harmonious cycle. If this harmonious cycle is interrupted, illness can result.

the tongue. The earth transformation phase is linked to the stomach and spleen. The metal transformation phase describes the delineation of the organism from its surroundings; accordingly, it is associated with the lungs and large intestine as well as the skin and nose. The water transformation phase is linked to the excretion organs, the kidneys and urinary bladder. Normally these phases of transformation exist in an internal balance. If this balance is disturbed, illness results.

The Wood Transformation Phase

The color of the wood transformation phase is the green of young leaves in spring. This phase is characterized by strong, changeable winds, as well as the outwardly oriented strengths of nature. Emotions associated with this phase are irritability, creativity, and anger. The wood element corresponds to the liver and gallbladder. The liver is the human organ in which the end results of the metabolism process are collected. At the same time, it has the fastest-healing tissue in the body. A common German turn of phrase refers to a "louse having run over someone's liver" to describe someone with a sudden change of mood. Similarly, a person who is easily irritated or angry is sometimes referred to as "galled." The body tissues corresponding to this transformation phase are the tendons and muscles.

The taste of this phase is sour, like unripe fruit in spring. The sensory organ of this phase is the eye. As alluded to above, certain types of people can be linked to the wood transformation phase. These types of people are extroverted, creative, and easily irritated. They have positive characteristics including courage, decisiveness, flexibility, and entrepreneurship. However, if these characteristics get out of control, they can lead to negative impulses including anger and aggression.

Associations with the Wood Transformation Phase

- Season: spring

- Climatic factor: wind

- Color: green

- Sensory organ: eye

- Body tissue: muscles and tendons

- Yin organ: liver

- Yang organ: gallbladder

- Emotion: excitability

- Positive characteristics: courage, initiative, creativity, entrepreneurship, ambition, openness to change, flexibility in thought and action

- Negative characteristics: anger, temper, aggression, irritability, impulsiveness

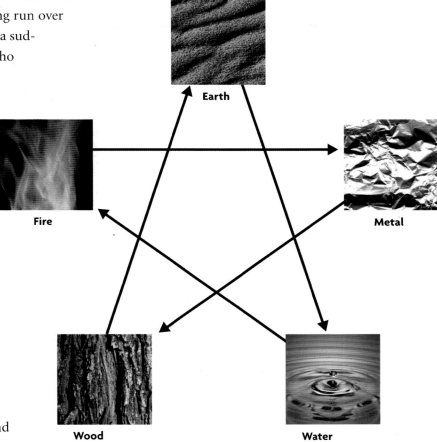

Earth

Fire

Metal

Wood

Water

The five transformation phases regulate one another in the control cycle. If this cycle is interrupted, illness can result.

The Fire Transformation Phase

The color of the fire transformation phase is red. The corresponding climatic factor is heat. The fire transformation phase is thus very clearly linked to the season of summer. The corresponding emotion is joy. The organs belonging to the fire transformation phase include the heart and small intestine (which are in turn linked to the soul and consciousness), the body tissues are the blood vessels, and the sensory organ is the tongue, as the organ of speech. The taste is "burned" or bitter.

Fire, heat, and the color red have always symbolized great quantities of energy. In the human body, joy causes the release of a lot of energy: circulation increases and the heart beats faster. An old proverb illustrates the connection between joy and fire's sensory organ, the tongue: "He whose heart is full, his mouth runs over." People of a fire constitution are warm and have a lively, infectious manner. They radiate energy and have the ability to liven up people around them and influence them in a positive way.

In fire's negative direction, these characteristics can lead people toward nervousness and a hectic and forgetful manner. Such people often suffer heart and blood problems such as hypertension; this condition is often accompanied by a reddened face.

The Earth Transformation Phase

The color of the earth transformation phase is yellow, like that of ripe fruit. The taste is sweet. The corresponding season is late summer, the time at which the harvest is brought in. The climatic factor is humidity. Nutrition, substance, and a closeness to the earth are associated with this phase.

Earth is linked to the spleen and stomach. The stomach is necessary for digestion, while according to the understanding of traditional Chinese medicine, the spleen takes up the good things out of food and transforms it into life energy (qi). Connective tissues and fat are the corresponding tissue types for this phase.

People with an earth constitution are characterized by being firmly grounded and having a reality-based approach to life. They have both feet firmly on the ground and enjoy comfort and good food. They are willing to pass their internal strength to other people and are always ready to help and care for others.

Ideally, earth people are balanced and pragmatic. They can think through things and promote change. Negative aspects of the earth constitution are laziness, overthinking, and concentration problems, as well as digestive problems or food allergies.

Associations with the Fire Transformation Phase

- Season: summer
- Climatic factor: heat
- Color: red
- Sensory organ: tongue
- Body tissue: blood vessels
- Yin organ: heart
- Yang organ: small intestine
- Emotion: happiness
- Positive characteristics: warmth, vitality
- Negative characteristics: stress, nervousness

Associations with the Earth Transformation Phase

- Season: late summer
- Climatic factor: humidity
- Color: yellow
- Sensory organ: mouth
- Body tissue: connective tissue, fat
- Yin organ: spleen
- Yang organ: stomach
- Emotion: pensiveness
- Positive characteristics: groundedness, reliability
- Negative characteristics: laziness, lack of concentration

The Metal Transformation Phase

The color of the metal transformation phase is white, like the first frost on grass or the shine of a steel weapon that one uses to defend oneself. Its taste is spicy. Its season is the fall. In central China fall is one of the driest seasons, which is why the metal transformation phase is also connected to dryness. In the fall the body has to mobilize its defenses. Organs linked to the metal transformation phase are the lungs and large intestine as well as the nose and skin. These are the areas in which people have the closest contact with their surroundings. With the lungs and nose we breathe in and out, while the large intestine makes use of food taken in from outside. Especially in these organs we find a large quantity of immune-system cells designed to resist possible negative external influences. The skin covers the organism like a protective shell. Often, problems in the large intestine such as food allergies lead to reactions on the skin, for example, in the form of a rash.

People of the metal constitution are alert, introverted, and attentive to detail. In their positive manifestations, these characteristics lead people to be sensitive and honest. In their exaggerated or negative form, they cause people to isolate themselves, to be hypersensitive, and to have a tendency toward sadness and depression.

The Water Transformation Phase

The water transformation phase is linked to winter, often referred to as the dark season; the corresponding color is black. In the cold of winter, nature takes a rest. The primary objective becomes not growth and procreation but guarding life functions. When ice and snow dominate the landscape, life seems to come to a stop. The organs linked to the water transformation phase are the kidneys and urinary bladder, which through excretion regulate the level of fluids in the body. At the same time, according to the principles of traditional Chinese medicine, life energy (qi) is stored in the kidneys. The ear too is linked to the water phase, since it is especially sensitive to disruptions in the level of fluids in the body (a fluid imbalance could, for example, lead to tinnitus). The bones, teeth, and nerve tissue are also linked to the water phase, as is the salty taste. The link between the salt content of our food and the fluid levels in our body we know from experience: salty meals leave us thirsty.

People of the water constitution type impress through their determination and stamina. In the positive sense, they are punctual, reliable, and respectful of tradition. In exaggerated form, these characteristics turn into obsessiveness, stubbornness, and a lack of flexibility as an expression of an excessive fear of change.

Associations with the Metal Transformation Phase

- Season: fall
- Climatic factor: dryness
- Color: white
- Sensory organ: nose
- Body tissue: skin
- Yin organ: lungs
- Yang organ: large intestine
- Emotion: grief
- Positive characteristics: sensitivity, honesty
- Negative characteristics: hypersensitivity, sadness

Associations with the Water Transformation Phase

- Season: winter
- Climatic factor: cold
- Color: black
- Sensory organ: ears
- Body tissue: bones, teeth, nerve tissue
- Yin organ: kidneys
- Yang organ: urinary bladder
- Emotion: fear
- Positive characteristics: determination, reliability, respect for traditions
- Negative characteristics: pedantry, stubbornness

Yin and Yang—Powers in Balance

Traditional Chinese medicine has its origins in the natural philosophy of Taoism. The Chinese word *tao* means "way" or "law of nature." Taoism says that both the world and human beings can exist only when two opposite but interdependent powers are balanced: yin and yang.

The Chinese characters for yin and yang depict the two sides of a mountain. Yin is the shady side of the mountain, while yang is the side under the sun. This example helps us understand the characteristics of yin and yang. The sunny side represents warmth, light, movement, and dryness, while the shady side represents the opposite: coldness, darkness, calm, and humidity. Only the balance of yin and yang makes the creation and maintenance of life possible. In this sense, yang is the creating and yin the maintaining power.

To visualize this concept, picture the hands of a clock. The second hand moves forward second by second. It is powered by a spring, whose tension corresponds to qi, or life energy. The movement of the second hand represents the yang phase, but the short break before the next jump is the yin phase. Both phases are necessary to move the hand forward.

Now look at the heart: each heartbeat provides the body with blood and thus with the energy necessary for life. Like the movement of the hands of the mechanical clock, the heartbeat occurs in two phases: first the heart expands and fills with blood (yin phase), then it quickly contracts and thus pumps the blood into the body (yang phase). Afterward the heart muscle relaxes and once again takes in blood. These phases always take turns.

Yin and yang are symbolized by two intertwined shapes that together form a circle. In this representation both shapes represent a cycle, each brought about by the other; neither could exist on its own. When they are in balance, a steady flow results: if one decreases, the other increases. In this symbol another basic principle can be seen: Each contains a small point of the other. The black area, for example, contains a white point. This means that one is always a component of the other. In yin there is always a little yang, and in yang always a little yin.

Together, yin and yang form a whole. Since all life is based on the presence of yin and yang, all things can be assigned to either yin or yang, in pairs of opposites that complete each other. Yin embodies the female, calmness, and steadiness, while yang embodies the male, movement, and action. The opposite pairs of yin and yang are in turn partial aspects of the whole. In this way, the principle of yin and yang extends throughout nature.

Left: Yin and yang correlate to the shady and sunny sides of a mountain.

Right: The symbol for yin and yang is also referred to as a monad: an indivisible center of energy from which all the physical properties of matter are derived.

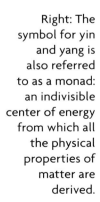

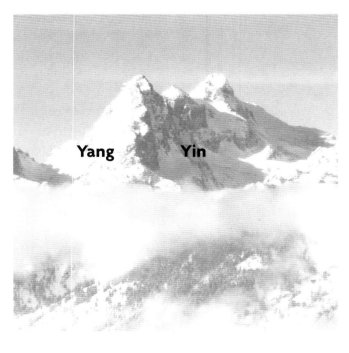

Yang   **Yin**

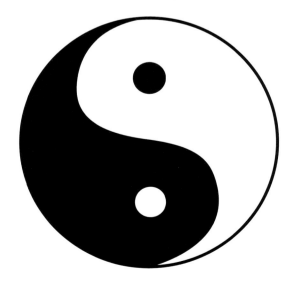

ASPECTS OF YIN AND YANG	
Yin	**Yang**
Girl, woman	Boy, man
Night	Day
Asleep, calm	Awake, active
Material	Spiritual
Static	Dynamic
Passive	Active
Chronic	Acute
Creeping	Sudden
Feeling of cold, need for warmth	Feeling of heat, need for coolness
Light urine, soft stool	Dark urine, constipation
Pale tongue	Red tongue
Weak pulse	Full pulse
Reducing, pulling together	Enlarging, spreading out
Exhaling	Inhaling
Inside the body	Body surface
Front of the body	Back of the body
Body substance	Body functions
Guarding, maintaining	Dynamic, energizing

These are only some aspects, but they serve to illustrate what yin and yang mean. Of course the principle of yin and yang can also be applied to the human body. Just as they do the cycles of the heartbeat, yin and yang encompass breathing and all other bodily processes of every person. Breathing in is active, strong, dynamic, or yang, while breathing out is passive and slow, or yin. The front of the body is yin (in the case of a four-footed animal, the front faces the ground and is hence in the shade), while the back is yang (in the case of a four-footed animal, the back is turned toward the sun). That is why the meridians that run across the back are assigned to yang, and the meridians on the front of the body to the yin (see pages 32–46).

The model of yin and yang also applies to symptoms and processes of illness. Usually yin and yang are in a harmonious balance in the body. An imbalance leads to illness. The goal of treatment is thus to recreate the balance. An excess of yin influence leads to a slow or chronic illness. Illnesses with a yang influence are characterized by a sudden onset and possibly signs of increased activity, such as redness or warmth of the skin. In traditional Chinese medicine diagnosis is based on judging patients and their characteristics—as well as the characteristics of their illness—according to the principles of yin and yang. A precondition for successful treatment is the correct assignment of illness indications according to these criteria.

An example will help illustrate this point. The pain characteristic of arthrosis (an illness characterized by the wearing down of joints) is steady and constant. It thus has yin character. The sudden, piercing pain of a migraine, in contrast, has yang character. Both illnesses are accompanied by pain, but they must be treated in fundamentally different ways.

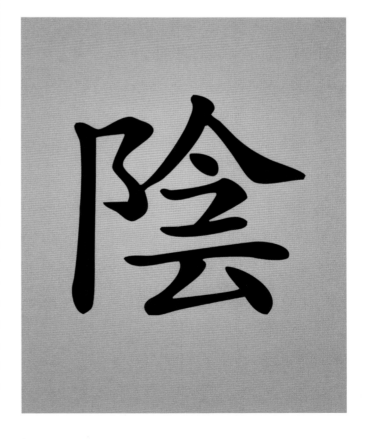

This illustration shows the Chinese character for the term *yin*.

The Five Basic Substances

According to the teachings of traditional Chinese medicine, five substances form the basis of all life processes, including physiological processes like digestion, blood formation and circulation, neurovegetative connections, and hereditary links. These basic substances are called *qi, xie, shen, jing*, and *jinye*. They consist of substance and energy in different ratios.

THE FIVE BASIC SUBSTANCES	
Qi	Life energy
Xie	Blood
Shen	Spirit
Jing	Life strength
Jinye	Body fluids

Qi—Life Energy

The Chinese character for qi (pronounced *chee*), life energy or "vitalizing breath," contains the terms for "raw rice" and "steam." In ancient China, cooked rice was the foundation of life for people. In that sense, the symbol expresses that the presence of qi is a necessary precondition for life. Life without qi is not only unthinkable but entirely impossible. The qi in the body circulates through the meridians.

Xie—Blood

Xie (pronounced *sheh*) is the blood, which carries the energy that nourishes, warms, and wets bones, muscles, tendons, and internal organs. Xie is formed by the Spleen from the food we eat and circulates in the blood vessels. It is moved by the heart and stored in the liver. Xie is the precondition for our organs being nourished and able to function.

Shen—Spirit

Shen (pronounced *shun*) is the spirit and resides in the Heart. Shen is a characteristic that is unique to humans and differentiates man from animals. It refers to the vitality in the human body. Shen steers thinking, memory, consciousness, and sleep. Looked at from the outside, shen can be seen in the eyes. Aside from its manifestation as spirit, shen also has a material aspect, since it can exist only in conjunction with a body.

Jing—Strength of Life

There are three types of jing (pronounced *jeeng*). The first is the constitution a person is born with, the sum of life strength that the child inherits from its two parents. In the case of insufficient nourishment the body increasingly uses these inborn reserves, which cannot be replenished.

The second type of jing is the essence the body forms after birth through the food it takes in. The right selection of food can strengthen this jing and can counteract a depletion of the inborn reserves.

The final type of jing is the individual strength of life. It is located in the kidneys and is used over the course of a lifetime. A decrease in jing expresses itself in aging symptoms such as graying hair or loss of teeth. In the case of poor-quality food or a lack of inborn reserves, these symptoms appear early in life.

Jinye—Body Fluids

The fifth basic substance, jinye (pronounced *jeen yeh*), is the bodily fluids that nourish and wet the individual cells. It has yin characteristics. According to traditional Chinese medicine, jinye encompasses both the fluid in the tissues as well as the digestive fluids, tears, saliva, breast milk, and sweat. In its name, the syllable *jin* refers to the light and clear body fluids, while the ending *ye* refers to the heavy and thick fluids.

The Eight Key Principles

The eight key diagnostic principles *(ba gang)* together form a simple schematic into which illness symptoms fit, thus providing the basic scaffolding for a diagnosis. This schematic ultimately aims to find the correct treatment for a disturbance in the energy balance. The eight key principles are the following pairs of opposites:

THE EIGHT KEY PRINCIPLES	
Yin	Yang
Inside	Outside
Emptiness	Fullness
Cold	Heat

The Yin-Yang Key Principle

The lead pair, yin and yang, creates an overarching diagnostic classification of an imbalance in the flow of energy. A disturbed condition is categorized based on its appearance of having either yang quality (external, fullness, heat, overfunction, acute) or yin quality (internal, emptiness, coldness, underfunction, slow or chronic onset).

YIN AND YANG QUALITIES		
Yin		**Yang**
Internal		External
Emptiness		Fullness
Cold		Hot
Underfunction		Overfunction
Slow onset or chronic state		Sudden onset

Yin Quality

Yin disturbances generally present as a weakness or lack of something. They are oriented inward, meaning they affect deep layers inside the body. They can be chronic and may be accompanied by signs of underfunctioning of organs or organ systems. They can be caused by deficiencies in various substances required by the body for healthy functioning. Examples include low blood pressure, exhaustion, slow metabolism, anemia, and increased sensitivity to cold. A depressive mood is also considered a yin quality. People who exhibit these symptoms tend to be thin and to have a weak, slow pulse and a pale tongue, often with a white coating. They can be helped with warmth and dryness.

Yang Quality

Yang disturbances describe the contrast to the symptoms listed above. They can present as an acute illness. They are characterized by hyperfunctioning and have external effects, meaning that they affect external layers of the body. Examples include hypertension and other illnesses that are accompanied by an increase in body temperature and reddening of the skin. Fever and a heightened sensitivity to warmth are also characteristic of yang disturbances. People who exhibit key yang characteristics tend to have a strong build, a strong, quick pulse, and a red, dry tongue, frequently with yellow coating. Coolness and calming exercises can help them.

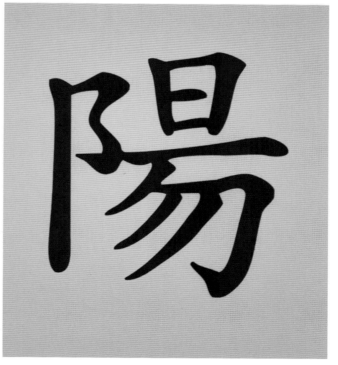

This illustration shows the Chinese character for the term *yang*.

Yin or Yang?

This table provides an overview of the different characteristics of yin and yang.

YIN AND YANG TENDENCIES		
	Yin	**Yang**
Constitution	Delicate to weak	Strong
Posture	Bent	Upright
Skin	Cool, moist	Warm, dry
Temperature sensitivity	Sensitive to cold	Sensitive to warmth
Mood	Tends toward depression	Is impulsive
Duration	Tends toward chronic ailments	Tends toward acute illnesses and fever
Pulse	Weak	Strong
Face	Pale	Rosy
Energy	Quickly fatigued	Has stamina

The Inside-Outside Key Principle

The difference between inside and outside disturbances is relatively easy to distinguish and helps differentiate the clinical picture between the internal organs and the external shell of the body. The assessment is made for the part of the body where the symptoms of the illness are located.

Inside

The inside principle applies when internal organs are affected by the illness. Such "inside" illnesses can be caused by internal as well as external influences. These illnesses begin slowly and last a long time.

Outside

In traditional Chinese medicine, the skin, muscles, and meridians form the surface, or the outside, of the body. Symptoms that involve the outside include:

- Sudden onset
- Fever
- Sore muscles
- Stiff neck

"Outside" illnesses are caused by external influences. In keeping with the metal transformation phase (see page 17), the skin and muscles are related to the Lungs and Large Intestine. Accordingly, the Lung meridian can be used to influence the outside.

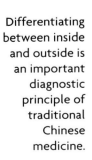

Differentiating between inside and outside is an important diagnostic principle of traditional Chinese medicine.

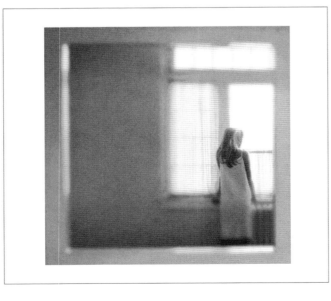

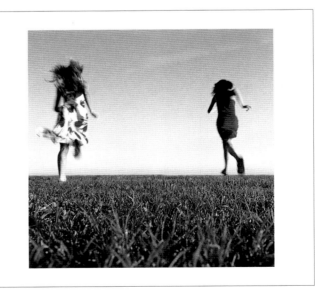

The Emptiness-Fullness Key Principle

The differentiation between emptiness and fullness is of decisive importance in categorizing symptoms of illness. Fullness means that an illness-causing factor is present in excess and is responsible for an energetic imbalance. Emptiness, in contrast, means that there is a lack of energy, due to which the internal organs are unable to function properly. The determination of whether a case of emptiness or fullness exists is made by observing the patient.

Emptiness

People experiencing emptiness symptoms speak with a low voice and appear indifferent, weak, and downtrodden. Their movements are careful and weak, their faces pale or even gray, their breathing flat, and their pulse weak. People experiencing an emptiness condition frequently suffer from sweating attacks, bladder fullness, and constipation. Such illnesses tend to be long-lived.

Fullness

Fullness conditions can be recognized by overall excitability, anxiety, a loud voice, and strong heat development (fever). People experiencing fullness conditions have large and strong movements. They often experience pain in the chest and abdomen that gets worse when pressure is applied. Their tongue usually has a thick coating and they need to urinate less frequently. Fullness conditions are often characterized by the sudden onset of an illness of short duration.

Differentiating between Emptiness and Fullness

It is helpful to compare the criteria of emptiness and fullness conditions against each other. This table shows the contrast of these two important key principles.

EMPTINESS AND FULLNESS TENDENCIES		
	Emptiness	**Fullness**
Constitution	Weak	Strong and robust
Illness	Creeping	Sudden and short
Mood	Little energy	Excited
Voice	Quiet	Loud
Color of the face	Pale	Quick to redden
Breathing	Weak	Heavy
Pulse	Weak	Strong
Blood pressure	Low	High
Urine amount	Lots	Little
Pain	Better through pressure	Worse through pressure
Tongue	Small	Large
	Little or no coat	Thick coat
Temperature	Cold hands and feet	Fever
	Better through warmth	Better through coolness

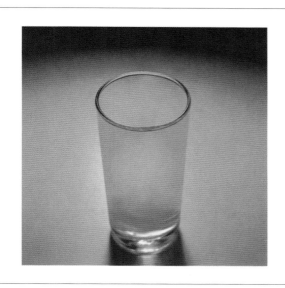

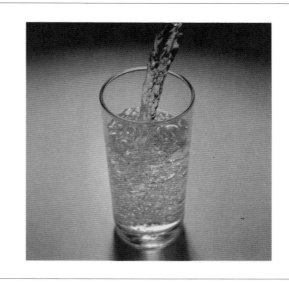

Another important principle is the distinction between emptiness and fullness.

The Cold-Heat Key Principle

Cold and heat are categories to which individual illness symptoms can be clearly assigned. Either condition can occur in combination with a fullness or emptiness condition. In other words, emptiness does not automatically equate to coldness, and fullness does not automatically equate to heat. A heat-fullness condition is present in cases of excess heat. Similarly, a cold-fullness condition is present in cases of excess cold. In the case of heat-emptiness or cold-emptiness, the illness-causing influence is encountering a weakness (emptiness) of the body.

Heat

The intrusion of an illness-causing heat influence causes a heat illness, such as sunstroke, sunburn, fever, or skin rash. The specific presentation depends on whether there is at the time an emptiness or fullness condition. Overall characteristics of an illness caused by heat are a reddened face, thirst, elevated temperature, and a red tongue with a yellow coating.

Cold

A cold disturbance is characterized by increased sensitivity to cold. People suffering from this feel cold, are pale, usually complain of cold hands and feet, and have soft stool and a lot of light-colored urine. Their tongue is pale with a white coating.

HEAT AND COLD TENDENCIES		
	Heat	**Cold**
Body	Feverish, dry	Cold, with cold extremities
Course of illness	Strong, sudden	Creeping
Mood	Irritable, angry	Withdrawn
Temperature sensitivity	Feels hot, desires cool drinks	Increased sensitivity to cold, desires hot drinks
Interactions	Talkative	Reserved, quiet
Face	Reddened, sometimes accompanied by a rash	Pale
Pulse	Quick	Slow
Need to urinate	Lots	Little
Pain	Burning	Pulling
Tongue	Red, with yellow coating	Pale, with white coating
Excretion	Dark yellow or green coloring of body fluids, constipation	Soft stool, light-colored urine
Complaints	Gastrointestinal problems, thirst, feverish infections	Joint pains, muscle tensions, stiffness
Improvement	Better through addition of cold	Better through addition of warmth

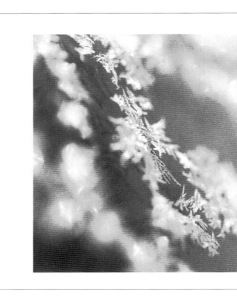

The diagnosis also takes into account cold and heat symptoms.

The Art of the Examination

The goal of examination in the framework of traditional Chinese medicine is to allow the therapist to quickly and precisely recognize the patient's condition as well as the causes for it. Examination of both the mental and the physical condition is always a component of diagnosis in traditional Chinese medicine. The different examination methods together allow a comprehensive description of the physical and mental condition of the patient. The picture that emerges from such examination points clearly to the correct comprehensive treatment. (The examination of a person suffering from illness should be undertaken by a therapist trained in the methodology of traditional Chinese medicine. As laypeople, readers are asked to proceed with extreme caution, and not to offer premature diagnoses.)

In traditional Chinese medicine, the following examination methods are used:

- Questioning
- Feeling the pulse
- Examining physical characteristics such as the tongue, posture, movement, voice, body odor, and so on.

Questioning

Through a questioning conversation (anamnesis), the therapist first compiles a comprehensive picture of the patient's mental, emotional, and physical situation. At this point the focus is on the patient rather than his or her illness. After evaluating the results, the therapist has a first impression whether this is a case of

- a weakness illness, for example, chronic back pain or burnout; or
- a fullness illness, for example, infection, hyperthyroidism, hypertension, or acne.

Feeling the Pulse

Examining the pulse requires a great deal of experience. The traditional Chinese method differentiates between different types of pulses occurring even on a single wrist. (See Kaptchuk 2001.) To feel the pulse, use your fingers to find the radial artery on the inside of the patient's wrist. Feel for a prominent bump at the top of the radial bone, called the styloid process, just under the base of the thumb. Set the tip of your middle finger just inside this bump; the radial pulse is strongest here. Set the tips of your index and ring fingers on either side of your middle finger to encompass the pulse area.

Observe the pulse for about one minute, registering both the quantity of beats and their quality (hard or soft, flat or strong).

> **Note**
>
> When taking the pulse, don't use your thumb to feel it, as you would then also feel your own pulse.

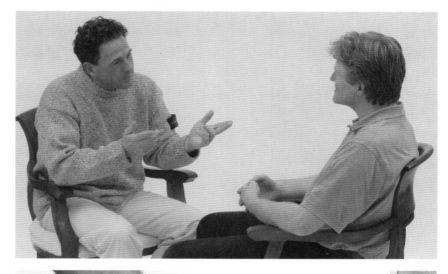

The examination begins with an in-depth interview of the patient by the therapist.

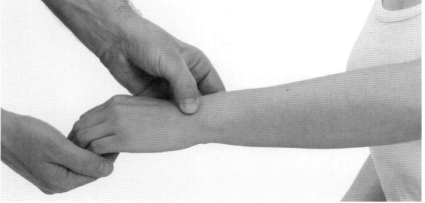

When feeling the pulse, pay attention not just to its frequency but also to its quality.

Observing and Examining

Simply by observing the patient, you can gain many indications about the root imbalance and its possible treatment. Traditional Chinese medicine has always placed special emphasis on the examination of the tongue. Also important are evaluations of the patient's appearance, posture, movement, and face.

Tongue Diagnostics

The appearance and makeup of the tongue are often the clearest and most reliable indicators of disharmony in the body. Experienced diagnosticians usually need only a short look to understand the type of problem the patient is experiencing. This explains the high priority assigned to tongue diagnostics in traditional Chinese medicine. The tongue offers information about:

- The current stage of illness
- The process of the illness
- Factors contributing to the illness
- Affected meridians

The size, shape, and color of the tongue are all evaluated. These criteria as well as the quality of the coating are used to determine the circulation of qi (life energy), xie (blood), jinye (bodily fluids), and jing (life strength)

and the relationship between yin and yang in the body.

In healthy people, the tongue is pale red and somewhat moist. A very pale tongue color can, for example, indicate a lack of blood, lack of qi, or an excess of cold.

FINDINGS IN TONGUE DIAGNOSTICS	
Size of the Tongue	
Small	Yin deficiency
Swollen	Excess fluids
Color of the Tongue	
Pale	Lack of qi or xie, intrusion of cold
Red	Excess heat
Dark red	Blood clot
Color and Quality of the Tongue Coating	
Whitish, thin	Normal, possibly slight coolness in temperature
Yellowish, thick	Excess heat
Dry	Lack of body fluids
Sticky	Problems with liquids or food trapped in stomach

Left: The size and shape of the tongue are evaluated from both the front and the side.

Right: The quality and color of the tongue's coating can offer important indications about the cause of the illness.

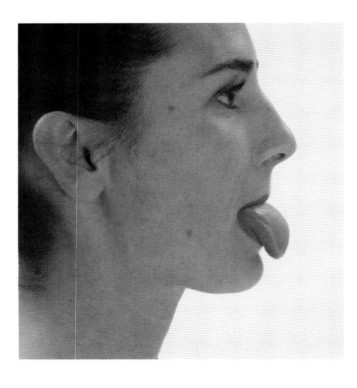

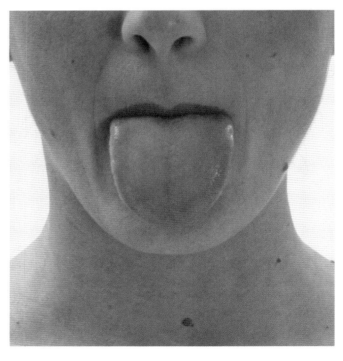

A clearly red tongue indicates an excess of heat, while a dark violet tongue suggests a blood-flow impediment.

The color and quality of the tongue coating are also very important in the diagnosis. A thick yellow coating suggests an excess of heat, while a sticky phlegm coating can be observed when the body has an excess of fluids. If these variations are confined to only small, discrete parts of the tongue, analysis of the affected body regions is relatively easy. The illustration below divides the tongue into the five areas that correspond to particular organs and organ groups. However, to draw accurate conclusions, the following rules need to be observed:

- The patient should not have ingested any falsifying foods such as sweets, coffee, tea, or coloring additives for one to two hours before the exam. The patient should not smoke before the exam.
- The examination of the patient's tongue should take place in good light, specifically white light or daylight.
- The tongue should be shown several times for short intervals, since prolonged extension (more than three seconds) causes changes in the makeup.
- The constitution of the patient must be taken into account. For example, small, slender people have smaller tongues than tall, strong people.

A rosy tongue with a light, thin white coat that shines and cannot be wiped off indicates a healthy condition.

Examining Appearance, Movement, and the Face

Examining the patient's overall appearance as well as facial color and movement allows the therapist to gain an overview of the condition and severity of the illness. For example, larger persons with a strong appearance are more likely to have strong organs that, in the case of illness, are prone to fullness syndromes. Tender, weak people tend to have smaller, weaker organs and are more prone to emptiness syndromes. The patient's overall appearance also offers hints about which meridians are affected. Try to classify the external appearance of the patient according to the yin and yang criteria. Observing and listening will help you get an impression of which meridians are affected by the illness. For this, you have to know that each meridian has either a yin or a yang quality and that each is assigned a particular transformation phase. You will find more about this in the discussion of the individual meridians. (See pages 32–46.)

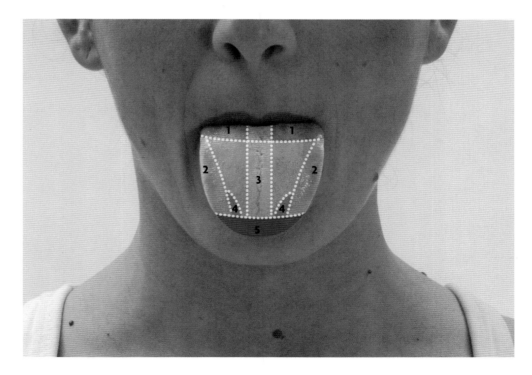

Changes in individual tongue areas indicate disruptions in the corresponding areas of the body:
1 kidneys and urinary bladder
2 liver and gallbladder
3 spleen and stomach
4 lungs
5 heart

EVALUATING FACIAL COLOR AND APPEARANCE

Facial Color

Pale	Coldness, emptiness
Red	Heat, fullness
Redness only in the cheeks	Heat, emptiness, lack of yin
Blue	Blood clot

Appearance

Thin, frail	Heat, emptiness, lack of yin
Fat	Lack of qi and yang, excess of liquids

Listening to the Voice

The sound of the voice is also part of Chinese diagnostics. A quiet voice indicates an emptiness condition, or a lack of yang. In contrast, a loud, strong voice suggests a fullness condition, or an excess of yang.

EVALUATING VOICE

Quiet voice	Emptiness, lack of yang
Loud voice	Fullness, excess of yang

The lungs/ large intestine, spleen/stomach, and liver/ gallbladder are referred to as organ pairs in traditional Chinese medicine.

The Twelve Organs

Traditional Chinese medicine describes twelve organs: lungs, large intestine, stomach, spleen, heart, small intestine, urinary bladder, kidney, pericardium (heart area), Triple Heater (the three body cavities of the Lungs, upper abdomen, and lower abdomen), gallbladder, and liver. These organs are divided into solid organs and hollow organs depending on their shape and function. Among the solid or storage organs are the lungs, pericardium, spleen, heart, kidneys, and liver. They produce, regulate, and store the basic substances of the body, thus fulfilling yin functions; for this reason they are also called yin organs. The hollow organs are the stomach, large intestine, small intestine, gallbladder, urinary bladder, and Triple Heater. Their function is to take in food, to break it down into its components, to separate useful ingredients from useless ones, and to excrete waste products. These functions are associated with yang, and they are thus called yang organs.

But of course yin and yang organs should not be viewed in isolation from one another. Both groups of organs work together, and each yin organ has a corresponding yang organ. There are thus six organ pairs, of which five are listed in the table on this page. They are sometimes referred to as function circles. The sixth

ORGAN CORRESPONDENCES

Transformation Phase	Organ	Association
Earth	Spleen	Yin
	Stomach	Yang
Metal	Lungs	Yin
	Large Intestine	Yang
Water	Kidney	Yin
	Urinary Bladder	Yang
Fire	Heart	Yin
	Small Intestine	Yang
Wood	Liver	Yin
	Gallbladder	Yang

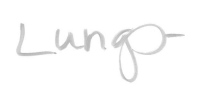

organ pair, pericardium–Triple Heater, is defined in very different ways in the literature. Each organ pair is associated with a transformation phase (see pages 14–17).

The Lungs and Large Intestine

The lungs create qi from the air that we breathe in. When we inhale, they take in external qi, and when we exhale they expel the used air. If our breathing is not regular, symptoms like cough or shortness of breath result. The large intestine has a similar function. It takes up the (clear) water from the intestinal contents and transports the (turbid) things that cannot be used to the organs of excretion. In other words the large intestine, like the lungs, via intake and excretion regulates the substances that can stay in the body and bring energy.

The Spleen and the Stomach

Traditional Chinese medicine views the spleen primarily as a digestive organ. It transforms nutrients into qi and blood. Beyond this, the spleen has a transportation function, distributing nutrients and clean water across the body. The stomach receives solid and liquid food and breaks it down into its components. In doing so, it separates the pure, good substances from waste components and sends them on to the spleen. The waste components are sent to the intestines for further processing.

THE LUNGS/LARGE INTESTINE ORGAN SYSTEM	
Main responsibility	The lungs are responsible for breathing. It is their job to control the flow of air and the flow of qi, or life energy. The lungs also send immune-system components from inside the body to the surface and open and close the pores. The large intestine is responsible for excretions. The lungs and large intestine are connected energetically. This is shown by the following example: the diaphragm, moving in rhythm with the lungs, massages the large intestine, thereby stimulating digestion.
Transformation phase	Metal
Damaging Influence	Dryness; also phlegm and cold
Emotions	Sadness, grief
Functions	**Signs of Disharmony**
Control of breathing	Weak voice, shortness of breath, sneezing, illnesses of the sinuses, weak sense of smell, loss of energy
Control of immune-system strength	Susceptibility to colds, allergies, insufficient distribution of body fluids and life energy
Regulation of digestion	Constipation

THE SPLEEN/STOMACH ORGAN SYSTEM	
Main responsibility	The spleen and stomach are responsible for digestion and for the distribution of nutrients and water. They separate "good" from "bad" nutrients by transporting the "good" nutrients upward and the "bad" nutrients downward to the intestines for excretion. In addition, the spleen ensures that body fluids (such as blood and sweat) remain at normal levels. Since the spleen is responsible for processing food, it also controls the growth and development of muscles. Moreover, the spleen is connected to the mouth, the organ that takes in food; therefore there is a connection between the health of the spleen and the state of the lips.
Transformation phase	Earth
Damaging influence	Wetness, phlegm, mental exertions (for example, learning)
Emotions	Worry, pondering, sense of responsibility
Functions	**Signs of Disharmony**
Control of digestion	Weak stool, flatulence
Transportation of nutrients	Diarrhea, organ failure
Control of body fluids	Suddenly appearing blue spots, sweating
Control of the muscles	Feeling of heaviness or weakness; weak muscles
Connection to the mouth	Dry, cracked lips

The Kidneys and Urinary Bladder

The urinary bladder and kidneys are assigned to the water phase. The kidneys are seen as the source of life and development. Here is located jing (life strength), which has the ability to differentiate yin and yang and to create life. The kidneys separate the good or "pure" bodily fluids from the "cloudy" or unusable ones. The pure fluids are transported upward, the cloudy ones down to the urinary bladder. The urinary bladder, as a hollow organ, receives the urine and ensures its excretion from the body.

The Liver and Gallbladder

The gallbladder and liver are assigned to the wood phase. The liver ensures a balanced, fluid movement of substances in the body, including qi and the emotions. An imbalance can lead to disharmonies in blood circulation as well as in digestion and the emotional state. The liver produces bile, a bitter, green-yellow liquid that is important for digestion in the small intestine. Bile is stored in and excreted from the gallbladder, whose function depends on a harmoniously functioning liver.

THE KIDNEYS/URINARY BLADDER ORGAN SYSTEM

Main responsibility	The kidneys are the seat of jing, or life strength. Their condition is reflected in that of the hair on the head, since the kidneys are linked to the hair. The kidneys regulate growth and reproduction and the production of bone and bone marrow. Together with the urinary bladder they regulate water levels in the body. The sensory organ most sensitive to changes in the body's water levels is the ear. For this reason the kidneys are also linked to the ears.
Transformation phase	Water
Damaging influence	Cold, dryness
Emotions	Fear, pedantry, narrow-mindedness

Functions	Signs of Disharmony
Home of jing (life energy)	Thin and weak hair, hair loss, premature graying of hair
Control of reproduction	Infertility, impotence, retarded physical development
Control of water levels	Malodorous and dark urine, need to urinate during nighttime, tendency toward constipation, bladder infections, Kidney stones
Control of the ears	Bad hearing, ringing in the ears, tinnitus, deafness
Associated with	Weakness of will, indecisiveness, stubbornness, insecurity

THE LIVER/GALLBLADDER ORGAN SYSTEM

Main responsibility	The liver controls the flow of blood and qi (life energy). It is responsible for the smooth functioning of all systems in the body and for releasing emotions. The liver also stores the blood. The condition of the liver is reflected in that of the muscles, tendons, and nails. The sensory organ linked to the liver is the eye (in the case of jaundice, the eye is the first to turn yellow).
Transformation phase	Wood
Damaging influence	Wind (also in the sense of internal wind, as from stress, frustration, or anger)
Emotions	Anger

Functions	Signs of Disharmony
Control of body functions, for example, function of the muscles	Cramps, stiffness, shaking
Control of the blood	Menstruation problems (pain because of "blood blockages")
Link to the nails	Dry, torn, or broken nails; grooves in the nails
Link to the eyes	Vision problems, eye problems (infections, sensitivity to light)
Associated with	Headaches, migraine, depression caused by "swallowing" of anger and rage, that is, qi blockage

The Heart and Small Intestine

The heart and small intestine are assigned to the fire phase. The heart is the seat of the psyche, of the intellect, and of consciousness. According to Chinese medicine, the heart is the "regent" of the body. When the heart is functioning normally, blood flow is steady and continuous, the pulse beats regularly, and the tongue retains its pale red color. If the heart does not transport enough blood, the tongue becomes very pale, just as a dark red tongue indicates blood congestion in the heart area.

The small intestine receives the processed food mix from the stomach and continues to separate this mix into "pure" and "cloudy" substances. It sends the pure substances to the spleen, while the cloudy substances are transported to the large intestine for excretion.

The Pericardium and Triple Heater

While Chinese medicine assigns the spirit and the psyche to the heart, the pericardium is linked to bodily functions of the heart, for example, pulse rate and blood pressure. For this reason, in the case of heart problems, the pericardium meridian is massaged.

The Triple Heater has an overarching energetic function: it is responsible for providing the organs of the three hollow parts of the body with energy. That is why points along the Triple Heater meridian can be massaged to harmonize and balance a wide range of problems.

THE HEART/SMALL INTESTINE ORGAN SYSTEM	
Main responsibility	The heart controls the blood and its flow through the blood vessels. It is the seat of shen (meaning the soul, personality, and consciousness) and controls speech. For that reason the heart is also linked to the mouth and tongue. The small intestine receives the food mix from the stomach. Its function is to separate "good" from "bad" nutrients.
Transformation phase	Fire
Damaging influence	Heat
Emotions	Happiness, vitality, joy for life
Functions	**Signs of Disharmony**
Control of blood and blood vessels	Slow or fast pulse, high or low blood pressure
Seat of the soul	Concentration problems, nervousness, excitement, insomnia, confusion, psychosomatic or psychological problems, fainting
Control of speech	Speech problems (for example, stuttering), speechlessness, or excessive talking
Associated with	Lack of will to live, heaviness, living in dreams rather than in reality

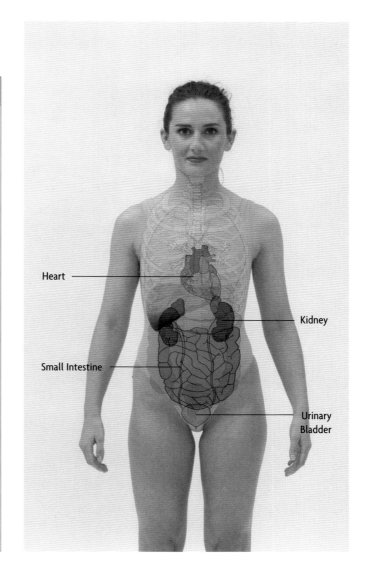

The heart/small intestine and kidney/urinary bladder make up one unit each as yin/yang organ pairs.

Meridians: The Body's Energy Pathways

A pillar of traditional Chinese medicine is the model that sees qi (life energy) circulating through the human body within a series of channels or meridians. Altogether there are twelve meridians that form a cycle through which qi circulates over a period of twenty-four hours. Lined up along the meridians like pearls on a string are the acupuncture or acupressure points. It is at these points that the meridians are connected to the surface of the body; by touching these points from the outside, energy can be moved.

A meridian has either a yin or a yang quality. To picture this, think of a person with arms extended upward. The following rules apply:

- The yin meridians run along the front of the body from bottom to top (from the ground to the body to the sky).
- The yang meridians—with one exception—run along the back of the body from top to bottom (from sky to the body to the earth).

MERIDIAN ROTATIONS	
Front	Lungs—Large Intestine—Stomach—Spleen
Back	Heart—Small Intestine—Urinary Bladder—Kidneys
Sides	Pericardium—Triple Heater—Gall Bladder—Liver

In this way traditional Chinese medicine sees each person as part of the energy circulation between the sky (yang) and the earth (yin).

The meridians are named after the internal organs as they are described in traditional Chinese medicine. A meridian, together with its corresponding organ and that organ's transformation phase, completes another functional circle. A yin meridian is always paired with a yang meridian, meaning that a disturbance in one meridian will have effects on the other. This is often described as an expanded functional circle.

There are three so-called rotations, or routes of four meridians each (yin-yang-yang-yin), one for each side of the body. (See the chart above.) During the course of a day qi runs through each rotation once. From this cycle we can determine certain times at which a meridian will have a maximum of energy flowing through it. Knowledge of these maximum-qi times is important when evaluating illness symptoms: Heart symptoms, for example, occur more frequently during the Heart time, which is between 11 AM and 1 PM, while biliary colic occurs most frequently between 11 PM and 1 AM.

Aside from the twelve main meridians there are two special meridians: the Conception Vessel and the Governor Vessel. These overarching meridians run along the center of the body on the front and the back and are directly related to yin and yang. Except for the Conception Vessel and Governor Vessel, each of the meridians manifests in two parts, one on each side of the body.

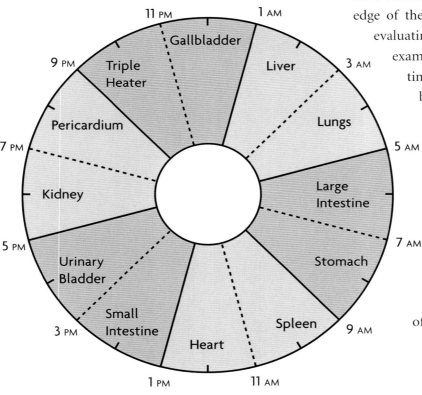

The organ clock shows the times at which the individual organs carry maximum qi. The yin organs are shaded in light blue, and the yang organs in orange.

The Lung Meridian

The Lung meridian is a yin pathway. This meridian is connected to the body surface at eleven points. The meridian starts at the upper front of the rib cage, in the space between the top ribs, with the point Lung 1. From there it reaches just slightly up and then across to the shoulder and then stretches down the inside of the upper arms, elbows, and lower arms and along the side of the thumb up to the thumbnail. The meridian ends on the edge of the nail furthest from the index finger, at the point Lung 11.

THE LUNG MERIDIAN	
Transformation phase	Metal
Color	White
Season	Fall
Emotion	Grief
Damaging influence	Dryness makes the lungs susceptible to external influences

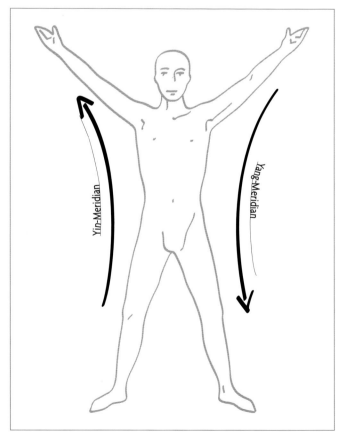

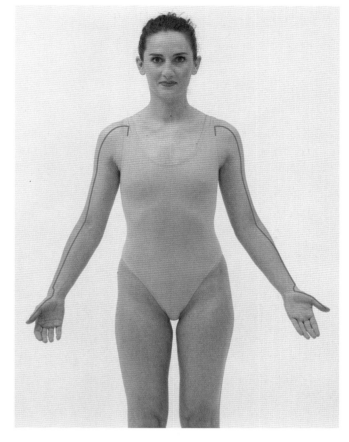

The Lung meridian runs from the shoulder to the thumb.

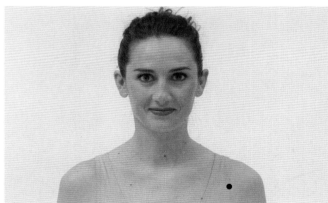

The first point of the Lung meridian, known as Lung 1, is in the front part of the shoulders.

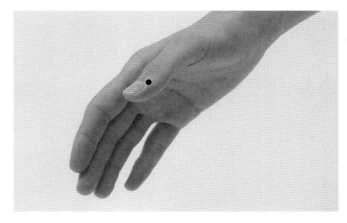

The endpoint of the Lung meridian, known as Lung 11, is located on the outer edge of the thumbnail.

The Large Intestine Meridian

The Large Intestine meridian is a yang pathway. It exhibits twenty points. The meridian begins on the nail of the index finger, on the side closest to the thumb, with the point Large Intestine 1. It continues along the index finger across the hand and wrist, along the outside of the lower arm and elbow, and along the upper arm up to the shoulder. From there it runs sideways along the neck up to the corner of the mouth. Above the mouth it crosses over the upper lip to the opposite side. The endpoint Large Intestine 20 is located here, in the skin fold alongside the nostril.

In the sense of the yin-yang pairing, the Large Intestine meridian is connected with the Lung meridian, meaning that it too belongs to the metal transformation phase.

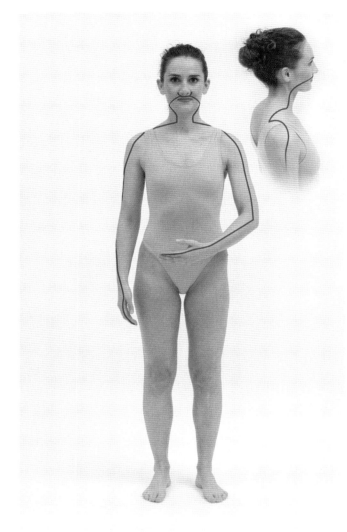

The Large Intestine meridian runs from the index finger along the outside of the arm to the face.

THE LARGE INTESTINE MERIDIAN	
Transformation phase	Metal
Color	White
Season	Fall
Emotion	Grief
Damaging influence	Dryness, for example, dry air

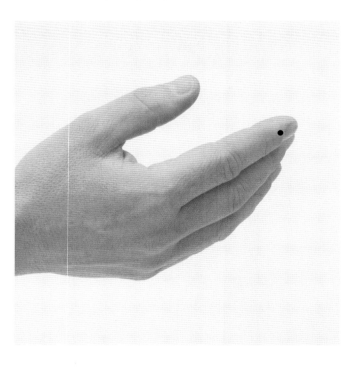

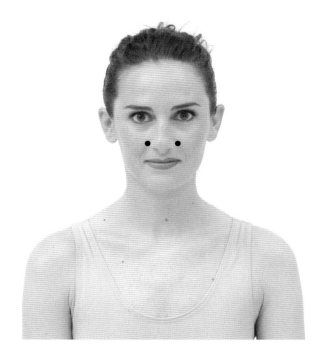

Left: The first point of the Large Intestine meridian is located on the edge of the nail of the index finger, on the side near the thumb.

Right: At the beginning of the nose–lip fold is Large Intestine 20, the endpoint of the Large Intestine meridian.

The Stomach Meridian

The Stomach meridian is the "yang in the yin"—it is the only yang meridian that crosses through the yin area of the front of the body. The point Stomach 1 is located at the center of the lower edge of the eye socket. From there the meridian runs vertically downward to the edges of the mouth and past the outside of the jaws. One branch of the meridian returns upward past the ear to the temple. The main meridian continues along the lower jaw to the upper collarbone and from there straight down to the chest. It continues along the edge of the main abdominal muscles to the groin. From there it passes along the thigh and calf to the top of the foot; it ends on the outer edge of the nail of the second toe. In keeping with a yang-yin pairing, the Stomach meridian is linked to the Spleen meridian.

THE STOMACH MERIDIAN	
Transformation phase	Earth
Color	Yellow
Season	Late summer
Emotion	Worry
Damaging influence	Humidity

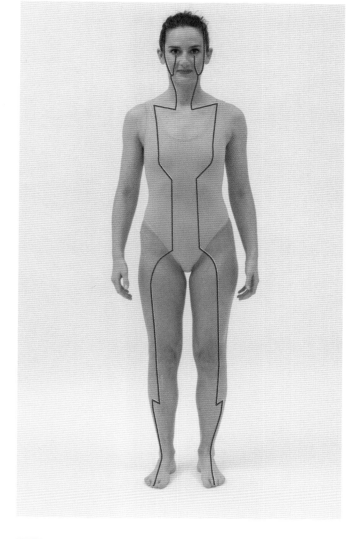

The Stomach meridian runs along the entire front of the body, from the face to the feet.

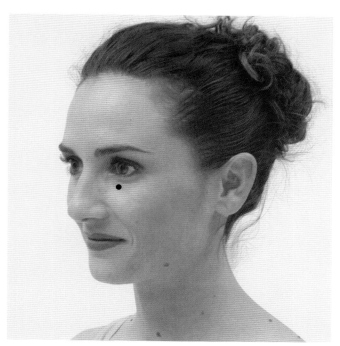

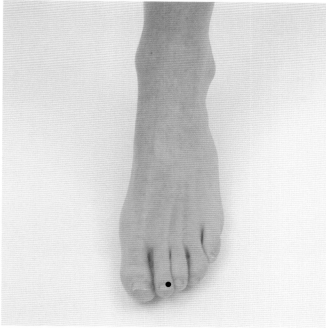

Left: The point Stomach 1 is located below the eye.

Right: The endpoint of the Stomach meridian is Stomach 45, located on the side of the second toenail.

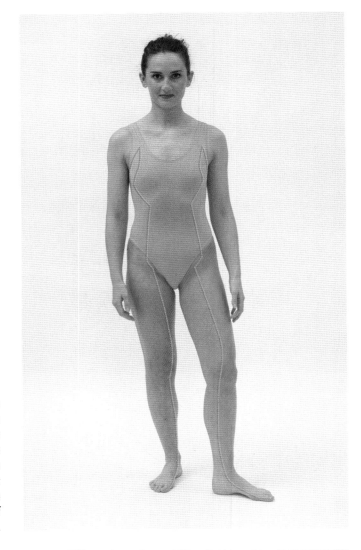

The Spleen meridian originates on the edge of the big toe and runs across the front of the body to the side of the chest.

The Spleen Meridian

The Spleen meridian is a yin pathway consisting of twenty-one points. It begins on the inside edge of the nail of the big toe and runs along the inside of the foot, past the inside of the ankle, and up to the inner calf and thigh. Running between the inside and front of the thigh, the meridian continues to the groin region. From there, it runs sideways and then up to the upper abdomen, marking point Spleen 16. From here it continues upward along the outside of the chest to the point Spleen 20, located in the space between the second and third ribs. From here the meridian turns downward along the side of the body. The endpoint of the meridian, Spleen 21, is located on the side of the body between the sixth and seventh ribs.

THE SPLEEN MERIDIAN	
Transformation phase	Earth
Color	Yellow
Season	Late summer
Emotion	Worry
Damaging influence	Humidity; a weakness of the spleen can lead to edema, diarrhea, or fatigue

Left: Spleen 1 is located on the inside edge of the nail of the big toe.

Right: The endpoint of the Spleen meridian is Spleen 21, located on the side of the chest area.

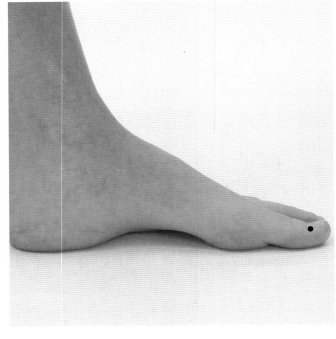

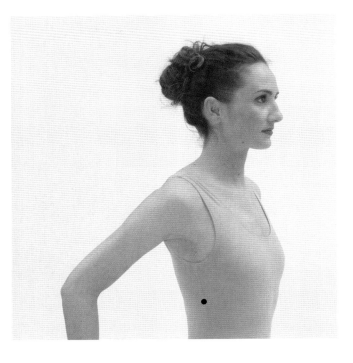

The Heart Meridian

The Heart meridian is a yin pathway along which lie nine points.

The meridian begins in the armpit at the point Heart 1 and runs along the inside of the arm and across the palm to the pinkie finger, where it ends at the inside edge of that finger's nail, at the point Heart 9. In the sense of yin-yang pairing, the Heart meridian is linked to the Small Intestine meridian.

THE HEART MERIDIAN	
Transformation phase	Fire
Color	Red
Season	Summer
Emotion	Happiness
Damaging influence	Heat

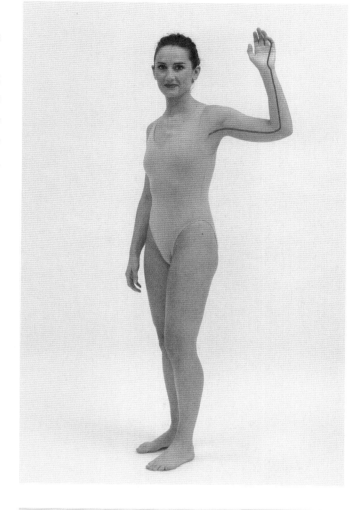

The Heart meridian runs from the armpit to the inner edge of the pinkie finger.

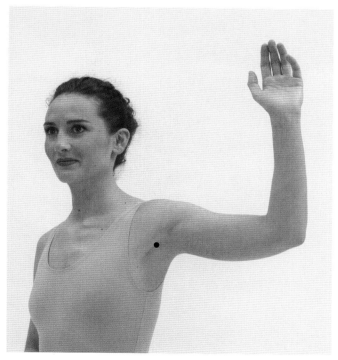

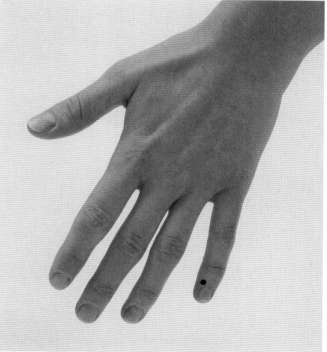

Left: Heart 1 is located in the armpit, exactly above the noticeable pulse of the armpit artery.

Right: The Heart meridian ends with Heart 9, located on the edge of the pinkie nail closest to the thumb.

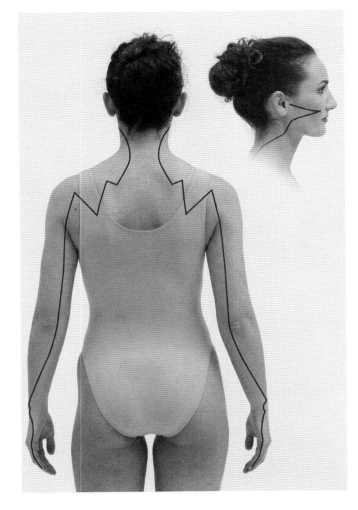

The Small Intestine meridian runs along both halves of the body from the hands along the backs of the arms up to the ears.

The Small Intestine Meridian

The Small Intestine meridian is a yang pathway along which are nineteen points. It begins at the outer edge of the nail of the pinkie finger with the point Small Intestine 1. From there it passes along the outer edge of the pinkie and hand and up the back of the arm to the back of the shoulder. Running in a zigzag pattern across the shoulder blade, the meridian then heads up the side of the neck and across the cheek to the cheekbone. Another zag turns the meridian upward once again, until it ends with the point Small Intestine 19, just in front of the ear. In the sense of a yin-yang pairing, the Small Intestine meridian is linked to the Heart meridian.

THE SMALL INTESTINE MERIDIAN	
Transformation phase	Fire
Color	Red
Season	Summer
Emotion	Happiness
Damaging influence	Heat

Left: The point Small Intestine 1 is located on the edge of the nail of the pinkie finger.

Right: The endpoint of the Small Intestine meridian, Small Intestine 19, can be located immediately in front of the ear.

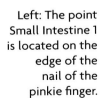
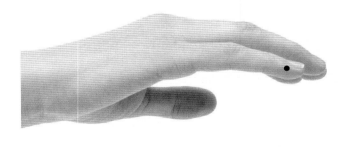
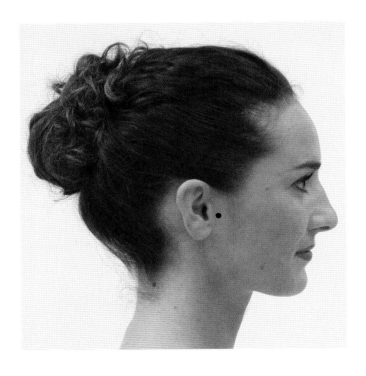

The Urinary Bladder Meridian

The Urinary Bladder meridian is a yang pathway, and with sixty-seven points it is the longest of the twelve main meridians. It begins on the inside edge of the eye socket and passes up to the hairline above the forehead. From here it turns sideways to the point Urinary Bladder 4, located at the front of the hairline. Just off to the side of the body's middle axis, it continues over the head to the point Urinary Bladder 10, located just under the back of the head at the top of the spine. From here it divides into two branches, which run down the back almost parallel to each other. The medial branch continues downward past the sacrum and the inside of the buttock to the back of the thigh. The lateral branch runs almost parallel across the middle of the buttock and along the back of the thigh to the knee. Here the two branches merge at the point Urinary Bladder 40. Crossing the back of the calf and the outer edge of the foot, the meridian ends at the small toe.

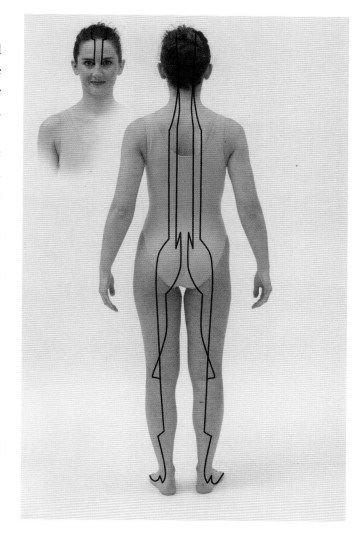

The Urinary Bladder meridian divides into two branches along the back of the body.

THE URINARY BLADDER MERIDIAN	
Transformation phase	Water
Color	Black
Season	Winter
Emotion	Fear
Damaging influence	Cold

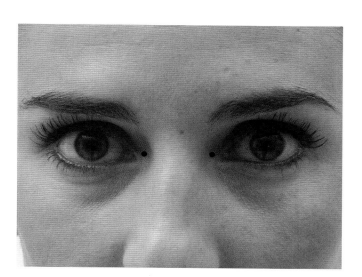

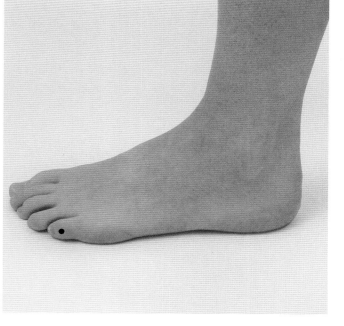

Left: The point Urinary Bladder 1 can be located on the inside corner of the eye.

Right: The Urinary Bladder meridian ends with the point Urinary Bladder 67, on the outside edge of the nail of the small toe.

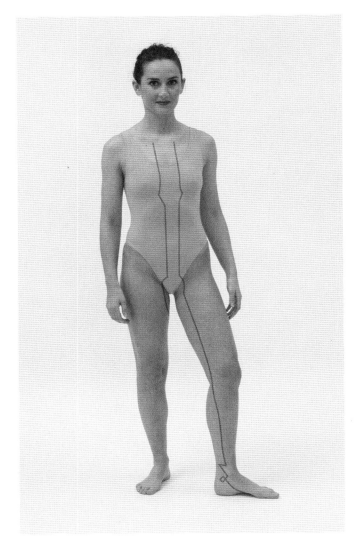

The Kidney meridian begins on the sole of the foot and runs up the front of the body to the collarbone.

The Kidney Meridian

The Kidney meridian is a yin pathway consisting of twenty-seven points. The pathway begins on the sole of the foot about one-third of the way down from the toes. From here it runs along the inner edge of the foot to a point between the Achilles tendon and inner ankle. There the meridian completes a loop around the ankle and continues up along the inside of the shin and thigh to the groin. From there it runs alongside the middle axis of the body up to the sternum and then widens on either side before resuming its run parallel to the middle axis up across the chest to the collarbone. The endpoint, Kidney 27, is located immediately beneath the collarbone, about two inches away from the middle axis.

THE KIDNEY MERIDIAN	
Transformation phase	Water
Color	Black
Season	Winter
Emotion	Fear
Damaging influence	Cold leads to a depletion of stored jing as well as yang, which is produced here

Left: The point Kidney 1 is located one-third of the way down the sole of the foot.

Right: Kidney 27 is immediately below the collarbone.

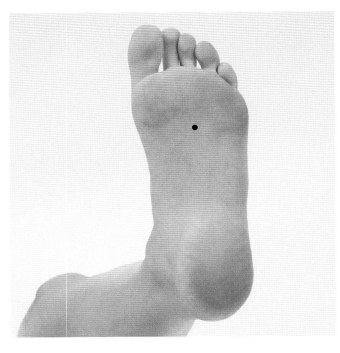

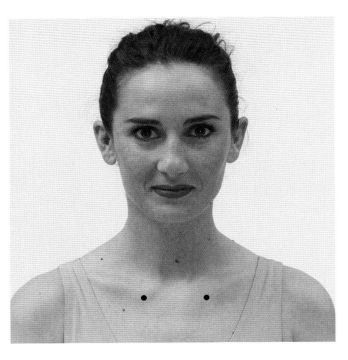

The Pericardium Meridian

The Pericardium meridian is a yin pathway with nine points that connect to the body's surface. It begins with the point Pericardium 1 in the fourth intercostal space about one inch toward the side from the nipple. From here the Pericardium meridian runs up along the front edge of the armpit and then down along the inside of the arm to the wrist. It continues along the palm to the tip of the middle finger, where it ends with the point Pericardium 9.

Like the Heart and the Small Intestine meridians, the Pericardium meridian is assigned to the fire transformation phase.

THE PERICARDIUM MERIDIAN	
Transformation phase	Fire
Color	Red
Season	Summer
Emotion	Happiness
Damaging influence	Heat

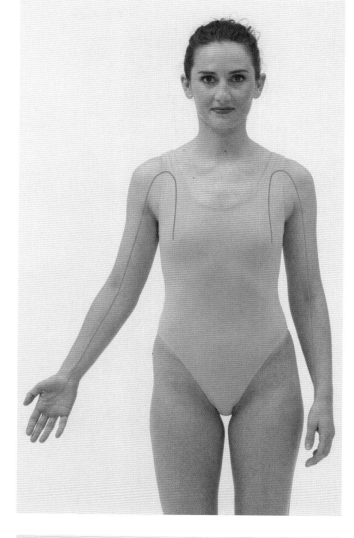

The Pericardium meridian begins on the chest and extends past the shoulder to the palm.

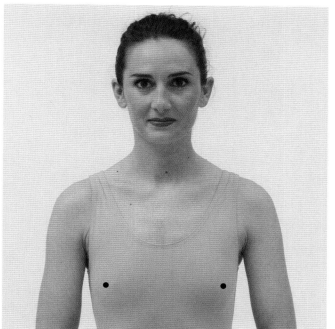

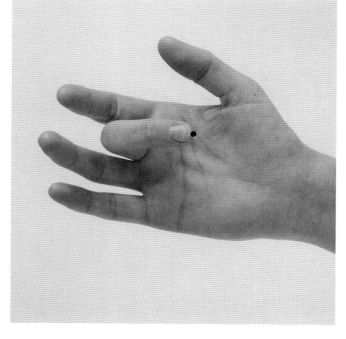

Left: The point Pericardium 1 is located to the side of the nipple.

Right: The Pericardium meridian ends in the point Pericardium 9, located at the tip of the middle finger.

The Triple Heater Meridian

The Triple Heater meridian is a yang pathway with twenty-three points. It begins on the edge of the nail of the ring finger with the point Triple Heater 1. From there it runs along the back of the hand and the back of the arm to the shoulder. It continues along the back of the shoulder and then up the neck, behind and around the ear, and past the temple, ending at the outer edge of the eyebrow with the point Triple Heater 23.

The Triple Heater meridian regulates the flow of energy in the three body cavities of the chest, upper abdomen, and lower abdomen. It is linked to the Pericardium meridian in a yin-yang pairing.

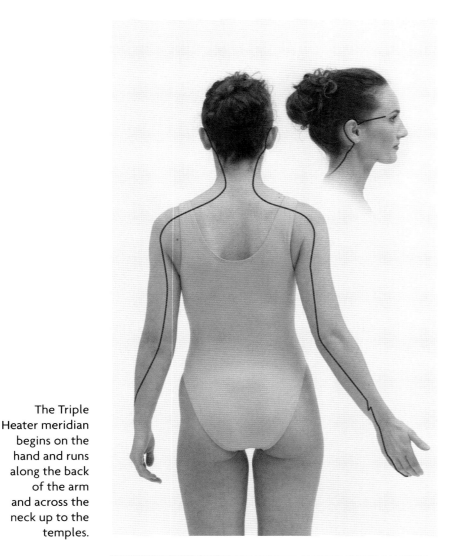

The Triple Heater meridian begins on the hand and runs along the back of the arm and across the neck up to the temples.

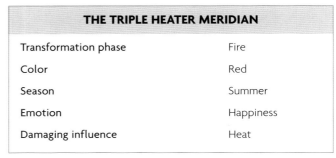

THE TRIPLE HEATER MERIDIAN	
Transformation phase	Fire
Color	Red
Season	Summer
Emotion	Happiness
Damaging influence	Heat

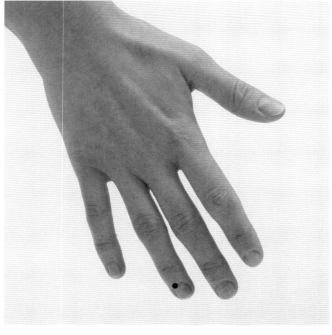

Left: The point Triple Heater 1 is located on the edge of the ring finger facing the pinkie.

Right: The point Triple Heater 23 is located in the indentation immediately next to the outside edge of the eyebrow.

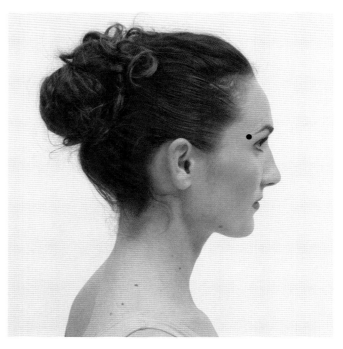

The Gall Bladder Meridian

This meridian is a yang pathway with forty-four points. It starts at the outer edge of the eye and runs in a descending line toward the ear. From there it rises to the temple and then drops down and circles the ear in a large arc. From the back of the ear the meridian arches along the side of the skull back to the forehead. Another arch runs back along the side of the head, down the neck, and along the shoulder muscles to the upper edge of the collarbone. From there the meridian arcs around the shoulder to the armpit and then zigzags down the side of the body past the buttock and thigh. It then continues along the outside of the leg to the foot, running along the top of the foot and ending at the point Gall Bladder 44, at the base of the nail of the fourth toe.

THE GALL BLADDER MERIDIAN	
Transformation phase	Wood
Color	Green
Season	Spring
Emotion	Anger, irritability
Damaging influence	Wind (also in the sense of internal wind, as from stress, frustration, or anger)

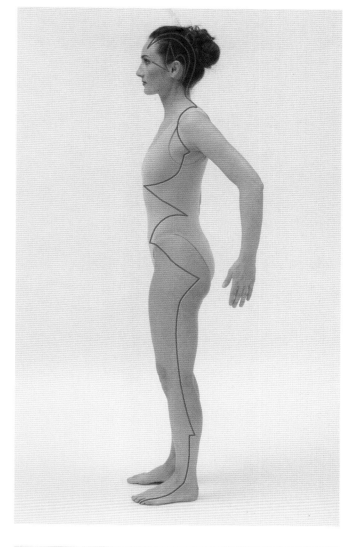

The Gall Bladder meridian frequently changes direction.

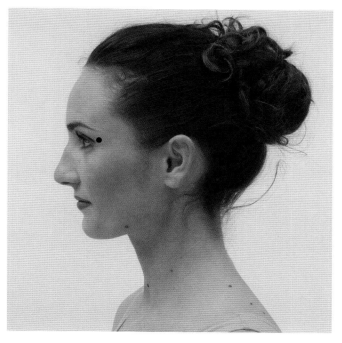

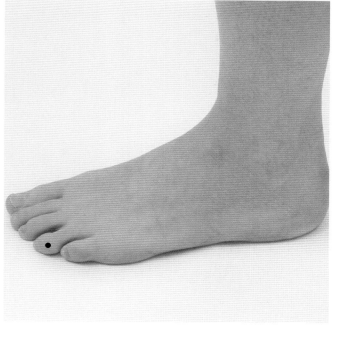

Left: The first point of the Gall Bladder meridian can be felt in an indentation on the edge of the bony eye socket.

Right: The point Gall Bladder 44 is located on the outside edge of the nail of the fourth toe.

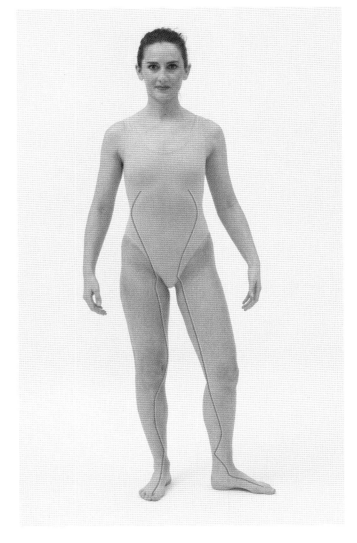

The Liver meridian starts at the big toe and runs up the inside of the leg, past the wall of the abdomen, and up to the chest.

The Liver Meridian

The Liver meridian is a yin pathway consisting of fourteen points. The meridian begins on the big toe with point Liver 1, at the lateral (meaning toward the outside of the body) edge of the toenail. From there it proceeds over the top of the foot to the inside of the ankle and up along the inside of the calf and thigh. At the level of the groin it passes points 12 and 13 of the Spleen meridian. The meridian skirts the genitals and moves up toward the ribs, where it ends in the sixth intercostal space, just beneath the nipple, with point Liver 14, which in traditional literature is named "Cycle Gate" or the "Gate of Hope."

THE LIVER MERIDIAN	
Transformation phase	Wood
Color	Green
Season	Spring
Emotion	Anger
Damaging influence	Wind; energy blocked by wind may be expressed through headache or neck pain

Left: The point Liver 1 is located on the bottom edge of the nail of the big toe.

Right: The Liver meridian ends with the point Liver 14, located below the nipple, between the sixth and seventh ribs.

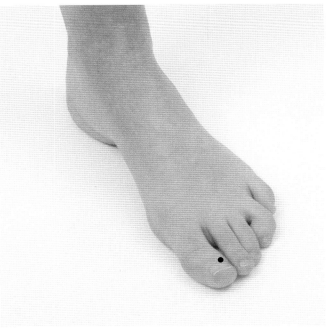

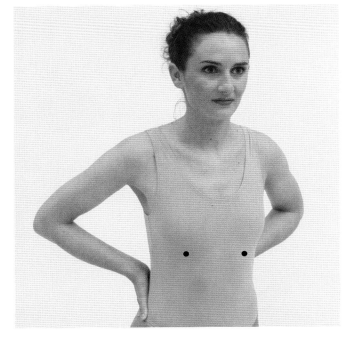

The Conception Vessel

The Conception Vessel is a yin pathway with twenty-four points. It begins between the legs and runs up over the genitals, continuing in a straight line up to the chin. It ends in the fold of skin between the chin and lips.

The Conception Vessel is sometimes known as the Sea of Yin. It controls sexual maturation and regulates qi in the Stomach and Lungs. Problems with the latter manifest as nausea, vomiting, or asthma. Points of the Conception Vessel can be massaged to address cardiovascular or respiratory ailments, problems in the mouth and throat area, facial nerve pain, and gastrointestinal problems as well as menstrual pain.

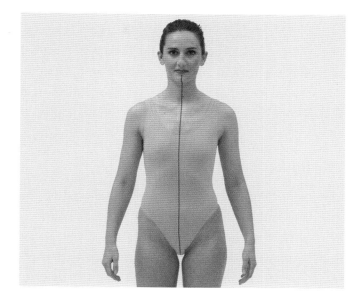

The Conception Vessel is a pathway that runs exactly along the middle axis of the front of the body.

The Governor Vessel

The Governor Vessel is a yang pathway with twenty-eight points. It begins between the anus and the tip of the coccyx and runs between the buttocks up in a straight line along the spine and over the head toward the mouth. It ends inside the mouth where the upper lip joins the gum at Governor Vessel 28. The points of the Governor Vessel can be massaged to address cases of fatigue or exhaustion, sexual dysfunction, weakness, spine problems, acute colds, and immune-system deficiencies. Points of the Governor Vessel can also be massaged to address cognitive problems such as mental development disabilities.

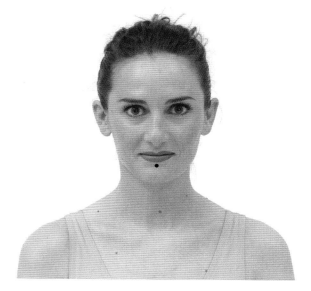

The endpoint of the Conception Vessel is just below the lower lip.

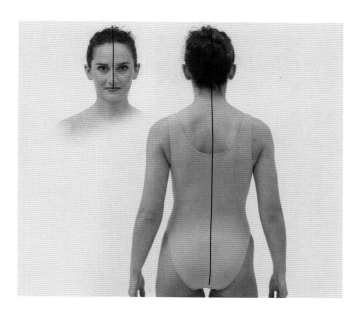

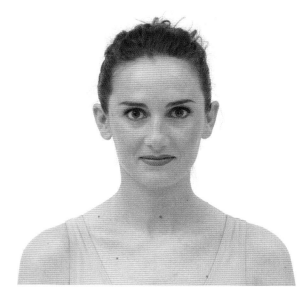

Left: The Governor Vessel runs along the middle axis of the body from the tailbone in an arch across the head to the face.

Right: The endpoint of the Governor Vessel is inside the mouth where the upper lip meets the gum.

How Acupressure Works

The points used in acupressure are the same points used in traditional acupuncture. Acupressure and acupuncture are both rooted in traditional Chinese medicine and are based on the same principles and methodologies.

The Points and Their Effects

The majority of acupressure points are located on the meridians and are distributed across the body's surface. They are often pressure-sensitive in those who suffer from an ailment or illness. Acupressure treats such painful points and zones with gentle pressure and massage techniques. In this way pain and ailments can be positively influenced.

> **Note**
> The points can be referred to both by their original Chinese names as well as by modern names. For example, the point He Gu (Valley of Union) is known in modern terms as Large Intestine 4. The modern names are used especially in medical practice. They increase a student's ability to understand the system, since aside from the precise location of the point, they refer to its link to a specific meridian. In the preceding example, *Large Intestine* tells us which meridian this point is found on, while the number 4 tells us it is the fourth point along this meridian.

Current Research into the Effectiveness of Acupressure

The many ways in which acupressure can be an effective therapy still have not been completely researched. Scientific work is concentrating especially on the some-

times spectacular effectiveness of acupressure on certain points to reduce pain. The possibility of reaching internal organs or entire areas of the body using seemingly distant acupuncture points has been explained by modern science as being linked to the body's embryonic development. During development of the embryo, a lot of tissue is created in one part of the body and then moves to its "correct" place. Today it is believed that each type of tissue can continue to communicate with other like tissue even in a fully developed human body.

The ability of acupuncture points to influence pain and illnesses and to indicate, for example, problems of internal organs through sensitivity to pressure shows this connection. As early as the beginning of the twentieth century, British neurologist Henry Head (1861–1940) discovered that problems in some organs can cause pain in body parts that are not in the immediate vicinity. For example, heart attacks can cause pain in the arm and hand. Without realizing it, Head had described a phenomenon that had been recognized in traditional Chinese medicine for hundreds of years: the fact that sensitivity to pain often runs along meridians associated with the affected internal organ.

Today we know that these sensations are transmitted via reflectory mechanisms of the spinal cord. Additional research has shown that many acupuncture points are marked by a nerve bundle surrounded by loose, water-rich connective tissue. This means that compared to the areas around them, the points have a high level of electrical conductivity. These nerve bundles pass from the surface to the depths of the body, where they connect to larger nerves and the autonomic nervous system. In

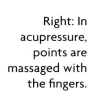

Left: Acupuncture uses very thin and fine needles.

Right: In acupressure, points are massaged with the fingers.

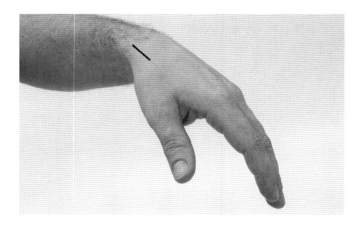

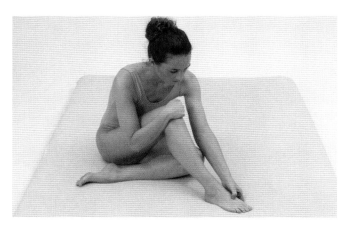

this way signals given via acupressure or acupuncture can reach and have positive effects on far-removed parts of the body.

Needling acupuncture points causes nerve endings to release endorphins, substances that block pain. This fact has been used to explain the effectiveness of acupuncture in treating pain. It is believed that similar effects come into play in acupressure. Positive influence on the male and female hormone system has also been noted; research has shown that the positive effects on male and female fertility through acupuncture were comparable to those of hormone therapy (see Kaptchuk 2001).

Using Acupressure

Acupressure is a treatment method that can be used successfully to treat a wide range of ailments. One of its most important uses is in counteracting pain. It is, however, important to remember that acupressure works by addressing energetic disruptions, restoring energetic balance. It is not suitable for counteracting organic changes.

Treatment Areas of Acupressure

Massaging yourself or a partner is a gentle way to counteract pain, ailments, or illnesses and to support the healing process. Please note, however, that pain is an alarm signal from our bodies. In the case of more serious illnesses accompanied by fever or continuing pain, acupressure cannot be the sole treatment. In these cases, consult a qualified health care practitioner who can form a diagnosis and, based on that diagnosis, decide on a course of treatment.

Suddenly occurring pain such as toothache or back pain as well as chronic pain and so-called functional disturbances can be treated equally well through acupressure. Functional disturbances are ailments whose causes remain unclear despite thorough medical examination. In addition to relieving these acute and chronic pains, acupressure is frequently effective in treating nonspecific problems such as nervousness, anxiety, stress, and sleeping problems. However, despite the tangible effectiveness of properly conducted acupressure for these ailments, it is not a panacea.

The Limits of Acupressure

Like any type of therapy, acupressure has its limits, which you should be familiar with. Areas of the body with localized damage, including injuries that have not completely healed, scars, infections, burns, varicose veins, and rheumatic pain should not be treated with acupressure. People with serious health problems such as cardiovascular problems, cancer, osteoporosis, or epilepsy should be treated only by experienced therapists. In the case of pregnant women, certain precautions should be taken and certain points avoided (as noted in the text

Caution

Do not carry out acupressure in the case of:
- Pregnancy
- Any kind of acute infection
- Acute injury of muscle, tendon, or bone
- Cold accompanied by fever
- Unclear and strong pain
- Slipped disc
- An artery ailment such as severe varicose veins, thrombosis, or circulation problems
- Heart attack
- Recent surgery
- Advanced osteoporosis
- Skin infection
- Burns
- Problems with blood clotting or while taking blood-thinning medication
- Cancer

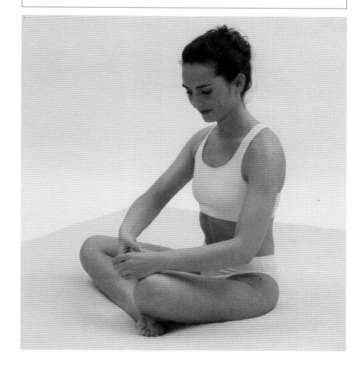

Most acupressure points are well suited for self-massage.

where appropriate), meaning that such massages should be carried out only by experienced therapists.

Duration and Frequency of Acupressure

The intensity, duration, and frequency of acupressure treatment depend on a range of factors. In the case of self-treatment, you will know best what is good for you. Note when the pressure is strong enough and determine the frequency of the massage based on your needs. If you want to massage others, the following contains a few rules of thumb about the duration and frequency of acupressure.

How frequently and how strongly you practice acupressure depends first and foremost on the person you are treating. Children, the elderly, and people in a weakened state generally can handle only a gentle massage of short duration. Strong people, in general, can be massaged for longer and more frequently.

Another factor for the intensity of the treatment is the type of ailment you are aiming to address. Chronic ailments are treated less frequently. For example, in the case of a chronic ailment of the respiratory passages, one or two acupressure sessions per week usually suffice. The duration of each treatment in this case should be between thirty and sixty minutes.

Acute ailments, on the other hand, can be treated

FREQUENCY AND DURATION OF ACUPRESSURE TREATMENT	
Acute ailments	Frequency: two or three treatments per day Duration: ten to fifteen minutes each
Chronic ailments	Frequency: one to two treatments per week Duration: thirty to sixty minutes

more frequently. For example, if you are aiming to treat a sudden-onset headache or acute back pain, up to three treatments a day can be given until the pain subsides. The duration of each treatment should be shorter, generally between ten and fifteen minutes.

During massage, some points may prove to be especially sensitive. Even light pressure will cause certain physical reactions, such as a burning, pulling, or pulsating feeling. These perceptions can extend along the part of the body being massaged and are referred to as the *de-qi* feeling. This reaction is normal and indeed desirable, as it indicates that you have correctly located the appropriate point of a meridian. If a point seems to be sensitive in this way, a shorter treatment duration than you would use for a less sensitive point is usually sufficient. Reddening skin shows that you have reached the maximum duration and pressure for the massage.

De-Qi Feeling

The *de-qi* feeling (pronounced *deh tschee*) occurs as soon as an acupressure point is correctly "hit." Typically it entails a blunt or cutting pain that spreads along the meridian, referred to as a feeling transferred through the meridian.

The de-qi feeling is generally experienced only on the arms and legs (not including the buttocks). It is a frequent occurrence but by no means present during the massage of every acupressure point. Thus, even if you cannot observe a de-qi feeling in your partner, you may, nevertheless, have correctly located the point.

Acupressure on Pregnant Women and Children

One frequently asked question is whether it is possible to use acupressure on pregnant women and children. This question can generally be answered in the affirmative, as long as certain rules are followed.

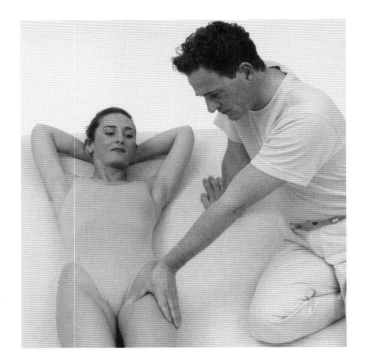

Always pay attention to the reactions of your partner. Acupressure should always be perceived as a pleasant therapy.

Acupressure during Pregnancy

Massage of some acupressure points has a stimulating effect on the uterus. Massaging these points during pregnancy carries the risk of causing contractions. For this reason, and especially in the first five months of pregnancy, pregnant women should avoid acupressure therapy. If you intend to practice acupressure on a pregnant woman, consult with a therapist who has been trained in acupuncture or acupressure. The therapist should show you exactly which points are safe to massage and which are not. And before undertaking the acupressure treatment, read the notes in this book about the individual points.

To relieve nausea and vomiting during pregnancy, the point Pericardium 6 (see page 122) can be massaged. This point does not affect the uterus and so is safe to massage.

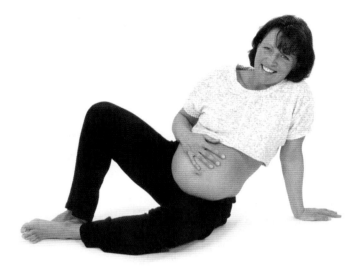

Special rules apply for acupressure during pregnancy.

> **Caution**
>
> The following points should not be treated during pregnancy, since they have a stimulating effect on the uterus and may cause contractions:
> - Large Intestine 4
> - Gall Bladder 21
> - Conception Vessel 4
> - Governor Vessel 3
> - Stomach 28
> - Spleen 6

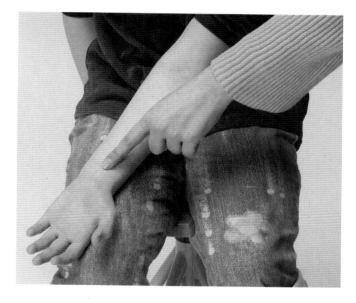

For acupressure on children, shorten the duration of treatment.

Acupressure for Children

In principle it is possible to practice acupressure with children. Indeed, children tend to respond particularly well to this type of therapy. It is important, however, that you do not make your own diagnoses. Ailments should always be diagnosed by a physician before you begin with acupressure massage. Please note that when massaging children, you have to reduce the orientation values given here regarding duration and pressure, which are based on adults.

Two acupressure points of particular use with children are Urinary Bladder 50, which is a very effective point to help with digestive problems in children, and Pericardium 6, which has proven effective in relieving motion sickness (see page 185).

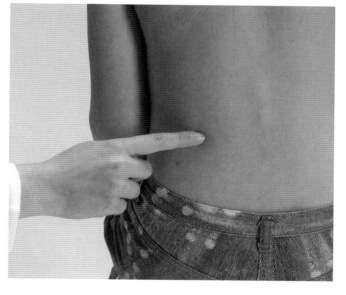

The point Urinary Bladder 50 can be massaged to address digestive problems in children.

Acupressure Step by Step

This book contains all the information you need to carry out an acupressure massage. This chapter contains the essential information you need to know before you begin giving acupressure massages. Before the massage, make sure there are no counterindications (see page 47). If you want to influence a specific ailment using acupressure massage, check to see whether the ailment is listed in the chapter "Targeting Ailments with Acupressure" (see pages 144–99); if it is, orient yourself in the proposed sequence. Many of the acupressure points listed in reference to a specific ailment are effective for multiple ailments and even support overall health. These points are therefore listed in more than one place. These points are described in full for each application, allowing you to follow each acupressure program in full without having to refer back to other sections. Readers may also be interested in taking a look at the most important points on the meridians to gain a systematic overview of the meridians and their points in this way.

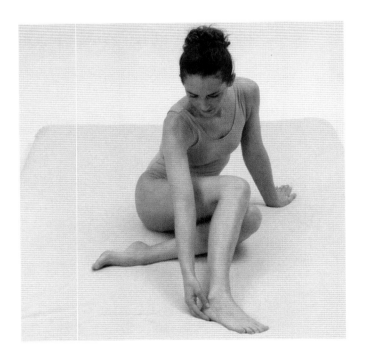

Take your time in locating the individual points.

Applying Acupressure

The success of an acupressure massage rests on two pillars. The first pillar is the general preparation, including the creation of a pleasant, relaxing atmosphere. The second pillar comprises the "tricks of the trade." This encompasses knowledge about the location and effects of the zones and points to be massaged, and about the technique and type of massage to use.

Preparation

Preparation is essential for the success of acupressure. If you are treating a partner this includes positioning yourself, enabling him or her to relax while you administer the massage. When massaging yourself, you should make sure to take up a relaxing and comfortable position.

Do not begin by applying maximum pressure on painful points along the meridians; instead, approach such zones carefully. It is ideal to loosen the muscles before acupressure massage, using soft strokes, gentle kneading, or shaking of the body part. A whole-body program (see page 200) that describes the use of these techniques is included in the chapter "Targeting Ailments with Acupressure." These techniques contain elements of classical Western massage. Remember that acupressure is one part of a large system called tui na. This term comes from the Chinese, with *tui* meaning "to push," and *na* "to grasp." Before a massage focuses on a specific point, it is thus always necessary to begin with an overall loosening of the body. Only the two elements together—the overall loosening and the acupressure of specific painful points—results in effective treatment.

The Room and Atmosphere

Carry out acupressure massage in an environment that is pleasant for both you and your partner. A room where you will not be disturbed is best. Relaxation is promoted by creating a pleasant atmosphere. This includes a comfortable temperature, dimmed or indirect light, and calm music (let yourself be guided in this by the preferences of your partner). Also make sure that you will not be interrupted by a ringing telephone or doorbell. You should have enough room to be able to move freely around the person being massaged. Your partner should take off any jewelry and other accessories and wear comfortable clothes. Clothes create a warming shell for the body, reducing the amount of energy needed to heat the skin.

Relaxation and Concentration

If you want to practice acupressure, it is important that you give yourself enough time and peace for this task. Focus your attention entirely on what you want to do. Concentrate on the points and zones you are treating. When you are treating yourself, observe your feelings.

What feeling spreads across the point you are treating? What is changing because of the treatment? Listen to your body. Practicing acupressure on yourself effectively is possible only if you focus your undivided attention on the treatment.

To do this, you will first need to learn the proper techniques. An acupressure massage during a quick break somewhere is not going to deliver the results you want. You will be able to take advantage of the positive effects of acupressure only if you have the opportunity to carefully search for and massage the right points.

The same principles apply to treating a partner. Before massaging somebody else, make sure you are comfortable with the techniques described in the book. You will be able to learn to find most points on your own body. When treating somebody else, concentrate entirely on the person you are massaging. Feel how your partner is receiving what you are doing. When treating a painful point, your partner may tense up or hold his or her breath. If this happens, it means that the pressure you are applying is too strong. Massage more gently, and take your time. Try to "see" with your hands. During acupressure massage, your hands receive a lot of information about your partner from

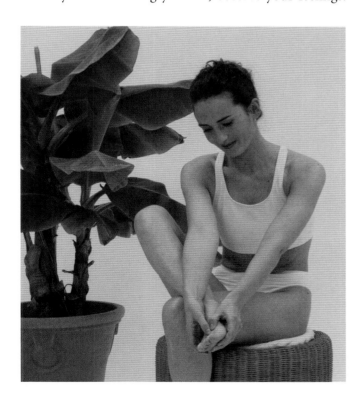

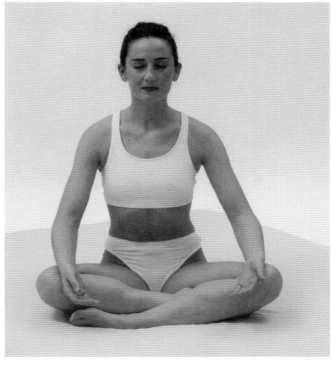

Left: A pleasant atmosphere and comfortable position are important conditions for the success of acupressure.

Right: Allow yourself a few minutes of reflection before longer acupressure treatments.

the temperature, moisture, and texture of the skin, from tension in the muscles, and from the reaction of his or her body to your massage. Take in this information and let it guide you in your acupressure massage.

Preparing Your Hands

The most important "tools" in acupressure are your hands. You use them to exert pressure and to feel how your partner is receiving your massage.

To carry out a good massage, your hands should be warm and relaxed. For this reason it makes sense to loosen the hand muscles before the massage: shake out your hands and then rub your palms together until you feel a cozy warmth between them.

More than a Pressure Tool

Hands are very important in acupressure massage. They should be warm and smooth. Your fingernails should not extend beyond your fingertips so that you will not accidentally injure your partner. Take off accessories like rings, bracelets, and watches before the massage.

Strengthening, Stretching, and Loosening

If you are new to the field of acupressure, it is possible that you will find the first massage treatments you give more exhausting than pleasant. For this reason, it makes sense to strengthen, stretch, and loosen the muscles in your hands with some simple exercises to prepare them for the massage.

To strengthen your muscles, take a small rubber ball that you can easily squeeze in one hand. (You can buy such balls at any toy store.) Squeeze the ball, hold the tension for seven to ten seconds, and then release. Carry out ten repetitions before switching to the other hand. During and after this strengthening exercise, you will feel your hands becoming warm and flexible.

To stretch the muscles of your palms, place your palms against each other in front of your chest, with your elbows pointing out. Keeping your palms together, move your hands downward, maintaining contact between the palms. You will now feel a slight pull in the muscles of your lower arms. If possible, maintain the tension for twenty to thirty seconds before releasing. Repeat this stretch three times.

Now stretch the bending muscles of your hands and lower arms. To do this, place your hands against a wall at

Left: Exercises with a soft rubber ball are very effective for strengthening your hands.

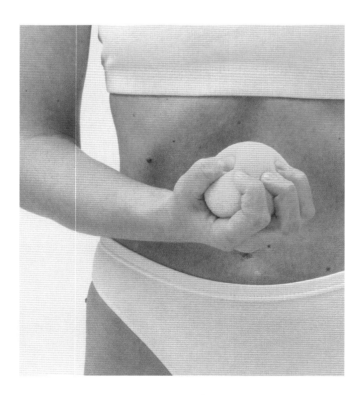

Right: Special exercises help stretch the muscles of the palm.

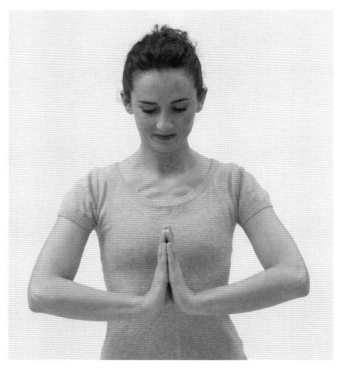

shoulder height and shoulder width apart. Spread your fingers straight and apart, and straighten your elbows. Now carefully press your wrists against the wall. When doing this exercise, keep your shoulders relaxed; make sure you don't pull them up. You can increase the stretch by slightly lifting up your fingers and palms while keeping your wrists against the wall. When doing this stretch you should feel a noticeable but not painful pull. Maintain the tension for twenty to thirty seconds before releasing, and repeat the exercise three times.

Feeling the Energy of the Hands

To increase the sensitivity of your hands, it helps to carry out the following simple but effective perception exercise after you have loosened and warmed up your hand muscles.

Close your eyes and breathe in and out regularly. Keep your shoulders relaxed. Bring your hands in front of your body, with your palms facing each other but not touching. Direct your attention toward your palms. Try to feel the warmth emanating from one palm to the other. Now imagine this feeling of warmth to be a flow of energy between your hands. As soon as you perceive this flow of energy, begin to play with it: Make small,

Summary
- Loosen your hand muscles by shaking your hands.
- Warm your hands by rubbing your palms together.
- Your fingernails should not extend past your fingertips, since they may otherwise cause injury during massage.
- Remove all jewelry from your hands.
- Strengthen your hand muscles by squeezing a small ball.
- Place your palms against each other in front of your chest and stretch them.
- Stretch your hands and lower arms against a wall.
- Through concentration, feel the flow of energy and warmth between your palms.

slow, circular movements in opposite directions with your hands. Increase the distance between your hands, but only to the point where you can still clearly feel the energy and flow of warmth. When you begin the acupressure massage, picture this energetic feeling passing into your partner during the course of the massage.

It is possible that at first you might find it difficult to feel the flow of warmth between your hands. Keep in mind that your hands have to be warm for this exercise. The more frequently you carry out this perception exercise, the more intensive and fine-tuned your perception will become.

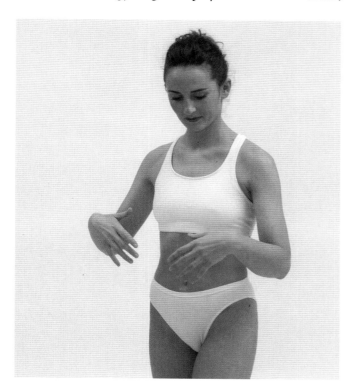

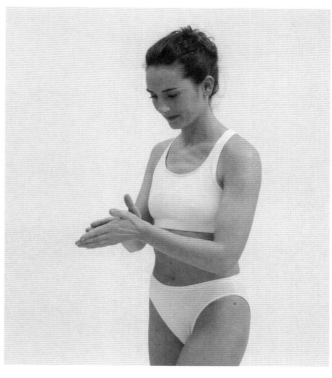

Left: Shaking the hands loosens the muscles.

Right: Rub your palms against each other to warm your hands.

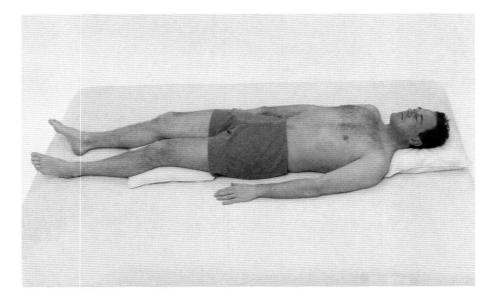

When your partner is lying on his or her back, the thighs and knees are elevated slightly to ensure that the lower spine remains in contact with the surface on which your partner is lying.

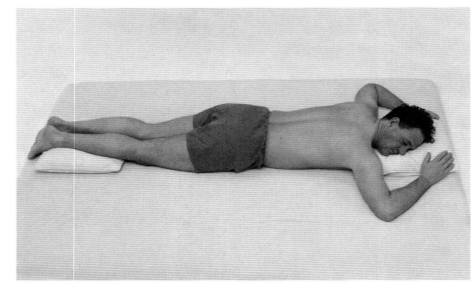

When your partner is lying on his or her stomach, the head and calves can be raised slightly on a soft surface, such as a pillow.

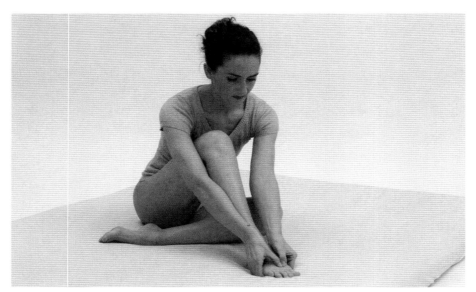

Self-massage is best done sitting down on a large, soft surface.

Body Posture and Positioning

If you are massaging yourself, take up a comfortable position. A comfortable position is a precondition for a successful acupressure treatment. Try a variety of different positions to find the one that is most comfortable for you. You should be able to reach all the acupressure points that you are planning to massage without any contortions. A comfortable chair or a soft mat on which you can sit or lie is good for this.

The same applies when you are massaging a partner. He or she should lie on a soft surface that is comfortable for both of you and helps your partner relax. When your partner lies on his or her back, you can place a small pillow under his or her knees, which helps relax the abdomen and promotes contact between the lower spine and the surface on which your partner is resting. If you want to massage the back area, have your partner lie on his or her stomach. Again, you can make this more comfortable using simple aids; for example, you can place a rolled-up blanket or a small pillow under your partner's feet, which ensures that the back and leg muscles are relaxed. A hollow in the back can be counterbalanced by placing a cushion under your partner's stomach.

The Basic Techniques

There are many techniques that can be used in Chinese acupressure, and it takes years to systematically learn them. For this reason we will limit ourselves here to basic techniques that can be used effectively with little practice.

Searching for and Locating Points

Acupressure focuses on points that—with a few exceptions—are located along the meridians. Each point has a unique and discrete location. Oftentimes points are located near noticeable areas like visible bones, skin folds, or the beginning of large muscle groups. All these characteristics can be used to measure and determine the location of the point in question. One measure used in locating points is hand width, which refers to the distance across the index, middle, ring, and pinkie fingers when held next to each other, at the level of the middle joints of the fingers.

For each application, the location of the point is described precisely. Try to follow this description. You will find that the points frequently are more sensitive than the tissue around them. This increased sensitivity to pain is a reliable indication that you have found the right point. Try to locate such sensitivities. Compare how these areas feel before and after the massage. Ideally the initial sensitivity to pressure should be noticeably reduced or even gone after the acupressure massage.

Cun—The Basic Measure

Cun (pronounced *tsun*) is the basic unit of measure for locating acupressure points on the body. It is not a preset distance but is based on the physical proportions of the person being massaged, or more precisely, on that person's finger width. This means that a cun is shorter for a small child than for an adult.

Note

One cun
- Is a proportional measure whose exact distance varies with each person
- Refers to the largest width of the thumb, usually at the level of the top joint

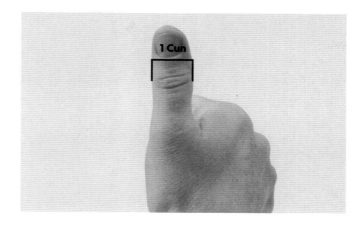

One cun is the width of the thumb at the level of the top joint.

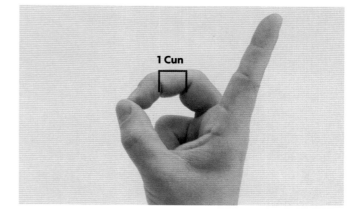

When the middle finger is placed against the thumb, the distance between the two joints of the middle finger also equals 1 cun.

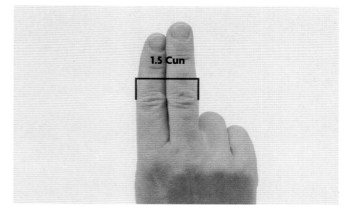

The width of index and middle fingers at the level of the middle joints is defined as 1.5 cun.

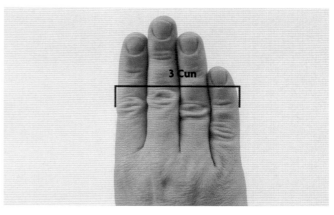

The width across the index, middle, ring, and pinkie fingers at the joint level is 3 cun.

One cun is equal to the distance across the widest point of the thumb of the person being massaged. When you massage a partner, it is important to compare your thumb with his or hers before you begin, so you can locate the points as you go along.

> **Note**
>
> Cun measurements refer to the body of the person being massaged. This means that for self-treatment, you should orient yourself on your own finger measurements. When you are massaging a partner, you have to use his or her finger measurements to locate the meridian points. On a grown person 3 cun is a longer distance than on a child. The location of points on a meridian is thus proportional to the size of the body.

Body Measures

To locate acupressure points, the measure of cun has to be determined for the person to be massaged. For this it is helpful to know that certain parts of the body always have the same proportions. For example, the distance between the navel and the upper edge of the pubic bone is five finger widths or 5 cun. You can divide this distance into five equal segments with four imaginary cross-lines along the way; each segment equates to 1 cun. In this way cun is related to the height of the patient; the distance from the navel to the upper edge of the pubic bone is 5 cun for every person, regardless of whether he or she is short or tall, with a big belly or not. The only difference between people is the absolute length of the individual segments.

You can measure the distance from the navel to the upper edge of the pubic bone using your four fingers as cross-lines. You could also use an elastic band divided into four parts, as is shown in the illustrations on the opposite page. Other fixed distances can also be measured. For example, it is 4 cun from the middle axis of the body to each nipple, and 8 cun from the navel to the tip of the sternum. The most important measures are given in the following tables.

Right and left: You can orient yourself to the cun measurements of the person to be massaged using these distances as guidelines.

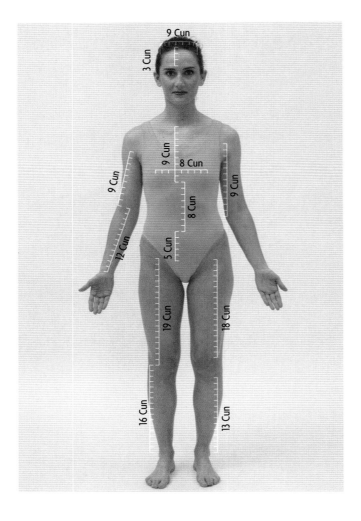

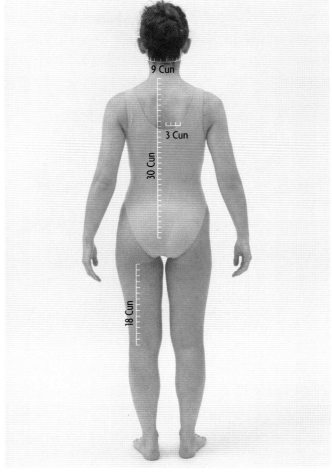

CUN MEASUREMENTS ON THE ARMS

From the top of the armpit to the inside of the elbow	9 cun
From the elbow to the wrist	12 cun

CUN MEASUREMENTS ON THE HEAD AND NECK

From Stomach 8 on one side to Stomach 8 on the other side	9 cun
On the middle axis, from between the eyebrows to the front of the hairline	3 cun
On the middle axis, from the ideal front of the hairline to the back of the hairline	12 cun
On the middle axis, from the back of the hairline to below the dorsal process of the seventh cervical vertebra	3 cun
From one mastoid process to the other	9 cun

CUN MEASUREMENTS ON THE TORSO

From one nipple to the other	8 cun
Length of the sternum	9 cun
From the lower edge of the sternum to the navel	8 cun
From the navel to the top edge of the pubic bone	5 cun
From the armpit in a vertical line down to the lower edge of the eleventh rib	12 cun
From the edge of the shoulder blade in a horizontal line to the dorsal process of the spine	3 cun
From the dorsal process of the first thoracic vertebra to the tip of the tailbone	30 cun

CUN MEASUREMENTS ON THE LEGS

From the top edge of the pubic bone to the top edge of the knee	18 cun
From the highest level of the buttock to the back of the knee	19 cun
From the knee to the highest rise on the outside of the ankle	16 cun
From the top of the shinbone to the highest rise on the inside of the ankle	13 cun
From the lower edge of the buttocks to the knee	18 cun

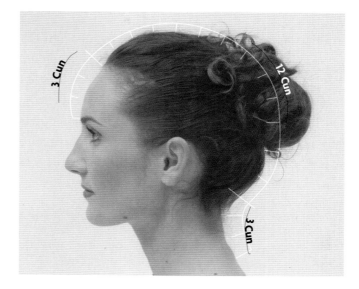

The forehead and neck measure 3 cun each, while the top and back of the head together measure about 12 cun.

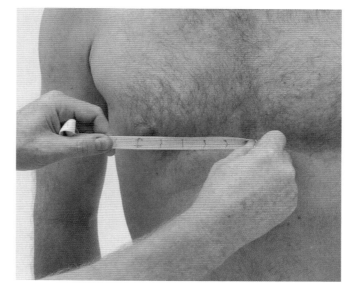

An elastic band with dividing marks can be helpful in locating the points.

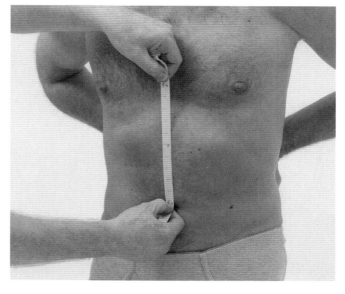

The distance from the navel to the sternum is 8 cun.

Breathing Properly during Acupressure

Make conscious use of your breathing during acupressure. A conscious breathing technique facilitates relaxation and contributes to the spread of relaxation throughout the entire body. When you are practicing self-treatment, once you have found the right acupressure point apply pressure while exhaling, and maintain pressure over several breathing cycles. If you want to increase the pressure, do this while exhaling. Reduce pressure while inhaling.

Use this same breathing technique when administering a massage to a partner. After you have located a point, apply pressure when your partner exhales, and maintain the pressure over several breathing cycles, releasing it when your partner inhales. In this way you will gradually adopt the breathing cycle of your partner, supporting the relaxing effects of the acupressure massage. Ideally your breathing rhythm will be synchronized with that of your partner to the point where you inhale and exhale together.

> **Note**
> - Make sure you adjust the strength of your pressure based on the comfort of your partner.
> - Be very careful in administering pressure. Especially when massaging older persons, apply only gentle pressure.
> - Do not use pressure techniques on areas that are injured or otherwise unhealthy.

Left: Apply pressure when your partner is exhaling.

Right: Pay attention to your breathing cycle during self-massage, increasing pressure while you are exhaling.

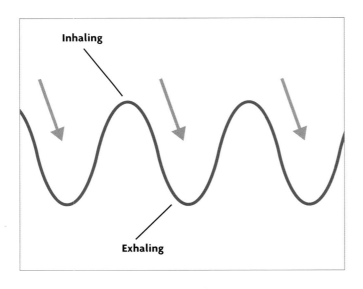

Inhaling

Exhaling

Pressure Points and Strength

When you first try acupressure, one question on your mind may be how to carry out these pressure techniques: where, for how long, and how hard are you supposed to press? Usually pressure is applied on specific points that are located predominantly along the meridians. The strength of the pressure depends on the sensitivity of your partner. Ask the person you are massaging how he or she feels about the pressure you are applying. At the same time pay attention yourself to your partner's reactions. If you are applying too much pressure, you will notice your partner's body tensing up.

Also pay attention to your partner's breathing. If you are pressing too hard and the pressure becomes uncomfortable for your partner, he or she will unconsciously hold his or her breath, interrupting the calm and relaxed flow of breathing.

Below the threshold at which pain becomes unpleasant is a type of pain that is still perceived as comfortable. This "wellness pain" is not characterized by the signals listed above; rather, it indicates that you have found the correct spot and are applying the correct pressure. This pain often extends along the line of the meridian, which also indicates that you are proceeding correctly.

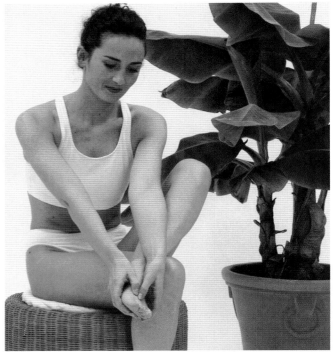

When using pressure techniques, do not begin with maximum pressure; instead, gradually build up to it. Begin with gentle pressure when your partner begins to exhale, increase it throughout his or her exhalation, and then maintain it for one complete breathing cycle until he or she exhales again.

Acupressure Techniques

Acupressure uses different techniques to treat specific points or areas. The most common ones are steady-pressure techniques using the fingertips, the whole hand, or other body parts. Other variations of steady pressure described in this book are applying circular pressure on meridian points and rubbing the skin. The latter is a good complementing connection between the different pressure techniques of a massage sequence.

We will also discuss kneading and shaking on the following pages. You can use all these techniques either on yourself or to massage a partner.

Steady Pressure (Figures 1 and 2)

Applying pressure with the tip of one or more fingers is a basic technique of acupressure. The pressure is applied to specific acupressure points with the finger bent and perpendicular to the surface of the skin. This positioning allows the most differentiated amounts of pressure. At the same time it prevents the finger joints from becoming overstretched while applying pressure. The effectiveness of the pressure depends on exactly locating the point in question. If a point is correctly located, you will often note a characteristic pull or burn, the de-qi feeling (see page 48).

How to Apply Steady Pressure

With your finger perpendicular to the surface of the skin, place the tip of your finger on the point and apply steady pressure. Be careful in the amount of pressure you apply: the pressure can cause a sensation like the poke of a needle; it can even be sharp or painful. If you find the pain uncomfortable and are becoming tense, you are

> **Note**
> - Use the tips of your fingers or thumb to massage points.
> - This book's instructions for which finger to use for massage are only suggestions. What's important is to use the finger with which you can best reach the point and most effectively exert pressure.

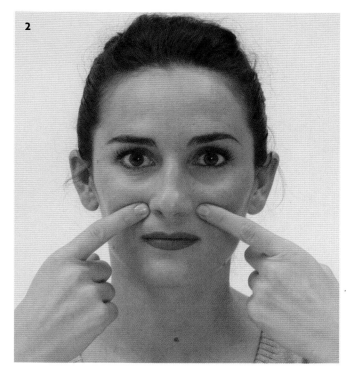

Left: To apply steady pressure, place the tip of a finger or thumb on the acupressure point. Use the other fingers to support the thumb.

Right: If the points are easily accessible, you can press two corresponding points at the same time.

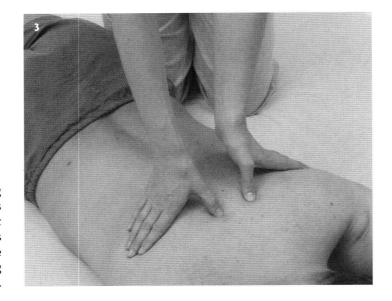

For circling pressure it is important that the fingers support the massaging thumbs.

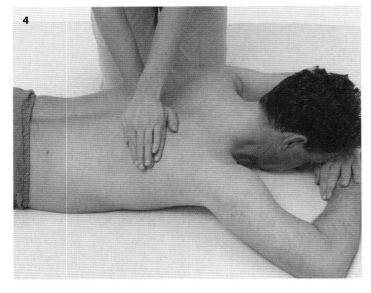

You can also apply circling pressure using the base of your hands.

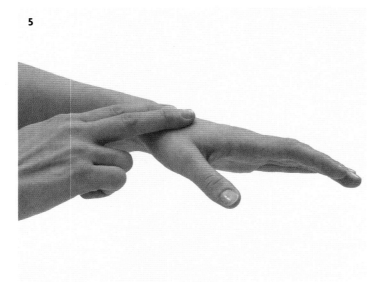

You can rub along the path of meridians, for example, on the hand above the point Large Intestine 4.

applying too much pressure. If you can hardly feel it all, you are applying too little. The de-qi feeling indicates that you've found the optimal amount.

Maintain pressure for several breathing cycles. In some techniques, strong pressure is maintained for two minutes and repeated five to ten times. Other acupressure techniques call for only one-time pressure, but for a duration of two to three minutes. How strongly and for how long you massage each point will be discussed in the Targeting Ailments with Acupressure chapter. As a rule of thumb, the more points you treat in a sequence, the shorter the duration of pressure.

Circular Pressure (Figures 3 and 4)

In many treatments pressure is applied with circular movements. Circular pressure is the most commonly used technique in acupressure. The circular movement has a relaxing and balancing effect and relaxes the muscles. Pressure can be exerted using the tips of the fingers or thumb, the palms, or the base of the hand.

How to Apply Circular Pressure

Apply steady pressure until you have found the right amount of pressure. Then begin to make small circular movements with your hand. As in other movements, apply pressure with your fingertips perpendicular to the skin surface. In this technique it is important not to move your fingertips or palms across the skin, but rather to move the skin itself.

It is important not to confuse circular pressure with rubbing. Especially in your first treatments, you should keep recalling to yourself that you are not aiming to rub the skin. The contact between your finger or palm and the body part you are massaging should not be interrupted. In this way you stimulate, depending on the pressure used, the lower layers of the skin as well as the muscles. Generally the tissues and organs react better when you apply pressure slowly and, most importantly, rhythmically.

Rubbing the Skin (Figures 5–7)

A good complementary measure in many treatment areas is rubbing the skin. With this technique you are not treating individual points but rather are massaging larger areas of skin and muscle groups. You can rub the skin with your fingertips, your palms, or the balls of your thumbs. When done gently and softly, the rubbing feels like a caress, with relaxing and calming effects. Strong rubbing, in contrast, warms and stimulates circulation in the body part being massaged. Which type of rubbing to use is detailed in the specific treatment instructions.

How to Carry Out Skin Rubbing

Place your fingertips or palms on the skin and carry out rubbing movements along the path of the meridian. For example, spend one to two minutes rubbing from the base of the hand up to the side of the tip of the index finger, following the path of the Large Intestine meridian. The skin will warm as you are doing this, and it may redden slightly. You can use your palms to rub larger areas; illustrations 6 and 7 on the right show the practitioner using her palms to rub the area of the Urinary Bladder meridian. The rubbing reddens and warms the skin.

Kneading (Figures 8–11)

Like rubbing, kneading is generally employed for larger body parts. While rubbing aims to stimulate only the surface of the skin, kneading stretches the muscles, leading to improved circulation and relaxation. Kneading usually encompasses several acupressure points and in the case of larger muscle groups is done using both hands. In those cases, the base of the one hand works with the fingers of the other to stretch the muscle perpendicular to its natural direction.

How to Knead

Place your hands flat on the body part to be massaged. With the fingers of your left hand, pull the muscles

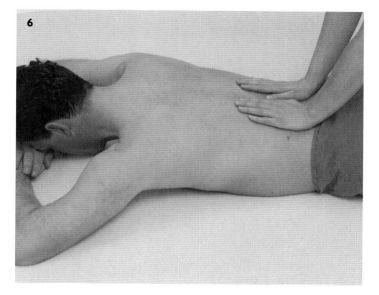

To massage along the path of the Urinary Bladder meridian, begin with rubbing the skin in the sacrum region . . .

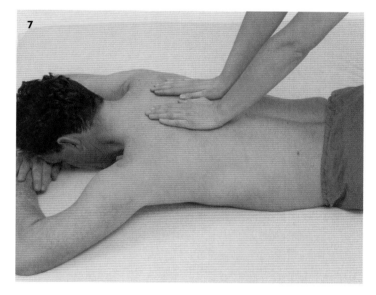

. . . and glide with the palms of your hands to the neck area.

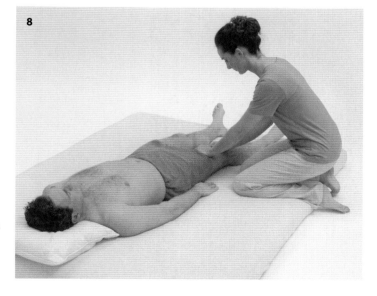

Kneading is good for the thigh muscles.

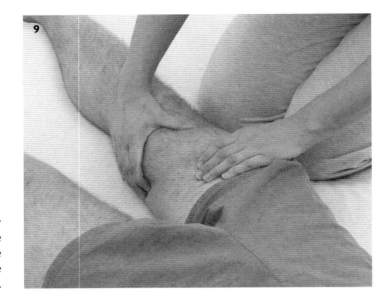

Begin by kneading the muscles on the inside of the thighs.

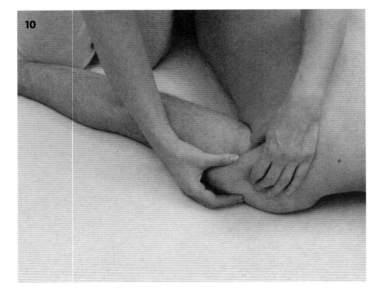

Kneading can be used on the large muscles in the shoulders and upper arms, including the deltoids . . .

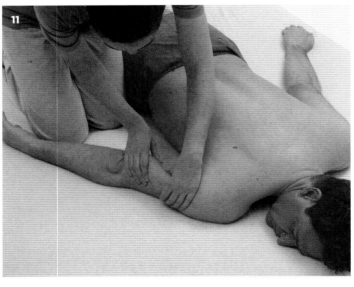

. . . and triceps.

against the thumb of your right hand. Follow this with the reverse movement: use the fingers of your right hand to pull the muscle against the thumb of your left hand. When you alternate these movements, you create a rhythmic, wavelike movement. You can also massage a muscle along its natural direction. In this case place both hands flat and next to each other on the thickest part of the muscle. With one hand press and lift the muscle toward your other hand, while that other hand relaxes. Follow with the reverse: use your other hand to press and lift the muscle while your first hand relaxes. When this movement is alternated between your hands, it creates a rhythmic, longitudinal kneading of the muscle.

Illustration 9 shows the practitioner kneading one part of the thigh muscles. To do this yourself, mentally divide the thigh into two parts. Begin touching the half that is closer to the inside of the leg. You will quickly notice that several muscles are located next to one another. These are the muscles that move the leg forward during walking and the ones that move it inward. Try to find the direction of one of these muscles and then place your hands flat on it. Now pull the muscle with the fingers of your left hand toward your right hand, and then repeat in the opposite direction. Repeat these movements several times slowly and steadily. Then increase the pressure by pressing the muscle with your left hand before moving it to your right hand. The right hand continues the movement and returns the muscle to the left hand. Rhythmically repeat these movements several times, and then focus on the next muscle.

You can use this same technique for the shoulders and upper arms. The deltoid muscles in the shoulders, in particular, are used a lot because they are active anytime we have to lift our upper arm. Kneading the deltoids as well as the triceps on the upper arms is thus a particular pleasure for the recipient.

Shaking (Figures 12–14)

Shaking has direct effects on muscles and tendons. Using this technique in a slow and rhythmic way helps relax your partner. It can improve circulation and thus the provision of oxygen to the tissues. Shaking is often recommended as a way to prepare body parts for acupressure. Long muscle groups are especially well suited for this technique, since they can be held easily. The preferred areas for shaking are the shoulders, the muscles of the upper arms, and the muscles of the thighs and calves. The larger the muscle or joint, the more strongly you can shake it.

How to Carry Out Shaking

Muscles should be shaken only when they are at rest and relaxed. Being sure not to stretch them, take the muscles you want to shake into your flat hand. Move the muscles gently but quickly perpendicular to their natural direction. Continue the movement until the muscles are relaxed.

You can shake the muscles of the upper arms while your partner is lying on his or her back or sitting up. The important thing is for your partner to keep his or her arms relaxed. Take one arm by the wrist and hold it at a ninety-degree angle to your partner's body. Place your other hand flat on the upper arm muscles, which can be easily felt, and shake these gently but quickly. Carry on shaking for at least one minute, and then switch to the other arm.

Shaking of the calf muscles is best done with your partner lying down and his or her knee bent. Use one hand to hold the leg at the bent knee and the other hand to carry out shaking movements of the calf muscles. This shaking is particularly pleasant for people who often suffer from muscle cramps in the calves. Switch to the other leg after one minute.

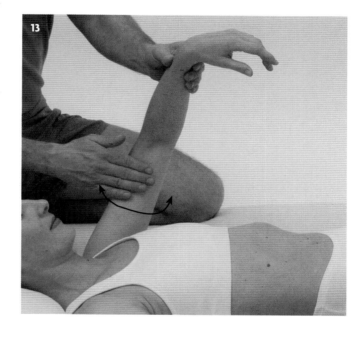

Before being shaken, the arm muscles should be completely relaxed.

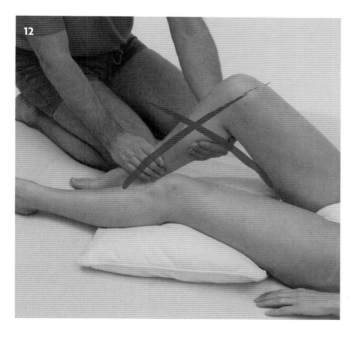

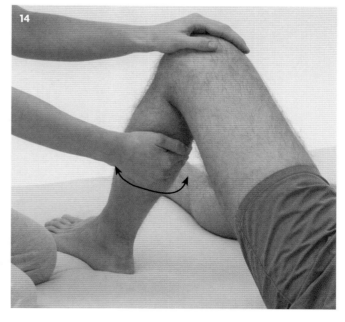

Left: This position is wrong. The calf is not fixed in place sufficiently and shaking will move the knee.

Right: This position is correct. Stabilize the knee, and then shake the calf muscles.

Ground Rules for Treating Yourself or a Partner

Acupressure is an effective method that can be used at any time and in many different surroundings. Its ease of application, however, should not let you forget that the success of the treatment depends on following several ground rules. These rules apply equally for self-treatment and for massages of a partner. When massaging a partner, several additional guidelines should be followed.

To begin, you should never attempt to treat a severe or chronic illness by practicing acupressure on yourself or a partner (see applications and limits, page 47). If you are not sure whether you can use acupressure in the case of a specific illness, consult a qualified health care practitioner. Do not make diagnoses or attempt treatment on yourself or a partner.

A basic precondition for giving all types of massages is that your hands be warm and clean. Cold hands can be warmed through rubbing or warm baths. Equally important is that the body parts you are planning to treat should also be warm. If your partner has cold hands or feet, make sure to warm them before beginning with acupressure massage. And since acupressure points on the body are often massaged with your fingertips, your fingernails should be short to avoid injuring the skin.

Adjust the pressure you use to the individual sensitivities of your partner. Keep in mind that the same amount of pressure can be perceived as pleasant by some people but as painful by others. Similarly, when massaging yourself you will note that pressure points on your body are more sensitive on some days than on others. In the same way, sensitivity to pressure will vary between body parts. On particularly strong muscle areas, for example, the thighs, you can apply more pressure than over sensitive bone areas or body parts that are covered by only a thin layer of skin, such as the head or neck. For these reasons, gradually build up your pressure to the desired maximum, keep up the pressure on each point for a specific amount of time, and then gradually reduce the pressure.

Factor in a resting period of about fifteen minutes both before and after the massage. Make sure that your treatment room is well ventilated and kept at a comfortable temperature. Carry out an acupressure massage only when you are feeling physically and emotionally fit and balanced. Excitement, anger, depression, or exhaustion can pose an obstacle to a successful massage. Do not give a massage when you are feeling hungry or immediately after eating a big meal. If possible, wait for at least two hours after a meal before giving an acupressure massage.

Aside from these rules, there are a few additional

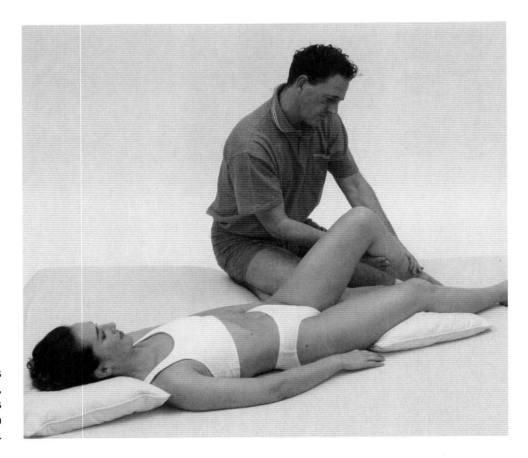

When the hands are warm, stroking feels good on tired legs.

considerations to follow if you are massaging a partner rather than yourself. Remember that the measurements that are given for locating the points are based on the body proportions of the person being massaged (see page 55). Also, inform your partner about the process of the acupressure massage. Explain that pressure on some points may be painful, and that a numbing or sharp feeling can emanate from the area being massaged to the body parts around it. This sensation is desirable, as it indicates that the correct point has been located.

If you already have experience administering pressure massages, you can use heat treatments on the points of different meridians to influence an illness. The next section describes how to apply a traditional heat treatment known as moxibustion.

Moxibustion

Specific skin zones and acupressure points are sometimes warmed in traditional Chinese medicine as a means of positively influencing qi, or life energy, as well as the blood and all substances and organs. The warmth is generated by burning dried and pressed mugwort *(Artemisia vulgaris)*. This type of focused warmth infusion is called moxibustion or moxa in traditional Chinese medicine.

Mugwort also has a rich tradition of use in Europe. Traditional homeopathy has a large number of mugwort recipes designed to, for example, alleviate foot pain after long walks or treat chronic diarrhea. In moxibustion the infused warmth stimulates the circulation and the functioning of the organs; warming up specific points stimulates the immune system. According to the *Huang Di Nei Jing*, moxibustion was in ancient times used especially to treat illnesses caused by cold or wetness.

Moxibustion can be helpful in the case of:
* Feelings of cold in the body, shivering, and paleness
* Fatigue and depression
* Pain that improves with the infusion of warmth
* Stiff joints
* Watery diarrhea

In the case of fever, infectious disease, or hypertension, however, you should not use moxibustion, since the infusion of warmth can make heat-related symptoms worse.

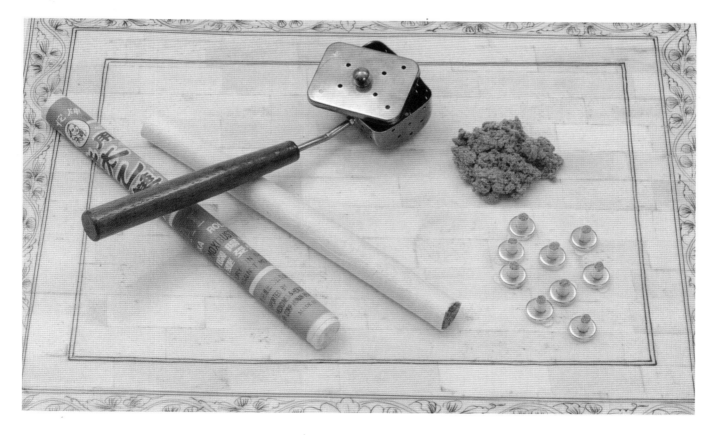

You can practice moxibustion using mugwort, special moxa cigars, or moxa pins.

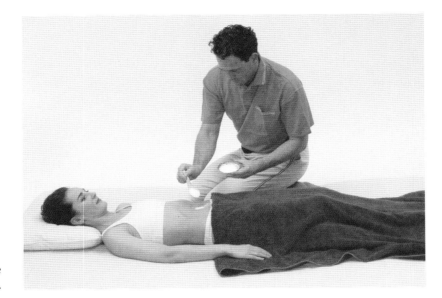

First place some salt in the navel.

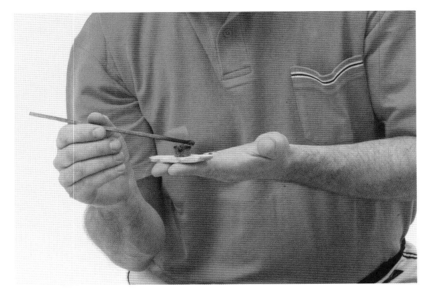

Light the moxa pin . . .

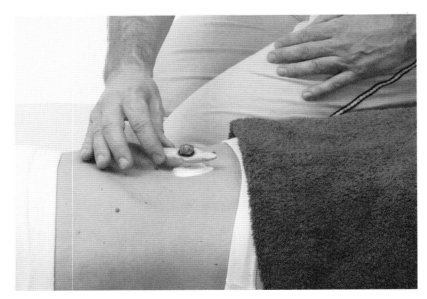

. . . and place it on top of a slice of ginger on the navel.

Applying Moxibustion

At the time of the *Huang Di Nei Jing*, a moxa pin was burned directly on the skin, a practice referred to as "direct moxibustion." Nowadays, a slice of ginger is often used to isolate the skin from the moxa pin. This technique, which you should employ to avoid injuries, is known as "gentle moxibustion" or "indirect moxibustion." An excellent application example is moxibustion above the navel, on acupressure point Conception Vessel 8. For this, put some salt in the navel and place a fresh slice of ginger, about 3 to 5 mm thick, on top. Light the moxa pin over the ginger slice. The pin will now emanate its warmth and generate a pleasant feeling of warmth that will spread through the abdomen. If the heat becomes too strong, you can carefully remove the moxa pin using tweezers.

Another method, and the safest one in terms of avoiding burns, is to warm an acupressure point using a moxa cigar. Light the mugwort stick on one end and slowly bring the lit end close to the point to be treated. Pull the stick back as soon as your partner senses its warmth. Repeatedly moving the moxa cigar toward and away from the body in this manner is called the "bird pecking" method. Keep it up for five to ten minutes, for example on the point Stomach 36. When practiced on a weekly basis, bird-pecking moxibustion has a vitalizing effect.

Larger areas of skin can be warmed using a moxa box, which is usually a metal case in which loose moxa (mugwort) leaves are burned. The moxa-box application is also good for use on the point Conception Vessel 8. Often the high level of relaxation it induces will lead the person being massaged to fall asleep. Always keep your partner under observation during moxibustion, since falling ashes can lead to skin injuries or even fires.

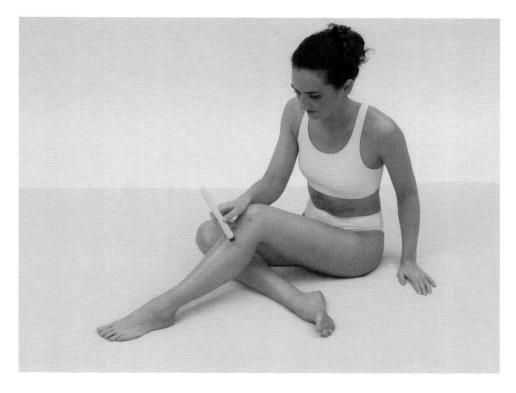

In the bird-pecking method, the moxa cigar is moved toward and away from the acupressure point.

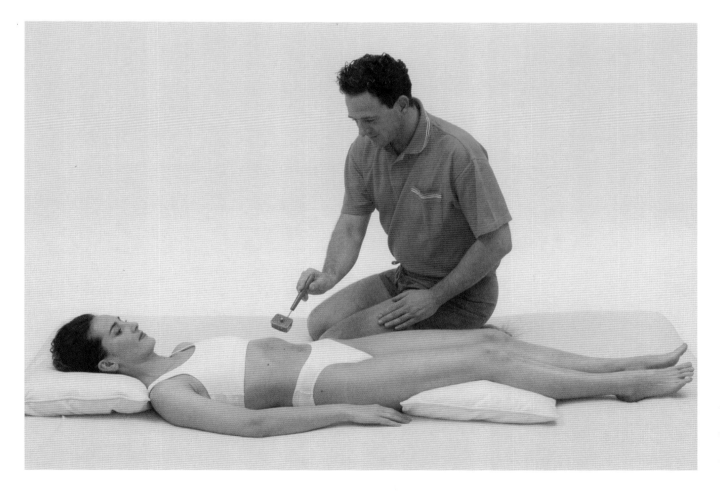

A moxa box is useful in treating the point Conception Vessel 8.

Acupressure on Different Parts of the Body

This section describes how to locate and massage the most important points on different parts of the body. This basic knowledge will enable you to design your own treatment plans.

The Points on the Face

On the face, the following meridian points are frequently massaged:

Yintang (an extra point), Gall Bladder 14, Urinary Bladder 2, Large Intestine 20, Small Intestine 18, and Governor Vessel 26.

Caution

Since the face is an especially sensitive area, you must be very careful when massaging points on it. You can treat points individually or as pairs.

Locating the Points on the Face

Aside from instructions on locating the points in the face, this section contains guidelines on which points should be massaged for what purpose. Be careful when massaging the points in the area around the eyes. It is important to keep an eye on your partner's facial expression to make sure you recognize any possible sensitivities to pressure.

Yintang—Hall of Seal

Yintang is an extra point, or a point that lies outside the meridians. Yintang is on the middle axis of the body, immediately between the eyebrows, at the root of the nose. Pressure on this point is said to alleviate pain and improve vision. Because of these qualities this point is frequently used to treat headache, dizziness, and confusion, as well as eye and nose problems.

Gall Bladder 14—Yang White

When you are looking straight ahead, Gall Bladder 14, referred to as Yang White in traditional Chinese medicine, is located straight up from the pupil, 1 cun above the eyebrow. This pain-relieving point is often used to treat ailments in the head area, such as headaches and infections of the sinuses. Eye ailments, including infections, redness, and night blindness and other vision problems, also can be positively influenced via this point.

Urinary Bladder 2—Bamboo Gathering

Urinary Bladder 2, also called Bamboo Gathering, is located on the inner edge of the eyebrow, in the slight indentation found there. It has the same effects as Gall Bladder 14 and is used to treat headaches in the forehead area, sinus infections, and eye problems including itchiness, redness, and sensitivity to light.

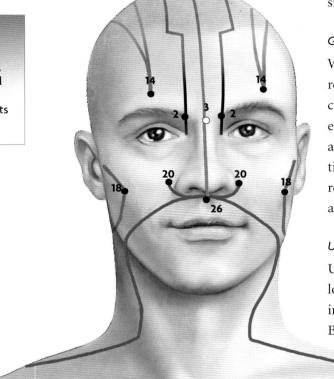

Five meridians run across the forehead and face. In addition, this area is home to extra points that are not located on meridians.

White	Extra point	Yintang
Dark green	Gall Bladder meridian	Gall Bladder 14
Black	Urinary Bladder meridian	Urinary Bladder 2
Dark blue	Large Intestine meridian	Large Intestine 20
Red	Small Intestine meridian	Small Intestine 18
Gray	Governor Vessel	Governor Vessel 26

Large Intestine 20—Welcome Fragrance

Large Intestine 20 is on the lower outer edge of the nostril. This point is treated primarily to address nose problems such as repeated nosebleeds, scent perception problems, and allergic reactions such as hay fever. It can also be used to treat facial paralysis, caused by the paralysis of certain nerves.

Small Intestine 18—Cheek Bone Hole

This point is located on a line below the outer edge of the eye in the indentation immediately below the zygomatic bone. It can be used to treat pain and cramps in the facial area, as well as facial nerve ailments such as facial paralysis, trigeminal neuralgia, and tics. This point is also effective in treating illnesses caused by wind or draft.

Governor Vessel 26—Water Trough

Governor Vessel 26 is located on the middle axis of the face between the nose and upper lip. It can be helpful in emergency situations, for example in cases of unconsciousness, stroke, shock, or epileptic seizure (after the administration of first aid and any other necessary medical procedures, of course). It can be massaged to alleviate psychological and psychosomatic problems, as well as fever, cramps, and acute pain in the lower back area.

Massaging the Points on the Face

Use the following instructions as a guide to massaging Yintang, Gall Bladder 14, Urinary Bladder 2, Large Intestine 20, Small Intestine 18, and Governor Vessel 26.

Yintang—Hall of Seal (Figure 1)

You can massage the extra point Yintang with your partner sitting up or lying down. If you are massaging yourself, a mirror can be helpful in locating the point. Find the point with the tip of your index finger, and apply first steady and then circular pressure for one to two minutes each.

Gall Bladder 14—Yang White (Figure 2)

Locate Gall Bladder 14 above the eyebrow using the tip of your thumb or index finger. Apply first steady and then circular pressure for one to two minutes each. Note that Gall Bladder 14 can be very sensitive to pressure in the case of gallbladder problems.

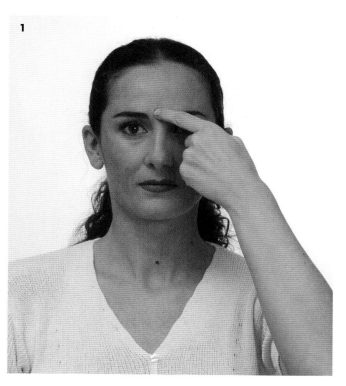

1

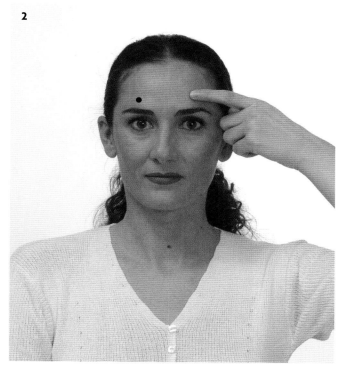

2

Left: Massage Hall of Seal point exactly on the middle axis, between the eyebrows.

Right: Gall Bladder 14 is located 1 cun above the eyebrow.

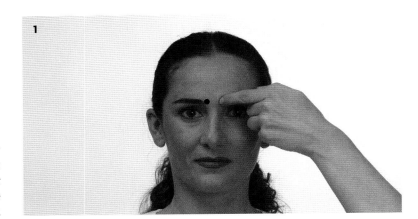

Urinary Bladder 2 is located in an indentation at the inside edge of the eyebrow.

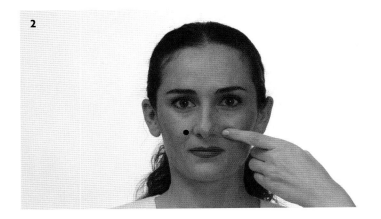

Large Intestine 20 is located at the beginning of the fold that runs from the nose to the edge of the mouth.

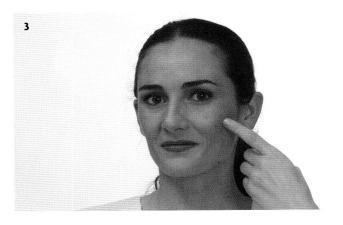

To locate Small Intestine 18, it helps to visualize a vertical line running down from the outside edge of the eye.

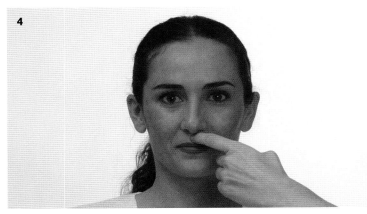

Governor Vessel 26 can be massaged as a complementary treatment for unconsciousness, for example, while waiting for medical help to arrive.

Urinary Bladder 2—Bamboo Gathering (Figure 1)

If you are massaging a partner, he or she can either sit up or lie down. You can massage the two Urinary Bladder 2 points one after the other, as shown in the photo, or at the same time. Place your finger on the inside edge of the eyebrows. Apply constant pressure for one to two minutes, then move your finger slightly farther out from the midline (no more than 1 cm) and apply stronger pressure. Release the pressure and move your finger back to Urinary Bladder 2, touching the skin gently without pressure.

Large Intestine 20—Welcome Fragrance (Figure 2)

The two Welcome Fragrance points are located on each side of the nostrils and can be massaged at the same time with your middle fingers, using first steady and then circling pressure for one to two minutes each.

Small Intestine 18—Cheek Bone Hole (Figure 3)

To massage Cheek Bone Hole, have your partner sit or lie down. If you are massaging yourself, you may want to sit in front of a mirror to help you locate the point. Using the tip of your thumb or index finger, locate the point below the edge of the zygomatic bone, below the outer edge of the eye. Massage the point using first steady and then circling pressure for one to two minutes each.

Governor Vessel 26—Water Trough (Figure 4)

Governor Vessel 26, also called Water Trough in traditional Chinese medicine, can be massaged with your partner either lying down or sitting up. Using the tip of your index finger, apply pressure below the nose on the middle axis, using first steady and then circling pressure for two to three minutes altogether.

Points on the Head

For acupressure treatment on the head rather than the face, different points are important. You will find these points on the top, sides, and back of the head.

In the case of headaches that are perceived as pain under the roof of the skull, massaging Governor Vessel 20 and 21 and Urinary Bladder 6, 7, and 8 can provide relief. Of these, the most important and effective point in controlling symptoms is Governor Vessel 21.

Locating the Points on Top of the Head

Governor Vessel 19—Behind the Vertex

Governor Vessel 19 is located on the middle axis of the body. Picture a line running from the front of the hairline to the back of the head. This point lies exactly 6.5 cun from the front of the hairline along that line. Acupressure on Governor Vessel 19 can have a calming and balancing effect on psychological and psychosomatic ailments. Massaging this point can also be helpful as a complementary treatment for hypertension.

Governor Vessel 20—Hundred Convergences

Governor Vessel 20 is also on the middle axis, 1.5 cun toward the front from Governor Vessel 19. You can locate this point by running your finger along the middle axis from the forehead toward the back of the head; Governor Vessel 20 is on the highest rise of the head. The most important treatment areas for this point are headaches, dizziness, and vision problems. Governor Vessel 20, though an important point in acupressure, should not be massaged in cases of high blood pressure, since this can cause headaches.

Governor Vessel 21—Before the Vertex

This point too is located exactly on the middle axis, being 3.5 cun toward the back from the front hairline. Applying pressure on this point is recommended as a complementary treatment in cases of hypertension or depression.

Governor Vessel 22—Fontanel Meeting

Governor Vessel 22, another important point, is also on the middle axis, 2 cun back from the front hairline. This point is massaged to relieve headaches.

Urinary Bladder 6—Light Guard

Light Guard is located on a line that runs parallel to the middle line but 1.5 cun away on either side. On this line, the point is located 2.5 cun back from the front hairline. Massaging this point can be helpful in the case of headaches.

Urinary Bladder 7—Celestial Connection

Urinary Bladder 7 is on the same line as Urinary Bladder 6, about 4 cun back from the front hairline. Treating this point is helpful in cases of headaches that are concentrated in the area under the roof of the skull. Urinary Bladder 7 can also be massaged in cases of illnesses relating to the nose.

Urinary Bladder 8—Declining Connection

Urinary Bladder 8 is located on the same line as Urinary Bladder 6 and 7. It is located 1.5 cun further toward the back of the head from Urinary Bladder 7. Acupressure on Urinary Bladder 8 is a beneficial complementary treatment in cases of hypertension as well as psychological and psychosomatic problems.

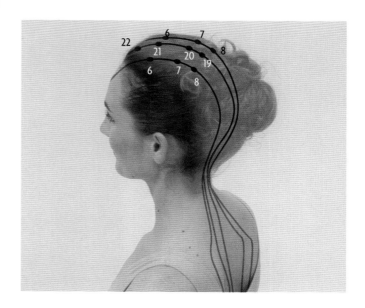

The Governor Vessel and Urinary Bladder meridians run along the head, neck, and back in close proximity to one another.

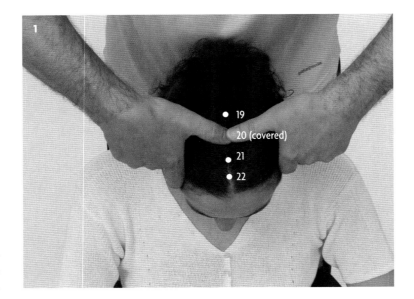

Governor Vessel 20 is used to treat headaches and dizziness.

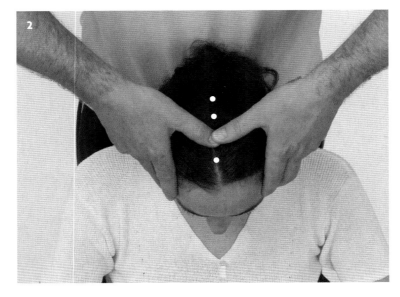

Governor Vessel 21 can be found by moving your thumbs 1.5 cun forward from Governor Vessel 20.

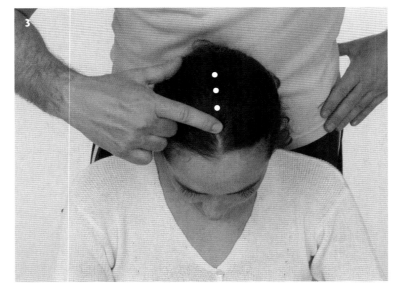

Governor Vessel 22 is 2 cun back from the front hairline on the middle axis of the head.

Massaging the Points on Top of the Head

The points on the top of the head are massaged using steady and circling pressure. Some of the points described here are more sensitive than others; these should be massaged for longer or more frequently.

Governor Vessel 19—Behind the Vertex

Governor Vessel 19 can be massaged with your partner either lying down or sitting up. Place the tip of one thumb on the middle axis at the hairline, and place the tip of your other thumb over the first. Move your thumbs 5.5 cun along the axis toward the back of the head. With your thumbs, press this point using first steady and then circular pressure for one to two minutes each.

Governor Vessel 20—Hundred Convergences (Figure 1)

Governor Vessel 20, also known as Hundred Convergences, is located on the middle axis, 1.5 cun from Governor Vessel 19, at the highest part of the head. Placing one thumb on top of the other, massage this point with first steady and then circular pressure for one to two minutes each.

Governor Vessel 21—Before the Vertex (Figure 2)

This point is also located on the middle axis, 1.5 cun toward the forehead from Governor Vessel 20. It can be massaged with your partner sitting up or lying down. Massage it using your thumbs, applying first steady and then circular pressure for one to two minutes each.

Governor Vessel 22—Fontanel Meeting (Figure 3)

Fontanel Meeting can be massaged with your partner either lying down or sitting up. Located on the middle axis, it is 2 cun from the hairline toward the back of the head. With your thumb or index finger, massage this point using first steady and then circular pressure for one to two minutes each.

Urinary Bladder 6—Light Guard (Figure 1)

Urinary Bladder 6, also known as Light Guard, can be massaged with your partner either sitting up or lying down. The point is located on the lines that run parallel to the middle axis, 1.5 cun away on either side; it is 2.5 cun back from the front hairline. Using both thumbs, as shown in the photo, massage Urinary Bladder 6 using first steady and then circular pressure for one to two minutes each.

Urinary Bladder 7—Celestial Connection (Figure 2)

Urinary Bladder 7, also known as Celestial Connection, is located on the same line as Urinary Bladder 6. It is located four finger widths, or 4 cun, back from the front hairline. You can massage Urinary Bladder 7 with your partner lying down or, as shown in the photo, sitting up. Let yourself be guided by your partner's preference in this. Using the tips of your thumbs or index or middle fingers, apply first steady and then circular pressure, for a total of two to three minutes.

Urinary Bladder 8—Declining Connection (Figure 3)

Declining Connection can be treated with your partner sitting up or lying down. This point, the eighth of the Urinary Bladder meridian, is located on the same line as the two Urinary Bladder points just described. Locate Urinary Bladder 8 by moving your fingers 5.5 cun back from the front hairline. Place your thumbs or, as shown in the photo, your index fingers on the two points. Treat them together with first steady and then circular pressure for one to three minutes each.

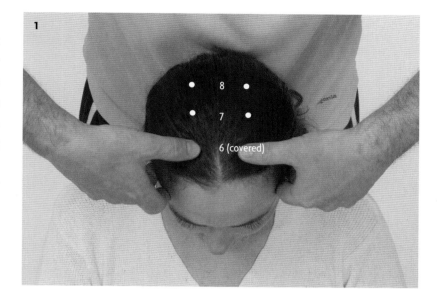

To massage Urinary Bladder 6, rest your fingers against your partner's temples.

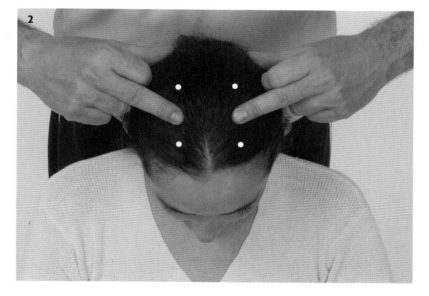

Urinary Bladder 7 is located 4 cun back from the front hairline.

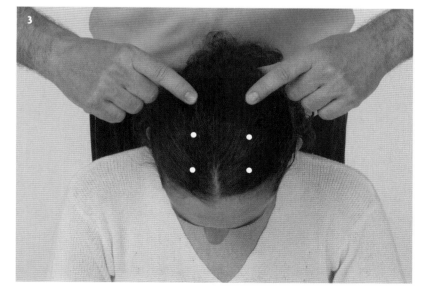

Urinary Bladder 8 is located 5.5 cun back from the front hairline.

Locating the Points on the Side of the Head

Three meridians run along the side of the head. These are the Gall Bladder meridian, which runs in a zigzag pattern along the temple area, the Triple Heater meridian, which circles the ear, and the Small Intestine meridian, whose end point is in front of the ear canal. On these meridians, the following points on the side of the head are massaged frequently: Gall Bladder 2, 3, 4, 7, and 8; Small Intestine 19; and Triple Heater 17, 21, and 23.

Note

For headaches on only one side of the head, massage the points:
- Gall Bladder 4
- Gall Bladder 7
- Triple Heater 23

To positively influence problems of the ear, massage the points:
- Gall Bladder 2
- Gall Bladder 3
- Small Intestine 19
- Triple Heater 17
- Triple Heater 21

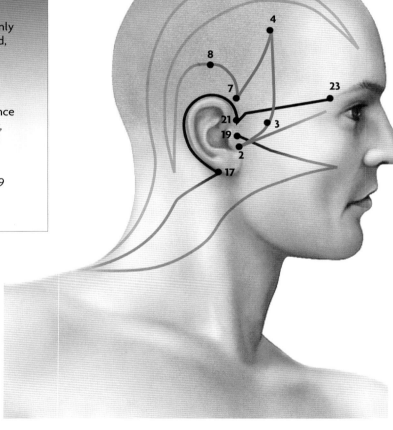

Because of the crisscrossing path of the Gall Bladder meridian, the meridians on the side of the head frequently intersect.

Dark green	Gall Bladder meridian	Gall Bladder 2–4
		Gall Bladder 7, 8
Red	Small Intestine meridian	Small Intestine 19
Purple	Triple Heater meridian	Triple Heater 17
		Triple Heater 21
		Triple Heater 23

Gall Bladder 2—Auditory Convergence

Gall Bladder 2 is located in an indentation in front of the ear. You can find this point by feeling your way along the lower edge of the zygomatic bone to the edge of the ear. Acupressure of this point is useful for treating headaches emanating from the side of the head, pain in the jaw, and toothaches. This point is also helpful in cases of ear problems, including hardness of hearing, deafness, ringing in the ear, and ear infections. (Gall Bladder 2 is one of three points that have special effects on the ear. The other two points are Small Intestine 19 and Triple Heater 21, which are described in detail on the following pages.)

Gall Bladder 3—Upper Gate

Upper Gate is located on the upper edge of the zygomatic bone, above Gall Bladder 2 and a little bit closer to the nose. Acupressure on Gall Bladder 3 is effective for treating ear ailments as well as toothaches in the upper jaw.

Gall Bladder 4—Forehead Fullness

Forehead Fullness is located on the side of the head, where the hairline recedes. This point is treated in cases of headaches on the side of the head and as a complementary treatment in the case of hypertension.

Gall Bladder 7—Temporal Hairline Curve

To locate this point, imagine two lines, one running horizontally at the height of the upper edge of the ear and the other running vertically directly in front of the ear. The point where these two lines cross is Gall Bladder 7. This point can be massaged to relieve headaches on the side of the head, as well as in cases of infection of the large parotid gland.

Gall Bladder 8—Valley Lead

Gall Bladder 8 is located 1.5 cun above the highest point of the ear. Massaging this point is helpful in cases of headaches on the side of the head and balance problems. It also can be helpful in treating hypertension.

Small Intestine 19—Auditory Palace

When your mouth is slightly open, Small Intestine 19 is located in an indentation in front of the ear drum; when your mouth is wide open, this point is located behind the jaw bone. Massage of this point can be used to treat ear problems such as hardness of hearing, ringing in the ear, or ear infections. The point is also effective in cases of facial nerve pain and pain in the jaw and teeth.

Triple Heater 17—Wind Screen

The point is located behind the earlobe, in a noticeable indentation between the mastoid process and the lower jaw bone. It can be used to treat ear problems such as hardness of hearing or ringing in the ear. Acupressure of this point can also be beneficial as a complementary therapy in the case of facial paralysis.

Triple Heater 21—Ear Gate

This point is located at the front edge of the ear, the crossing point between the upper edge of the zygomatic bone and the ear. Massage of this point can be used to treat ailments of the ear and infection of facial nerves.

Triple Heater 23—Silk Bamboo Hole

This point, the endpoint of the Triple Heater meridian, is located on the outer edge of the eyebrow, near the noticeable bony edge of the eye socket. Acupressure of this point is helpful especially in treating headaches in the area of the temples, eye problems including infection of the cornea, and tics in the eye area. Triple Heater 23 is an important point in the treatment of eye problems.

Massaging the Points on the Side of the Head

Points on the side of the head are generally effective for treating headaches that are located on the sides of the head and ear problems.

Gall Bladder 2—Auditory Convergence (Figure 1)

Gall Bladder 2 can be treated with your partner lying down or sitting up. Massage the point with the tip of your thumb or middle finger using first steady and then circular pressure for a total of two to three minutes.

Gall Bladder 3—Upper Gate (Figure 2)

Upper Gate can be treated with your partner lying down or sitting up. Locate the point with the tip of your thumb or middle finger in the indentation on the upper edge of the zygomatic bone. Apply first steady and then circling pressure for a total of two to three minutes.

1

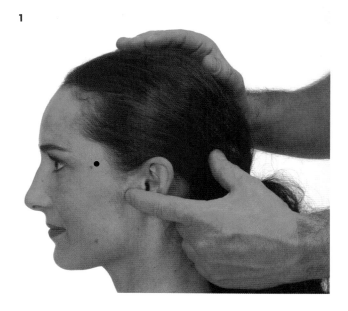

2

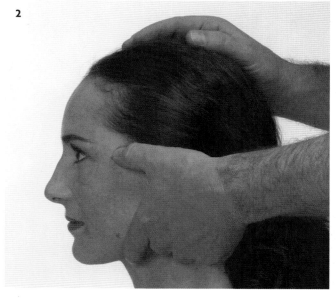

Left and right: When massaging the points on the side of the head, stabilize the top of the head with your free hand.

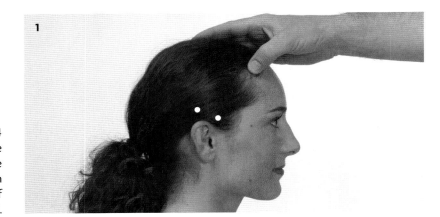

Gall Bladder 4 is located at the hairline in the temple region on both sides of the head.

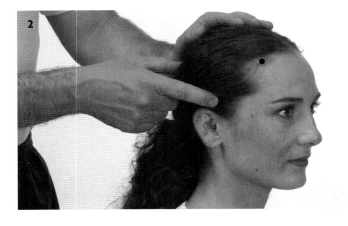

Gall Bladder 7 is located at the intersection of two imaginary lines running horizontally above and vertically in front of the ear.

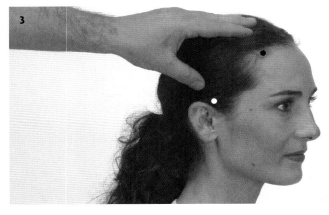

When massaging Gall Bladder 8 with your thumb, rest your other fingers against the top of the head.

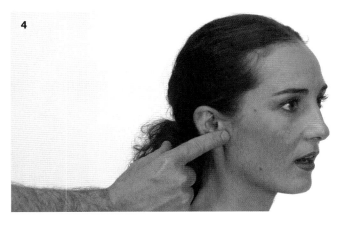

It is easiest to locate Small Intestine 19 when your partner's mouth is open.

Gall Bladder 4— Forehead Fullness (Figure 1)

Gall Bladder 4 can be massaged with your partner lying down or, as shown in the photo, sitting up. If you are massaging yourself for the first time, it helps to sit in front of a mirror to locate the point. Massage with the tip of your thumb or index finger, using first steady and then circular pressure for a total of one to three minutes or for as long as it feels good when massaging yourself.

Gall Bladder 7—Temporal Hairline Curve (Figure 2)

Temporal Hairline Curve can also be massaged with your partner lying down or sitting up. Massage with the tip of your thumb or index finger, using first steady and then circling pressure. You can massage the two Gall Bladder 7 points at the same time or separately for a total of one to three minutes or longer when massaging yourself.

Gall Bladder 8—Valley Lead (Figure 3)

Gall Bladder 8, also known as Valley Lead, can be treated with your partner lying down or sitting up. Massage the point with the tip of your thumb or index finger, using first steady and then circular pressure for a total of one to two minutes. You can also apply moxibustion to this point (see page 65).

Small Intestine 19—Auditory Palace (Figure 4)

Small Intestine 19 can be treated with your partner lying down or sitting up. Locate the point between the ear and the jaw joint. With your thumb or index finger, massage this point using first steady and then circular pressure for a total of two to three minutes. You can also apply moxibustion to this point.

Triple Heater 17—Wind Screen (Figure 1)

Wind Screen can be treated with your partner lying down or sitting up. Massage the point with the tip of your thumb or index finger, using first steady and then circular pressure for a total of two to three minutes. You can also apply moxibustion to this point.

Triple Heater 21—Ear Gate (Figure 2)

Triple Heater 21, also known as Ear Gate, can be treated with your partner lying down or sitting up. Massage the point with the tip of your thumb or index finger, using first steady and then circular pressure for a total of two to three minutes. You can also apply moxibustion to this point.

Triple Heater 23—Silk Bamboo Hole (Figure 3)

Triple Heater 23, also known as Silk Bamboo Hole, can be treated with your partner lying down or sitting up. Massage the point with your thumb or index finger, using first steady and then circular pressure for a total of one to two minutes. You can also apply moxibustion to this point.

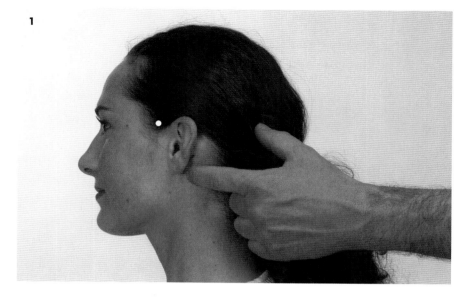

1

Triple Heater 17 is located behind the earlobe in an indentation between the mastoid process and the lower jaw.

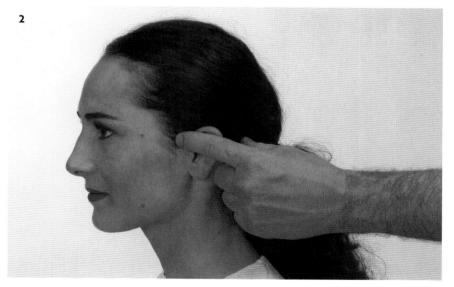

2

Triple Heater 21 can be massaged to treat problems in the ears.

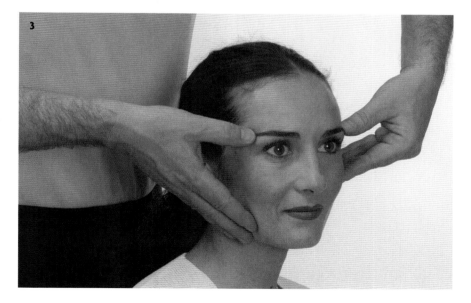

3

Triple Heater 23 can be massaged to treat headaches and eye problems, among others.

Locating the Points on the Back of the Head

Acupressure of the points on the back of the head is helpful in treating headaches in the back of the head and the neck. In this area the points Governor Vessel 16, Gall Bladder 12 and 20, and Urinary Bladder 10 are of special importance.

Governor Vessel 16—Wind Mansion

Governor Vessel 16 is located exactly on the middle axis of the body, 1 cun above the hairline on the neck. If you move your fingers up along the middle axis from the hairline on the neck, you encounter a small bump of bone.

Note

Massage of the points on the back of the head is especially pleasurable when done by a partner, since this allows the recipient to relax more. When massaging this area, make sure to respect your partner's sensitivity to pressure.

The Governor Vessel and the Urinary Bladder and Gall Bladder meridians run almost parallel to each other on the back of the head and the neck.

Gray	Governor Vessel	Governor Vessel 16
Green	Gall Bladder meridian	Gall Bladder 12, 20
Black	Urinary Bladder meridian	Urinary Bladder 10

Governor Vessel 16 is located just beneath this bump.

This point has a wide range of applications. It can be used to treat headaches emanating from the neck, migraines, and dizziness. It is also effective in treating infection accompanied by fever, as well as infection of the sinuses or throat. Moreover, Governor Vessel 16 is helpful as a complementary therapy in cases of cramps, circulation problems in the head, and psychological problems.

Note the following peculiarity: this point is especially effective in treating ailments caused by wind or draft.

Gall Bladder 12—Completion Bone

The Gall Bladder meridian runs in a zigzag along the side of the body. On one end of the zag is the point Gall Bladder 12. Behind the ear it is easy to find a bony bump, which is called the mastoid process. Gall Bladder 12 is at the back of this bump, in a small indentation. This point is used to treat headaches in the side of the head, ailments in the neck area of the spine, and circulation problems in the blood vessels that supply the brain.

Gall Bladder 20—Wind Pool

Gall Bladder 20 is a neighbor to Gall Bladder 12, being just to its side at almost exactly the same height on the back of the head. Gall Bladder 20 is one of the points with a wide range of application possibilities. It is especially beneficial in treating illnesses caused by wind, such as the flu and infections of the sinuses. This point is also effective in treating headaches, migraines, and tension in the neck area of the spine, as well as infections of the upper respiratory passages, hypertension, and circulation problems in the blood vessels that supply the brain.

Urinary Bladder 10—Celestial Pillar

Urinary Bladder 10, also known as Celestial Pillar, is located 1.5 cun to the side of the middle axis, in an indentation just under the bony edge of the back of the head. It is used to treat headaches, sleeping problems and ailments in the cervical spine (the neck part of the spine).

Massaging the Points on the Back of the Head

In this area the points Governor Vessel 16, Gall Bladder 12 and 20, and Urinary Bladder 10 are massaged one after the other.

Governor Vessel 16—Wind Mansion (Figure 1)

Governor Vessel 16 can be massaged with your partner sitting up or lying on his or her stomach. With the tip of your thumb or index finger, apply first steady and then circling pressure for a total of two to four minutes.

Gall Bladder 12—Completion Bone (Figure 2)

Treat Gall Bladder 12 with your partner sitting up or lying on his or her stomach. With the tip of your thumb or index finger, apply first steady and then circular pressure for one to two minutes each.

Gall Bladder 20—Wind Pool (Figure 3)

The point can be treated with your partner sitting up or lying down. With the tip of your thumb or index finger, apply first steady and then circular pressure for two to three minutes.

Urinary Bladder 10—Celestial Pillar (Figure 4)

Urinary Bladder 10 is easiest to massage when your partner is sitting up or lying on his or her stomach. With the tip of your thumb or index finger, apply first steady and then circular pressure for two to three minutes.

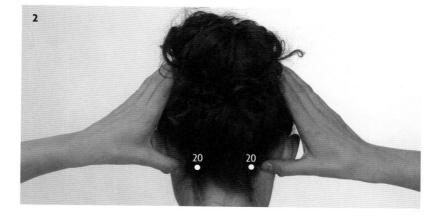

Governor Vessel 16 is located approximately 1 cun above the back hairline on the body's middle axis.

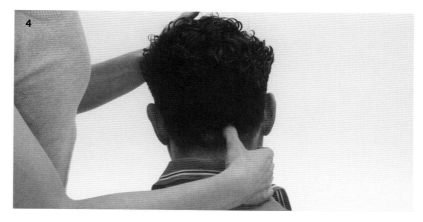

Gall Bladder 12 is located in an indentation behind the mastoid process.

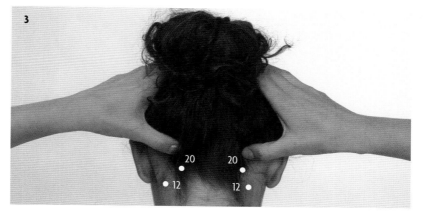

Gall Bladder 20 is located about 1 cun closer to the middle axis than Gall Bladder 12.

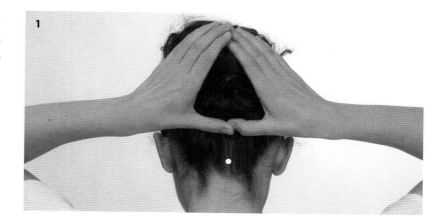

Urinary Bladder 10 is located 1.5 cun to the side of the middle axis, just below the base of the skull.

The Points on the Shoulders and Neck

Six meridians run across the shoulder and neck area. This section discusses the most important individual points in this area and introduces some massage techniques for the back, muscles, and skin that can be used effectively to treat pain in the shoulders and back. These techniques have effects on several points or chains of points.

Locating the Points in the Shoulder-Neck Area

The most important individual points in the shoulder-neck area link to the Governor Vessel, Gall Bladder meridian, Small Intestine meridian, Triple Heater meridian, and Large Intestine meridian.

Caution

Since the twenty-first point of the Gall Bladder meridian has effects on uterine contractions, this point must not be massaged during pregnancy. No moxibustion may be applied to this point during pregnancy either!

Governor Vessel 14—Great Hammer

Governor Vessel 14 is located on the middle axis of the back, in an indentation under the dorsal process of the seventh cervical vertebrae. This point can be used to treat problems in the shoulders as well as the cervical spine (the neck part of the spine). In addition, this point has holistic effects—it can be activated effectively to treat high and continuous fever as well as a range of colds and flus.

Urinary Bladder 41—Attached Branch

Urinary Bladder 41, traditionally known as Attached Branch, is located three finger widths, or 3 cun, to the side of the dorsal process of the second thoracic vertebra. This point can be used to treat pain in the shoulders, neck, and back.

Gall Bladder 21—Shoulder Well

Gall Bladder 21, also known as Shoulder Well, can be found by picturing an imaginary line from the dorsal process of the seventh cervical vertebra to the end of the upper shoulder blade. This point is located exactly in the middle of this line. Gall Bladder 21 is used to treat pain in the shoulders and back. It can also be massaged as a complementary therapy in cases of infections of the mammary gland. Do not massage this point during pregnancy.

Small Intestine 9—True Shoulder

This point is easiest to locate with the arm at rest, hanging down. In this position, Small Intestine 9 is located 1 cun above the back of the armpit fold. This point is used to treat pain in the shoulder joints and upper arms. It is also used to treat problems in lymph flow in the neck, throat, and armpit area.

Six of the fourteen meridians run along the shoulder and neck area.

Gray	Governor Vessel	Governor Vessel 14
Black	Urinary Bladder meridian	Urinary Bladder 41
Green	Gall Bladder meridian	Gall Bladder 21
Red	Small Intestine meridian	Small Intestine 9–15
Purple	Triple Heater meridian	Triple Heater 15, 16
Blue	Large Intestine meridian	Large Intestine 16

Small Intestine 10—Upper Arm Shu

To locate this point, move upward along the Small Intestine meridian from Small Intestine 9 until you come to a bony protrusion, the upper end of the shoulder blade. Directly below this protrusion is Small Intestine 10. It can be used to treat pain in the shoulder joints and upper arms as well as disruptions of the lymph flow in the neck and throat area.

Small Intestine 11—Celestial Gathering

This point can be found by imagining the shoulder blade divided horizontally into three equal sections; Small Intestine 11 is in the center of the line that divides the top third from the middle third. This point is used to treat pain in the neck, shoulders, and elbows. Acupressure of Small Intestine 11 is also helpful in treating pain that emanates from the back and outside of the upper arms. Finally, it can be used as a complementary therapy to facilitate easier breathing in cases of lung ailments that constrict respiratory passages, such as asthma.

Small Intestine 12—Grasping the Wind

Starting from Small Intestine 11, feel your way up in a straight line past the edge of the shoulder blade. There you will find a small indentation—this is the point Small Intestine 12. Acupressure on this point can alleviate pain in the neck, shoulders, and upper arms.

Small Intestine 13—Crooked Wall

To locate this point, feel your way horizontally along the bony upper shoulder blade; Small Intestine 13 is at the inner end of this bone. Massage of this point can be used to treat pain in the shoulders and neck and to relax the tendons and muscles there.

Small Intestine 14—Outer Shoulder Shu

Small Intestine 14 is located at the level of the gap between the first and second thoracic vertebrae, 3 cun to either side. This point can be massaged to treat pain in the neck and shoulders as well as to relax the muscles and tendons throughout the body.

Small Intestine 15—Central Shoulder Shu

Small Intestine 15 is located at the level of the gap between the seventh cervical vertebra and the first thoracic vertebra, 2 cun to either side. Applying pressure on this point can be helpful in relieving pain in the neck area, but its main effect is alleviating problems in the respiratory passages. Acupressure of this point can serve as a complementary therapy in the treatment of coughs resulting from infection of the upper respiratory passages.

Triple Heater 15—Celestial Bone Hole

To locate this point, feel your way along the upper shoulder blade toward the spine. Triple Heater 15 is located about 1 cun up from the end of this bone, between Gall Bladder 21 and Small Intestine 13. It can be used to treat pain in the shoulder area as well as pain resulting in limited range of motion in the cervical spine.

Triple Heater 16—Celestial Window

This point is located slightly below the mastoid process, on the sternocleidomastoid muscle (the large muscle that runs from the clavicle in the front to the mastoid process behind the ear and that is used to nod the head). It can be used to alleviate overall pain and to treat local problems in the throat and neck area. It also has positive effects on hearing and can be used as a complementary therapy in treatments for hearing loss.

Large Intestine 16—Great Bone

Large Intestine 16, also known as Great Bone, is located on the shoulder, at the spot where the collarbone and upper shoulder blade meet. This point is used to treat pain in the shoulders, back, and arms. It also has effects on the thyroid and can be used as a complementary therapy for treatment of thyroid problems.

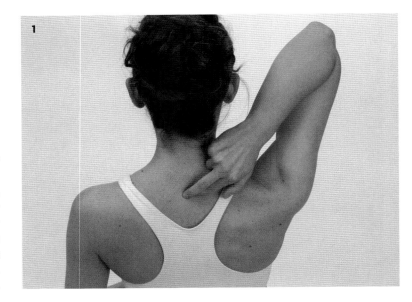

The dorsal processes of individual vertebrae can be felt as bony lumps. Governor Vessel 14 is just below the seventh cervical dorsal process.

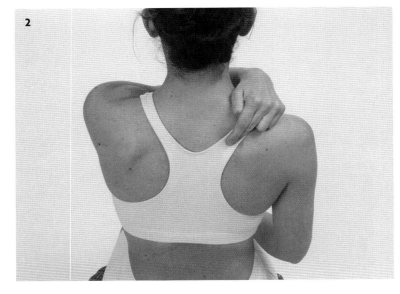

Urinary Bladder 41 is located about 3 cun to the side of the middle axis of the body.

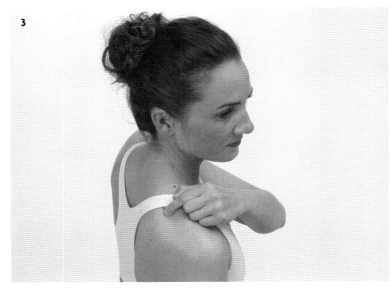

Gall Bladder 21 is located halfway between the highest rise of the shoulder and the seventh cervical vertebra.

Massaging the Points in the Shoulder-Neck Area

Systematically locate the points in the shoulder and neck area that you want to treat and check their sensitivity to pressure. Then massage the points using first steady and then circling pressure.

Governor Vessel 14—Great Hammer (Figure 1)

To locate this point, find one of the slightly protruding dorsal processes of the spine at chest level. Now follow the spine, dorsal process by dorsal process, up toward the head until you reach one dorsal process that protrudes slightly more than the others; this is the dorsal process of the seventh cervical vertebra. You will feel this protrusion even more clearly when your partner bends forward, curving his or her spine. Governor Vessel 14 is just below this protrusion on the middle axis of the body.

With the tip of your index finger over the tip of your middle finger, apply first steady and then circular pressure to this point for two to three minutes.

Urinary Bladder 41—Attached Branch (Figure 2)

You can locate this point in a similar manner to locating Governor Vessel 14. First find the protruding dorsal process of the seventh cervical vertebra. From there, move down two vertebrae. At a level just below that of the second thoracic vertebra and 3 cun to either side of the middle axis is Urinary Bladder 41. If it is sensitive to pressure you can massage it on both sides at the same time using your fingertips. Massage this point for two to three minutes using first steady and then circling pressure, focusing your pressure on the depths of the body.

Gall Bladder 21—Shoulder Well (Figure 3)

Gall Bladder 21 can be massaged with your partner sitting up or lying down. It is located at the spot midway between the highest rise at the outside edge of the shoulder and the seventh cervical vertebra. Touch the muscle knot above the point with your hand and apply as much pressure as you can withstand without feeling pain. Knead and rub the muscle area for two to three minutes. Then massage Gall Bladder 21 using your fingertips, applying first steady and then circular pressure for one to two minutes.

Small Intestine 9—True Shoulder (Figure 1)

For massage of Small Intestine 9, the arm should hang loosely to the side of the body. In this position, you will find Small Intestine 9 located 1 cun above the back of the armpit fold. With the tip of your index finger over the tip of your middle finger, apply first steady and then circling pressure for two to three minutes, focusing pressure on the center of the body and the head, meaning slightly upward.

Small Intestine 10—Upper Arm Shu (Figure 2)

Small Intestine 10 is located below the bony protrusion of the shoulder blade. With the tip of your index finger over the tip of your middle finger, apply first steady and then circling pressure for two to three minutes. Aside from pressure, you can also treat this point with warmth, using one of the special means of moxibustion.

Small Intestine 11—Celestial Gathering (Figure 3)

Have your partner lie on his or her stomach; if you're practicing self-massage, you should sit up. With the tip of your index finger over the tip of your middle finger, apply first steady and then circling pressure for two to three minutes. Aside from pressure, you can also treat this point with warmth, using one of the special means of moxibustion.

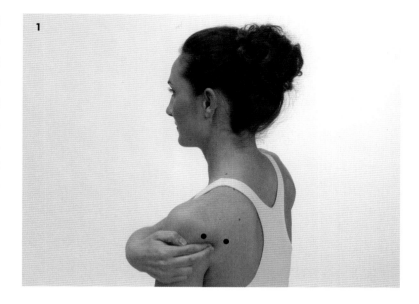

Small Intestine 9 is located 1 cun above the back of the armpit fold.

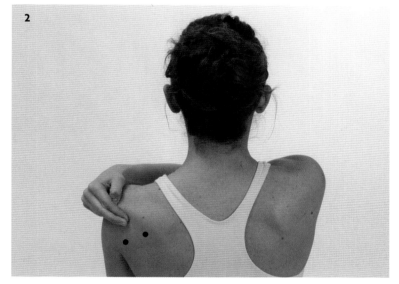

Small Intestine 10 can be massaged to alleviate pain in the shoulders and upper arms.

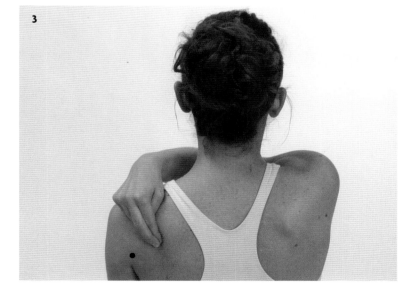

Small Intestine 11 can be massaged to treat lung ailments and pain in the neck, shoulders, and upper arms.

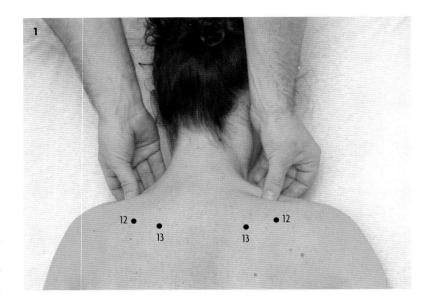

Small Intestine 12 is treated above the upper shoulder blade.

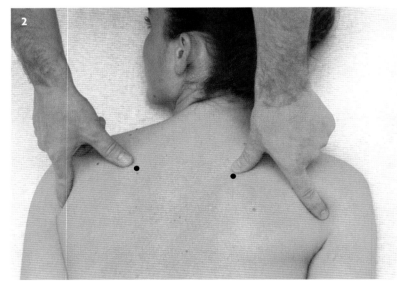

Small Intestine 13 is located at the inside edge of the upper shoulder blade.

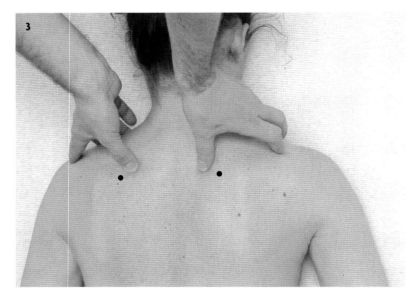

Small Intestine 14 can be massaged to treat pain in the shoulders and back.

Small Intestine 12—Grasping the Wind (Figure 1)

Locate this point above the bony horizontal protrusion of the shoulder blade, straight up from Small Intestine 11. Massage this point using the tip of your thumb or index finger, applying first steady and then circling pressure for two to three minutes. You can massage the two points of Small Intestine 12 at the same time or one after the other. You can also treat this point with moxibustion.

Small Intestine 13—Crooked Wall (Figure 2)

Locate Small Intestine 13 at the inner edge of the upper shoulder blade. With the tip of your thumb or index finger, apply first steady and then circling pressure for two to three minutes. You can also treat this point with a heat infusion using a moxa cigar, pin, or loose moxa.

Small Intestine 14—Outer Shoulder Shu (Figure 3)

This point is easiest to massage if your partner lies down; if you're practicing self-massage, you should sit up. To locate Small Intestine 14, feel for the protruding dorsal process of the seventh cervical vertebra. From here, work your way down to the dorsal process of the vertebra below; this is the first thoracic vertebra. Feel for the gap between the first and second thoracic vertebrae. Small Intestine 14 is 3 cun to either side of this gap. This point can be massaged with the tips of your thumbs as shown in the photo, or with your index fingers. Apply first steady and then circling pressure for two to three minutes. You can also use moxibustion on this point.

Small Intestine 15—Central Shoulder Shu (Figure 1)

This point can be located by first finding the protruding dorsal process of the seventh cervical vertebrae. From there, move your fingers two finger widths, or 2 cun, outward. Massage Small Intestine 15 with your thumbs or, as shown in the photo, index fingers, applying first steady and then circling pressure for two to three minutes.

Triple Heater 15—Celestial Bone Hole (Figure 2)

Triple Heater 15 can be massaged with your partner sitting up or lying down. With the tip of your thumb or index finger, apply first steady and then circling pressure for two to three minutes. You can also apply moxibustion to this point.

Triple Heater 16—Celestial Window (Figure 3)

Triple Heater 16 can be massaged with your partner sitting up or lying down. To find the point, locate the mastoid process behind the ear. At the back edge of the mastoid process, toward the neck, you will find the sternocleidomastoid muscle (the large muscle that runs from the clavicle in the front to the mastoid behind the ear and that is used to nod the head). Triple Heater 16 is at the edge of this muscle. Massage this point with the tip of your thumb or index finger, using first steady and then circling pressure for two to three minutes.

Large Intestine 16—Great Bone (Figure 4)

Locate this point in the corner between the collarbone and the upper shoulder blade. With the tip of your thumb, apply first steady and then circling pressure for two to three minutes. You can also apply moxibustion to this point.

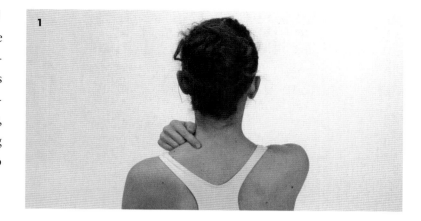

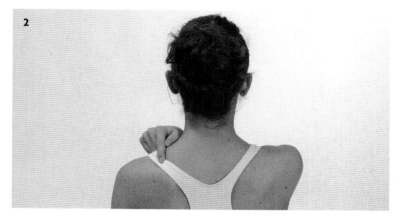

Small Intestine 15 is located slightly above Small Intestine 14, about 2 cun away from the body's middle axis.

Triple Heater 15 can be massaged to alleviate pain in the neck area of the spine.

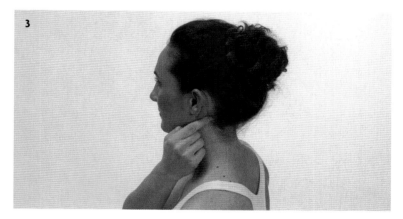

Triple Heater 16 can be massaged to treat pain in the neck area of the spine as well as hearing loss.

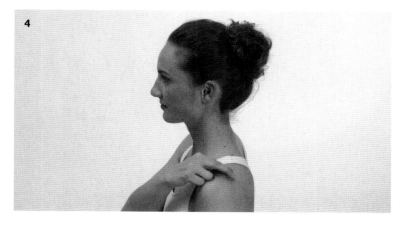

Large Intestine 16 is located in an indentation at the place where the collarbone meets the upper shoulder blade.

The Points on the Back

Two meridians run along the back from top to bottom: the Governor Vessel and the Urinary Bladder meridian. This section describes the points of the Urinary Bladder meridian.

Note

In addition to applying pressure, you can also apply a traditional moxibustion treatment to the points Urinary Bladder 11 through Urinary Bladder 25. Use only the specific aids for moxibustion described on pages 65–67.

The Urinary Bladder meridian is the longest of the fourteen meridians.

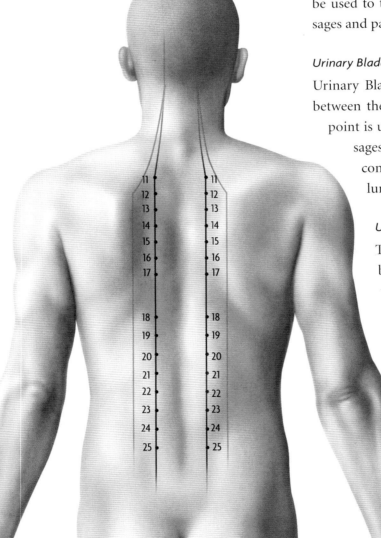

| Black | Urinary Bladder meridian | Urinary Bladder 11–17 |
| | | Urinary Bladder 18–25 |

Locating the Points on the Inner Branch

The Urinary Bladder meridian has two branches, one closer to and one further from the spine. We will first look at the points of the branch closer to the spine, known as the medial branch. The two facets of the medial branch run parallel to the middle axis of the body, 1.5 cun to either side.

Urinary Bladder 11—Great Shuttle

Great Shuttle is located at the level of the gap between the first and second thoracic vertebrae. This point can be used to treat illnesses in the upper respiratory passages and pain in the throat.

Urinary Bladder 12—Wind Gate

Urinary Bladder 12 is located at the level of the gap between the third and fourth thoracic vertebrae. This point is used to treat illnesses of the respiratory passages such as asthma. It can also be used as a complementary therapy in cases of infectious lung diseases such as pneumonia.

Urinary Bladder 13—Lung Shu

This point is located at the level of the gap between the third and fourth thoracic vertebrae. The most important uses of this point relate to problems in the respiratory passages, such as bronchial asthma. In addition, acupressure of this point can be used as a complementary therapy in cases of lung infections such as pneumonia.

Urinary Bladder 14—Pericardium Shu

Urinary Bladder 14 is located at the level of the space between the fourth and fifth thoracic vertebrae. It can be massaged to alleviate coughs or as a complementary therapy in cases of cardiovascular problems.

Urinary Bladder 15—Heart Shu

Heart Shu is located at the level of the gap between the fifth and sixth thoracic vertebrae. Acupressure of this point is used as a complementary therapy in cases of cardiovascular problems. In traditional Chinese medicine this point is said to bring about peace of mind, and thus it is also a good complementary treatment in cases of psychosomatic and psychological ailments.

Urinary Bladder 16—Governing Shu

Urinary Bladder 16 is located at the level of the gap between the sixth and seventh thoracic vertebrae. Acupressure of this point has positive effects on stomachaches and other pain in the abdominal area; it also can serve as a complementary therapy in cases of cardiovascular problems.

Urinary Bladder 17—Diaphragm Shu

This point is at the level of the gap between the seventh and eighth thoracic vertebrae and is used to treat asthma, nosebleeds, and hiccups. Traditional Chinese medicine sees this point as filling and calming the blood; this point can thus also be helpful in treating anemia.

Urinary Bladder 18—Liver Shu

This point is located at the level of the gap between the ninth and tenth thoracic vertebrae. It is used to treat illnesses of the liver and gallbladder as well as eye conditions and psychological and psychosomatic problems.

Urinary Bladder 19—Gall Bladder Shu

This point is located at the level of the gap between the tenth and eleventh thoracic vertebrae. It is used to treat illnesses of the gallbladder, such as infections or gallstones.

Urinary Bladder 20—Spleen Shu

This point is located at the level of the gap between the eleventh and twelfth thoracic vertebrae. It can be used

Caution

Remember that acupressure can only *complement* medical treatment; it is not a substitute for it.

to treat chronic infections of the mucous membranes of the stomach as well as digestive problems such as diarrhea.

Urinary Bladder 21—Stomach Shu

Urinary Bladder 21 is located at the level of the gap between the twelfth thoracic vertebra and first lumbar vertebra. This point is used to treat stomachaches and acute and chronic infections in the stomach.

Urinary Bladder 22—Triple Heater Shu

Urinary Bladder 22 is located at the level of the gap between the first and second lumbar vertebrae. Acupressure of this point has positive effects for acute and chronic stomach infections and digestive problems.

Urinary Bladder 23—Kidney Shu

This point is located at the level of the gap between the second and third lumbar vertebrae. Acupressure of this point is used to treat sexual dysfunctions, as well as menstruation problems and pain in the lower back.

Urinary Bladder 24—Sea of Qi Shu

This point is located at the level of the gap between the third and fourth lumbar vertebrae. It can be used to treat pain in the lower back as well as pain during menstruation.

Urinary Bladder 25—Large Intestine Shu

This point is located at the level of the gap between the fourth and fifth lumbar vertebrae. It can be used to treat pain in the lower back as well as digestive problems.

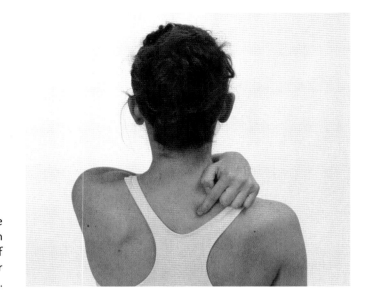

Begin the sequence with acupressure of Urinary Bladder 11 . . .

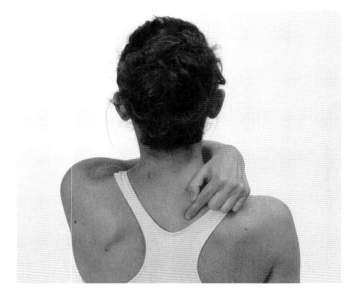

. . . and continue by moving your finger to the next point on the Urinary Bladder meridian.

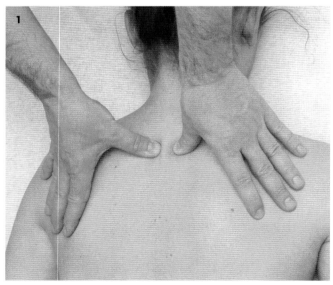

Lift the skin slightly by moving the points on the Urinary Bladder meridian together using the tips of your thumbs.

Massaging the Points on the Medial Branch

The points on the medial branch of the Urinary Bladder meridian are massaged from top to bottom.

Urinary Bladder 11 to 25

Massage these points with your partner lying down; if you are massaging yourself, you should sit up. You can massage the points on both sides of the spine at the same time. If you are new to acupressure, you can practice by massaging first one side and then the other. Applying pressure in sync with your partner's breathing (or your own, if you are massaging yourself), massage with first steady and then circling pressure. Slightly increase the pressure when your partner exhales, and decrease it when he or she inhales. In the area of the thoracic spine, that is, on the upper back, you can apply slightly stronger pressure, while in the lower back area, starting at about Urinary Bladder 18, use lighter pressure.

When you have finished massaging one pair of points, keep your fingers on them. Use your fingers to move each point toward the other horizontally, and then let them return to their natural position. Keep your fingers in contact with the skin as you move them down to the next pair of points.

Use this rhythm—pressing, circling, moving—to massage the points from top to bottom down to Urinary Bladder 25. Once there, lift your hands and place them again on Urinary Bladder 11. Begin anew from the top. Massage these points five times in this way.

Lifting the Skin (Figure 1)

Another way to massage the points is to lift the skin above them. To do this, place your index fingers or, as shown in the photo, thumbs on the points. Move your fingers toward each other, creating a fold of skin between them. Pull this fold upward. Here, too, keep your movements in sync with your partner's or your own breathing, lifting the skin during the exhalation and releasing it during the inhalation. This technique treats the points on both sides of the spine.

Locating the Points on the Lateral Branch

The lateral branch of the Urinary Bladder meridian runs parallel to the medial branch down the entire length of the back; it is 1.5 cun away from the medial branch, or 3 cun away from the middle axis of the body. The points on the lateral branch are located parallel to the ones of the medial branch.

Urinary Bladder 41—Attached Branch

Urinary Bladder 41, known traditionally as Attached Branch, is located at the level of the gap between the second and third thoracic vertebrae. Acupressure of this point is helpful in cases of pain in the shoulder, neck, and back area.

Urinary Bladder 42—Po Door

This point is located at the level of the gap between the third and fourth thoracic vertebrae. It can be massaged in cases of lung ailments such as bronchitis or asthma and pain in the shoulder, neck, and back.

Urinary Bladder 43—Gao Huang Shu

This point is located at the level of the gap between the fourth and fifth thoracic vertebrae. It is used to treat pain in the shoulder, neck, and back area as well as chronic bronchitis.

Urinary Bladder 44—Spirit Hall

Urinary Bladder 44 is located at the level of the gap between the fifth and sixth thoracic vertebrae. It is used to treat acute or chronic bronchitis as well as bronchial asthma.

Urinary Bladder 45—Yi Xi (Ow, That Hurts!)

This point is located at the level of the gap between the sixth and seventh thoracic vertebrae and has the same effects as Urinary Bladder 44.

Urinary Bladder 46—Diaphragm Pass

This point is located at the level of the gap between the seventh and eighth thoracic vertebrae. It is massaged to treat chronic gastrointestinal problems, as a complement to medical treatment.

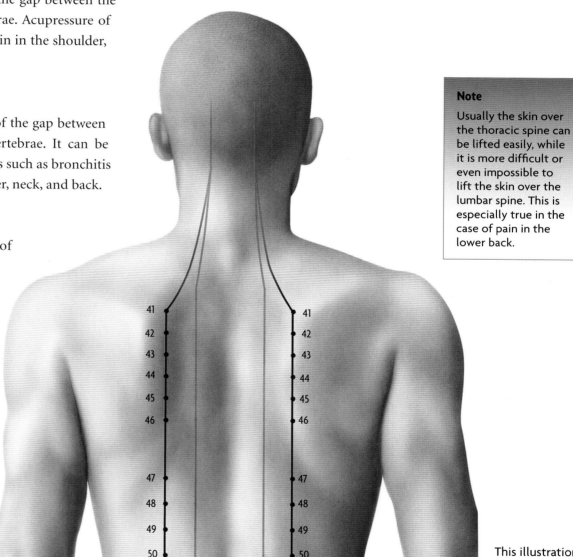

Note

Usually the skin over the thoracic spine can be lifted easily, while it is more difficult or even impossible to lift the skin over the lumbar spine. This is especially true in the case of pain in the lower back.

This illustration shows the upper part of the Urinary Bladder meridian, which runs along the entire back.

| Black | Urinary Bladder meridian | Urinary Bladder 41–46 |
| | | Urinary Bladder 47–50 |

Urinary Bladder 47—Hun Gate

Urinary Bladder 47, known as Hun Gate in traditional Chinese medicine, is located at the level of the gap between the ninth and tenth thoracic vertebrae. It can be massaged to treat both acute and chronic gastrointestinal infections.

Urinary Bladder 48—Yang Headrope

Urinary Bladder 48, also known as Yang Headrope, is located at the level of the gap between the tenth and eleventh thoracic vertebrae. It can be massaged to treat acute and chronic gastrointestinal infections, as well as infections of the gallbladder.

Urinary Bladder 49—Reflection Abode

Urinary Bladder 49, called Reflection Abode in traditional Chinese medicine, is located at the level of the gap between the eleventh and twelfth thoracic vertebrae. Like Urinary Bladder 47, this point is used to treat both acute and chronic gastrointestinal infections.

Urinary Bladder 50—Stomach Granary

This point, called Stomach Granary in traditional Chinese medicine, is located at the level of the gap between the twelfth thoracic vertebra and the first lumbar vertebra. Because of its harmonizing effects on the stomach, Urinary Bladder 50 is used to treat acute and chronic gastrointestinal infections, as well as digestive problems in children.

Urinary Bladder 51—Huang Gate

Urinary Bladder 51, known as Huang Gate in traditional Chinese medicine, is located at the level of the gap between the first and second lumbar vertebrae. It is said to have the ability to regulate the qi (life energy) and to reduce the swelling of edema. It is used to treat chronic constipation as well as swelling in the liver or spleen.

Urinary Bladder 52—Will Chamber

This point, called Will Chamber in traditional Chinese medicine, is located at the level of the gap between the second and third lumbar vertebrae. It is massaged to treat problems in male sexual functions, urinary tract infections, and pain in the lower back. According to traditional Chinese medicine, treating Urinary Bladder 52 clears and mobilizes both heat and humidity. This makes it useful in treating illnesses related to excess heat (see page 24), for example in the case of acute illnesses or fever, or excess of water, for example edema.

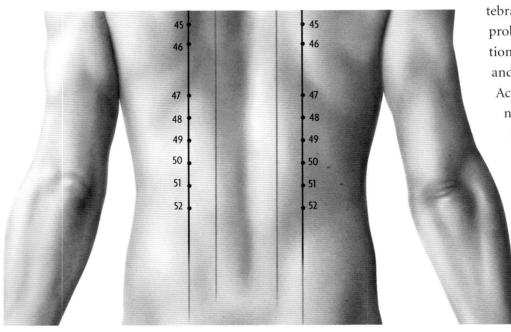

The lower part of the Urinary Bladder meridian contains the points Urinary Bladder 47 to 52.

| Black | Urinary Bladder meridian | Urinary Bladder 46 |
| | | Urinary Bladder 47–52 |

Massaging the Points on the Lateral Branch

The points on the lateral branch of the Urinary Bladder meridian can be massaged to treat a wide variety of health problems. In addition, acupressure of these points can be pleasant for the recipient in the context of a wellness massage or to relieve back pain. The points are massaged from top to bottom.

Urinary Bladder 41 to 52 (Figures 1–3)

Acupressure of these points is done with your partner lying on his or her stomach. Begin the massage with the Urinary Bladder 41 pair of points, at the level of the gap between the second and third thoracic vertebrae. It is easiest to massage both points, one on each side of the spine, at the same time if you use your thumbs. Apply light pressure to the points at first, and slowly increase it. Be guided by the breathing of your partner: slightly increase pressure as your partner exhales, and decrease pressure as she or he inhales. Apply steady pressure for one to two minutes, then apply circular pressure for about one minute, finally reducing the radius of your circles and letting your thumbs come to a rest on the points.

Once you have finished with one pair of points, move on to the next pair. Make sure your thumbs don't lose contact with your partner's skin while you're moving your hands. Rather, glide or push your thumbs to the next pair of points, keeping them in steady contact with your partner's skin. Massage the next pair of points in the same way described above. All points of the lateral branch of the Urinary Bladder meridian should be massaged according to this pattern: pressing, circling, and sliding in synchrony with your partner's breathing. After you have finished massaging Urinary Bladder 52, you can now lift your thumbs from your partner's skin and place them again on point Urinary Bladder 41, beginning the massage anew. Altogether, you should carry out this process five times.

Interrupt the massage if your partner feels uncomfortable. If, on the other hand, your partner is responding well to the treatment, you can increase the duration of the massage for individual points by as long as you like. Note, however, that certain points on the lateral branch of the Urinary Bladder meridian are best massaged in several repetitions.

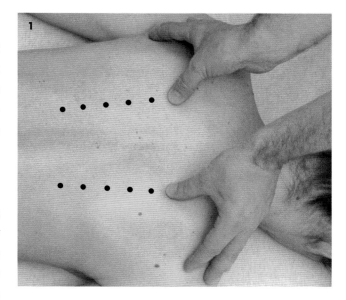

Begin massaging the lateral branch of the Urinary Bladder meridian with Urinary Bladder 41 . . .

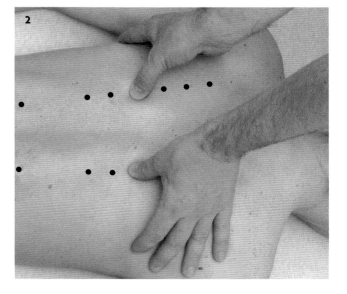

. . . and continue along the course of the meridian . . .

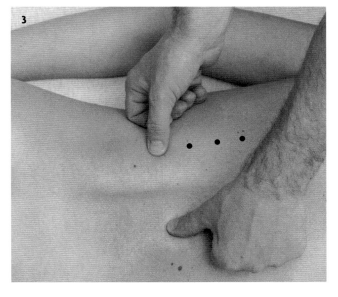

. . . until you reach Urinary Bladder 52.

The Points on the Sacrum and Buttocks

In the area of the sacrum and the buttocks muscles are several points that can be massaged to alleviate severe back pain as well as ailments of the urinary system.

Locating the Points of the Sacrum and Buttocks

The following introduces each point in the area of the sacrum and buttocks, along with their uses in acupressure.

Urinary Bladder 31—Upper Bone Hole

Upper Bone Hole is located on the sacrum at the height of the first sacral foramen (hole in the bone). This point can be massaged to treat sexual dysfunctions in men and gynecological problems, including difficulties of menstruation, in women.

Urinary Bladder 32—Second Bone Hole

This point is located below Urinary Bladder 31, on the sacrum at the second foramen. This point can be mas-

saged to treat gynecological problems, such as those related to menstruation, as well as infections in the abdomen and as a complementary treatment for paralysis of the legs.

Urinary Bladder 33—Central Bone Hole

Urinary Bladder 33, also known as Central Bone Hole, is located below Urinary Bladder 31, at the third sacral foramen. It can be massaged in cases of pain in the sacral region as well as gynecological conditions such as uterine infections and menstruation problems.

Urinary Bladder 34—Lower Bone Hole

Urinary Bladder 34 is located below point Urinary Bladder 33 on the fourth sacral foramen. It is used to treat acute and chronic intestinal infections as well as anuria.

Urinary Bladder 54—Sequential Limit

This point is located 3 cun to the side of the middle axis of the body, at the same level as Urinary Bladder 34. It can be massaged to treat pain along the course of the sciatic nerve (ischialgia, lumbago, sciatica), prostate problems, and hemorrhoids.

Gall Bladder 30—Jumping Round

It is easiest to locate this point with your partner on his or her side and his or her hip joint bent. Imagine a line running from the bottom of the sacrum (at the top of the seam between the buttocks) to the greater trochanter (a prominence at the top of the femur). If you divide the line into three equal parts, Gall Bladder 30 is located at the spot that divides the middle from the outer third. Massage of this point is effective against pain in legs, feet, and lower back.

Governor Vessel 3—Lumbar Yang Pass

This point is located on the body's middle axis, just below the fourth lumbar vertebra at the same level as the upper edge of the pelvic bone. It can be used to treat pain in the lumbar region and in the legs.

> **Caution**
>
> The points Urinary Bladder 31 through 34 must not be massaged during pregnancy!

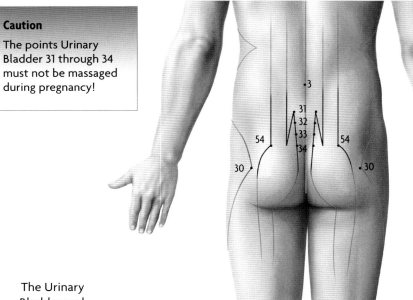

The Urinary Bladder and Gall Bladder meridians as well as the Governor Vessel all run along the buttocks and sacrum.

Black	Urinary Bladder meridian	Urinary Bladder 31–34 Urinary Bladder 54
Dark green	Gall Bladder meridian	Gall Bladder 30
Gray	Governor Vessel	Governor Vessel 3

Massaging the Points on the Sacrum and the Buttocks

These points are massaged one after the other. Acupressure of these points is helpful in treating a range of lower-body ailments, especially in the case of pain along the course of the sciatic nerve.

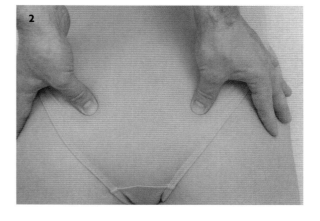

Massage Urinary Bladder 31 to 34 for one to two minutes.

Urinary Bladder 31 to 34 (Figure 1)

The points Urinary Bladder 31 to 34 occur as pairs; both points in each pair are massaged at the same time. Have your partner lie down. Use the tips of your thumbs to locate Urinary Bladder 31 on both sides of the spine; these points are above the exit points of nerves from the first sacral foramina (bone holes), which you can feel with your fingers. Maintaining contact with the skin, apply steady pressure on these points in sync with your partner's breathing, slightly increasing the pressure as he or she exhales, and releasing it as he or she inhales. Then apply circling pressure. When you have finished massaging this pair, move your thumbs down to Urinary Bladder 32, being sure to maintain contact with the skin as you move. Massage Urinary Bladder 32, 33, and 34 as just described. Then repeat the treatment, starting again with Urinary Bladder 31, for a total of five repetitions.

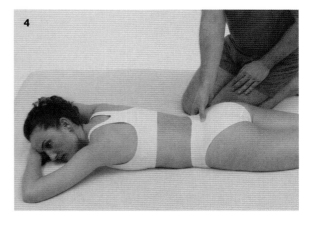

Use the tips of your thumbs to massage Urinary Bladder 54, which is 3 cun away from the middle axis on either side.

Urinary Bladder 54—Sequential Limit (Figure 2)

Urinary Bladder 54 is also massaged with your partner lying down. With the tips of your thumbs, find the two points of Urinary Bladder 54 on either side of the spine. Apply first steady and then circling pressure for a total of two to three minutes. Note that this point is frequently sensitive to pressure and painful. The point can be helpful when massaged in cases of hemorrhoids, prostate problems, or pain along the course of the sciatic nerve.

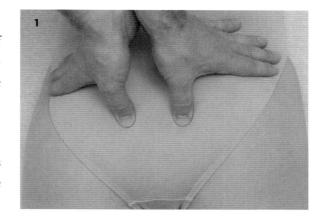

You can use your palm to massage Gall Bladder 30.

Gall Bladder 30—Jumping Round (Figure 3)

This point, too, is massaged with your partner lying down. It's helpful to have your partner lie on his or her side. Use the ball of your hand to massage this point with first steady and then circling pressure for two to three minutes. (The pressure should not be so strong that your partner has to counterbalance it by clenching his or her buttocks muscles.)

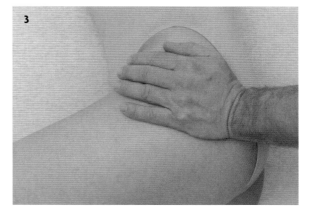

The massage of Governor Vessel 3 is especially pleasurable when done by a partner.

Governor Vessel 3—Lumbar Yang Pass (Figure 4)

Massage this point with your partner lying down, applying circular pressure for two to three minutes. Aside from applying pressure, you can also apply moxibustion to this point.

The Points on the Throat and Chest

In the case of localized throat problems, accupressure of the points of the Stomach meridian can be an effective treatment.

Locating the Points on the Throat and Chest

Two lines of the Stomach meridian, running to the left and right of the body's middle axis, can be found in the throat and chest area. Several of meridian's points in this area are important in acupressure. In addition, Conception Vessel runs through this area exactly on the middle axis; on this meridian, points 17 and 22 are of significance.

Stomach 9—Man's Prognosis

Stomach 9, known as Man's Prognosis in traditional Chinese medicine, is located at the level of the top of the Adam's apple, 1.5 cun away from the middle axis of the body (where the pulse of the carotid is usually felt). It is used to treat throat infections and can also be helpful in treating problems of the respiratory passages such as bronchitis and asthma.

Stomach 10—Water Prominence

Stomach 10 is located at the front edge of the sterno-cleidomastoid muscle (the large muscle that runs from the clavicle in the front to the mastoid behind the ear and that is used to nod the head), at the level of the bottom of the Adam's apple. It is used to treat infections in the throat or the respiratory passages, including acute tonsillitis, coughing, and shortness of breath.

Stomach 11—Qi Abode

Stomach 11 is located directly below Stomach 10, just above the collarbone. This point is used to treat acute infections in the throat as well as illnesses related to the respiratory passages such as asthma.

Conception Vessel 17—Chest Center

This point is located on the middle axis of the front of the body, at the same level as the nipples. Massage of this point causes the chest cavity to expand, which is why it is used to treat asthma. Conception Vessel 17 can also be massaged to stimulate the flow of milk after childbirth.

Conception Vessel 22—Celestial Chimney

This point is located on the middle axis of the front of the body, above the bony limit of the sternum. It is used to treat problems in the respi-

Caution

Because the points Stomach 9, 10, and 11 are located very close to the carotid artery, pressure should not be applied to these points!

The Stomach meridian and Conception Vessel run along the neck and middle of the chest.

Green	Stomach meridian	Stomach 9–11
Gray	Conception Vessel	Conception Vessel 17, 22

ratory passages, including asthma, and problems in the throat and mouth, such as hoarseness or loss of voice.

> **Note**
>
> To locate the points on the front edge of the sternocleidomastoid (head-nodding) muscle, it helps to have your partner turn his or her head in the opposite direction and slightly bend his or her head forward. This will help you see and feel the muscle.

Massaging the Points on the Throat and Chest

Because of the location of these points, the acupressure technique to be used in their massage is different from the techniques described up to this point. Please note the special instructions.

The points in the throat and chest area are treated primarily for problems in the throat, such as hoarseness, sudden loss of voice, tonsil infections, and illnesses of the upper respiratory passages.

Stomach 9 to 11 (Figures 1 and 2)

Massage points 9 to 11 of the Stomach meridian with your partner lying down. Place the tip of your index finger lightly on Stomach 9, and pull it gently across Stomach 10 to Stomach 11. Massage these three points with this stroking movement five times, first on one side of the throat and then on the other side.

Because these points are located close to the carotid artery and are especially sensitive to pressure, be sure not to exert pressure on them.

Conception Vessel 17 and 22 (Figure 3)

With your partner lying down, use the tip of your index finger to locate the point Conception Vessel 22 and apply circling pressure for one to two minutes. Then slide the tip of your finger along the sternum and down the middle axis of the body to Conception Vessel 17. Once there, lift your fingertip, place it again on Conception Vessel 22, and repeat the sliding motion down to point 17. Repeat this process four or five times. Then massage Conception Vessel 17 with steady or circling pressure for one to two minutes.

Note: Do not massage Conception Vessel 17 on a woman who is pregnant.

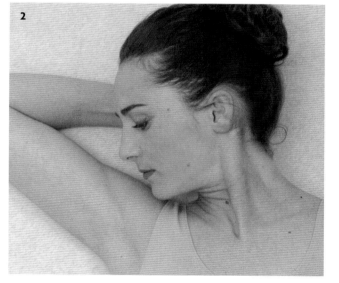

Stomach 9, 10, and 11 are located to the left and right of the trachea. Do not apply pressure to these points.

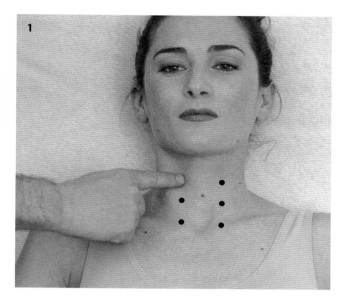

The sternocleidomastoid (head-nodding) muscle is most noticeable with the head turned to the side. Finding this muscle will help you locate the points on the Stomach meridian.

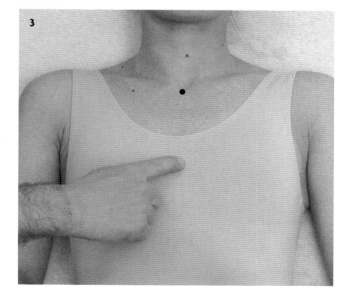

Conception Vessel 17 and 22 are massaged along the body's middle axis.

The Points on the Chest

The Spleen meridian runs on both sides of the body's middle axis, along the sides of the chest. The Lung and Pericardium meridians also originate in this part of the body.

Locating the Points on the Sides of the Chest

Several points located on the sides of the chest cavity are used frequently in acupressure.

Caution

Remember that in the case of cardiovascular ailments, acupressure of Pericardium 1 should be considered only a complementary measure to medical treatment. In this situation, you should consult with a doctor.

Pericardium 1—Celestial Pool

This point is located at the level of the gap between the fourth and fifth ribs, 5 cun to the side of the middle axis on the front of the body. Pericardium 1 is used to treat illnesses of the respiratory passages such as coughs and asthma. Massage of this point can also be used as a complementary treatment to modern therapies in cases of cardiovascular problems.

Lung 1—Central Treasury

Lung 1 is 6 cun to the side of the middle axis and 1 cun below the collarbone. It is treated in the case of problems in the respiratory passages or chest cavity, such as bronchitis, asthma, coughing, and shortness of breath. The point can also be used to treat pain along the Lung meridian, such as in the area of the shoulder and arm.

Lung 2—Cloud Gate

Lung 2 is located 6 cun to the side of the middle axis in an indentation below the collarbone and above Lung 1. The indentation can be felt with your fingers. This point has the same application range as Lung 1.

Spleen 17—Food Hole

Spleen 17 is located at the level of the gap between the fifth and sixth ribs, 6 cun to the side of the middle axis. The point is used to treat pain in the chest area, such as intercostal neuralgia, and difficulty swallowing.

Spleen 18—Celestial Ravine

Spleen 18, also known as Celestial Ravine, is located above Spleen 17 at the level of the gap between the fourth and fifth ribs, 6 cun to the side of the middle axis. It is used primarily to treat pain in the chest area but can also be massaged to stimulate milk production after childbirth.

The Pericardium, Lung, and Spleen meridians run along the sides of the chest.

Purple	Pericardium meridian	Pericardium 1
Blue	Lung meridian	Lung 1, 2
Green	Spleen meridian	Spleen 17–20

Spleen 19—Chest Village

This point is located at the level of the gap between the third and fourth ribs, 6 cun to the side of the body's middle axis. It is used to treat pain in the chest area.

Spleen 20—All-Round Flourishing

Spleen 20 is located at the level of the gap between the second and third ribs, 6 cun to the side of the body's middle axis. It is used to treat lung ailments and alleviates associated problems, including coughing and shortness of breath.

Massaging the Points on the Sides of the Chest

Pericardium 1, Lung 1 and 2, and the Spleen points lie along two almost parallel lines and can be massaged one after the other.

Pericardium 1 (Figure 1)

Massage Pericardium 1 using the tip of your thumb or index finger. If you are experienced in acupressure, you can massage the points on both sides of the body at the same time. Apply first steady and then circling pressure for a total of two to three minutes.

Lung 1 and 2 (Figure 2)

These points are massaged with your partner lying down. Lung 1 and 2 can be massaged together and on both sides of the body at the same time. Locate Lung 2 with the tips of your index fingers and Lung 1 with the tips of your thumbs. Apply steady or circling pressure for one to two minutes.

Spleen 17 to 20 (Figures 3 and 4)

Begin with Spleen 20 on both sides of the body. With the tips of your thumbs, apply first steady and then circling pressure in rhythm with your partner's breathing, slightly increasing pressure when your partner exhales, and decreasing pressure when he or she inhales. Then, applying circling pressure on both sides of the body, let your thumbs glide down to Spleen 19. Massage this point, and Spleen 18 and 17 below it, in the same way. After you have massaged Spleen 17, return to Spleen 20. Altogether these points should be massaged five times each.

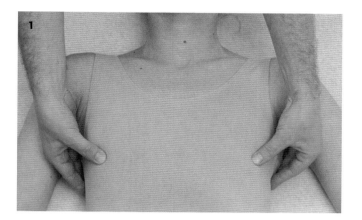

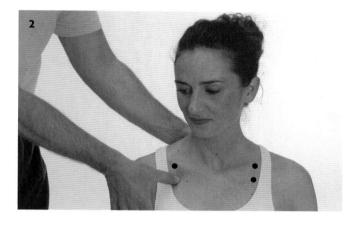

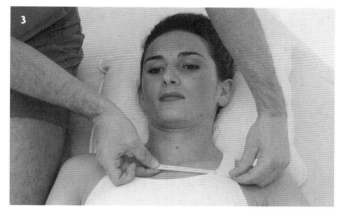

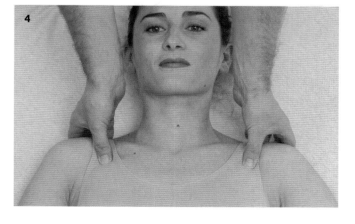

Massage Pericardium 1 using the tips of your thumbs.

Here, the thumb is used to massage Lung 1.

The points of the Spleen meridian are located in the chest area along a line 6 cun from the body's middle axis.

Begin acupressure of the Spleen meridian with Spleen 20.

Locating the Points on the Front of the Chest

The Kidney meridian runs along the front of the chest in two lines, one on each side, parallel to the body's middle axis. The Kidney meridian contains important and powerful points that can be massaged to alleviate problems in the chest. These points are described below.

Note

The points discussed here can be massaged one after the other, first on one side of the chest and then on the other, or you can massage each pair of points simultaneously, using two fingers.

In addition, you can apply a traditional Chinese warmth treatment (see page 65) to the points described here, Kidney 22 to 27.

Acupressure of Kidney points 22 to 27 can be especially helpful in alleviating respiratory and chest ailments.

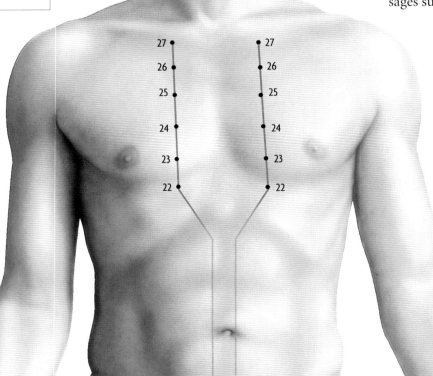

| Gray | Kidney meridian | Kidney 22–27 |

Kidney 22—Corridor Walk

Kidney 22 is located at the level of the gap between the fifth and sixth ribs, 2 cun to the side of the body's middle axis. It is used to treat pain in the chest area as well as acute and chronic infections of the respiratory passages.

Kidney 23—Spirit Seal

Kidney 23 is located at the level of the gap between the fourth and fifth ribs, 2 cun to the side of the body's middle axis. This point is used to treat pain in the chest area as well as infections of the respiratory passages such as asthma or bronchitis. It can also be massaged as a complement to medical treatment for infections of the mammary glands.

Kidney 24—Spirit Ruins

Kidney 24 is located at the level of the gap between the third and fourth ribs, 2 cun to the side of the middle axis. It is used to treat infections of the respiratory passages such as asthma and chronic bronchitis.

Kidney 25—Spirit Storehouse

Kidney 25 is located at the level of the gap between the second and third ribs, 2 cun to the side of the middle axis. It is massaged to treat pain in the chest as well as acute and chronic infections of the respiratory passages.

Kidney 26—Lively Center

This point is located at the level of the gap between the first and second ribs—that is, the first noticeable intercostal space—2 cun to the side of the middle axis. Massage of this point alleviates coughing and shortness of breath, and it is used to treat acute and chronic infections of the respiratory passages.

Kidney 27—Shu Mansion

Kidney 27 is located exactly at the lower edge of the collarbone, 2 cun to the side of the body's middle axis. This point is massaged in the case of pain in the chest area as well as in the case of acute or chronic infections of the respiratory passages.

Massaging the Points on the Front of the Chest

The points of the Kidney meridian on the front of the chest are massaged with the thumbs one after the other, from bottom to top. Both points in each pair, one on each side of the middle axis, are massaged at the same time.

Kidney 22 to 27 (Figures 1–3)

The massage is given with your partner lying down. Locate the pair of Kidney 22 points (one on each side of the middle axis) on the rib cage with your thumbs. Using your thumbs, apply steady pressure in rhythm with your partner's breathing: slightly increase the pressure as your partner exhales, and decrease it as he or she inhales. After four or five breathing cycles, switch to a circling application of pressure. Then guide both your thumbs slightly outward, applying light pressure. For Kidney 22 this means that your thumbs are following the lower edge of the rib cage. Now lift your thumbs and place them on the next point, Kidney 23. Massage this point in the same way, using first steady and then circling pressure. Then slowly move your thumbs outward along the space between the ribs, applying light pressure, before lifting them and proceeding to the next point. Massage the six points of the Kidney meridian one after the other from bottom to top in this way.

When you have finished massaging Kidney 27, begin again with Kidney 22. Massage all of these points a total of five times.

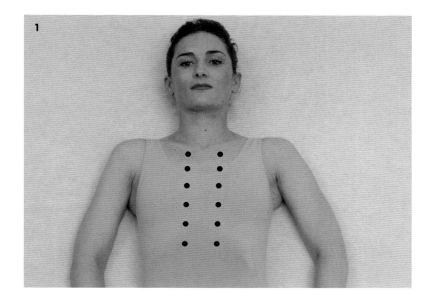

Six pairs of points on the Kidney meridian are found in the chest area.

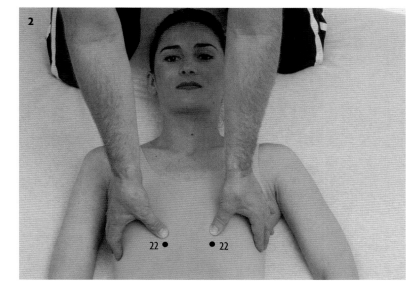

Begin the massage at Kidney 22.

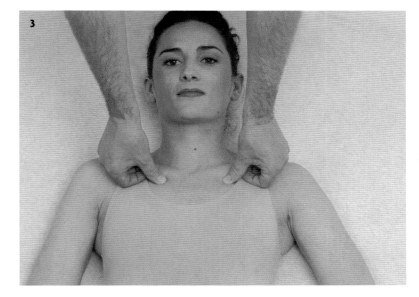

When you have finished massaging Kidney 27, begin the sequence anew.

The Points on the Abdomen

Six meridians run vertically across the upper and lower abdomen: the Stomach, Liver, Kidney, Gall Bladder, Spleen, and Conception Vessel. The points on these meridians that are important in acupressure are described in this section.

Locating the Points on the Upper Abdomen

The upper abdomen is home predominantly to points of the Conception Vessel, Stomach, and Liver meridians.

Liver 13—Camphorwood Gate

Feel along the side of the chest to the lowest curve of the ribs, where the eleventh rib is located. On its lower edge you will find Liver 13. This point can be used to treat acute and chronic gastrointestinal problems as well as liver and gallbladder problems.

Caution

Please note that Stomach 26, 27, and 28 and Kidney 15 and 16 must not be massaged during pregnancy!

The Stomach meridian and Conception Vessel run straight down along the abdominal wall. The Liver meridian runs in an arch along the sides.

Light green	Liver meridian	Liver 13
Dark green	Stomach meridian	Stomach 22–28
Gray	Conception Vessel	Conception Vessel 8

Stomach 22—Pass Gate

Pass Gate is located 3 cun above the level of the navel and 2 cun to the side of the body's middle axis. It is used to treat acute and chronic gastrointestinal problems.

Stomach 23—Supreme Unity

Stomach 23 is located 2 cun above the level of the navel and 2 cun to the side of the body's middle axis. Because of its calming effects, this point can be massaged to treat both stomachaches and psychosomatic problems.

Stomach 24—Slippery Flesh Gate

This point is located 1 cun above the level of the navel and 2 cun to the side of the body's middle axis. It has the same range of application possibilities as Stomach 23.

Stomach 25—Celestial Pivot

Celestial Pivot is located at the level of the navel, 2 cun to the side of the body's middle axis. It is used to treat stomachaches, digestive problems, flatulence, and constipation. It can also be massaged to alleviate menstrual problems or pain.

Stomach 26—Outer Mound

Stomach 26, also known as Outer Mound, is located below the navel, 2 cun to the side of the middle axis. This point can be massaged to address stomachaches and painful menstruation. It must not be massaged during pregnancy.

Stomach 27—Great Gigantic

This point, known as Great Gigantic in traditional Chinese medicine, is located 2 cun below the level of the navel and 2 cun to the side of the middle axis. It can be massaged to alleviate flatulence and to stimulate urination. This point must not be massaged during pregnancy.

Stomach 28—Waterway

Stomach 28, also called Waterway, is located 3 cun below the level of the navel and 2 cun to the side of the body's middle axis. It can be massaged to stimulate urination and alleviate constipation and painful menstruation. This point must not be massaged during pregnancy.

Conception Vessel 8—Spirit Gate

This point is located exactly in the center of the navel. It is helpful for treating pain in the navel area as well as acute and chronic intestinal infections.

Kidney 15—Central Flow

Kidney 15 is located 2 cun below the level of the navel and 0.5 cun to the side of the body's middle axis. It can be massaged to relieve constipation and menstrual problems. This point must not be massaged during pregnancy.

Kidney 16—Huang Shu

This point is located at the level of the navel, 0.5 cun to the side of the body's middle axis. It can be massaged to relieve bloating or tension in the abdominal area. This point must not be massaged during pregnancy.

Kidney 17—Shang Bend

Shang Bend is located 2 cun above the level of the navel and 0.5 cun to the side of the middle axis. Since this point has harmonizing effects on the stomach and stimulates digestion, it is often massaged to treat gastrointestinal and digestive problems.

Kidney 18—Stone Pass

Stone Pass is located 3 cun above the level of the navel and 0.5 cun to the side of the body's middle axis. It can be massaged to treat problems in the upper abdomen and acute gastrointestinal problems.

Kidney 19—Yin Metropolis

Kidney 19 is located 4 cun above the level of the navel and 0.5 cun to the side of the body's middle axis. It has the same application range as Kidney 18.

Kidney 20—Open Valley

Kidney 20, also called Open Valley, is located 5 cun above the level of the navel and 0.5 cun to the side of the body's middle axis. It can be massaged to treat cases of acute or chronic infections of the stomach's mucous membranes.

Kidney 21—Dark Gate (Pylorus)

Kidney 21, also called Dark Gate, is located 6 cun above the level of the navel and 0.5 cun to the side of the body's middle axis. It can be massaged to treat acute and chronic infections of the stomach or the esophagus, as well as to get rid of hiccups.

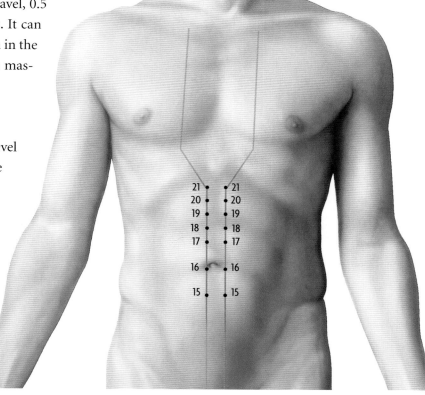

| Gray | Kidney meridian | Kidney 15–21 |

The Kidney meridian runs along the front of the abdomen, close to the body's middle axis.

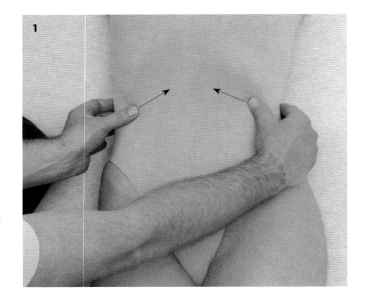

When you have finished massaging the Liver 13 pair of points, move your thumbs to the Stomach 22 pair of points.

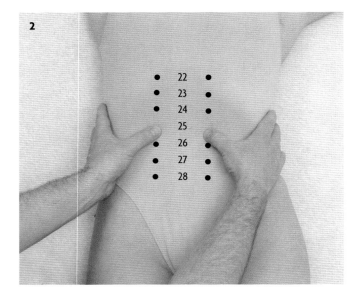

The individual points of the Stomach meridian are massaged in a sequence. Here, the thumbs rest on Stomach 25.

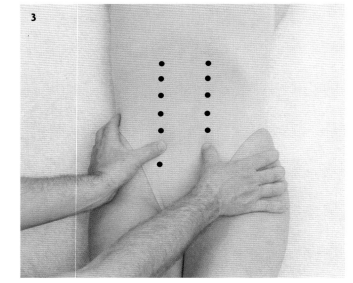

Left: Glide to the next pair of points without lifting your thumbs.

Right: With some practice, you will even be able to massage several points of a meridian at once.

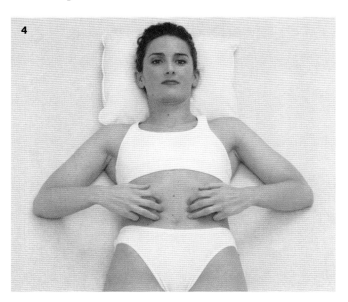

Massaging the Points on the Upper Abdomen

The points of the Liver, Stomach, and Kidney meridians occur in pairs. Both points in each pair, one on each side of the body's middle axis, are massaged at the same time with the thumbs.

Liver 13—Camphorwood Gate (Figure 1)

Massage the Liver 13 pair of points with your partner lying down. Liver 13 is massaged in three stages: First, use the tips of your thumbs to apply steady pressure on the two points. Next, apply circling pressure in synchrony with your partner's breathing, slightly increasing the pressure as your partner exhales, and decreasing it as he or she inhales, for three to four breathing cycles. Finally, slide the tips of your thumbs with slight pressure across the upper abdomen to Stomach 22.

Stomach 22 to 28 (Figures 2–4)

These points are also massaged in three phases: First, use the tips of your thumbs to apply steady pressure on the Stomach 22 pair of points. Next, apply circling pressure in synchrony with your partner's breathing for three or four breathing cycles. Finally, slide your thumbs down to Stomach 23. Massage this and the following points of the Stomach meridian in the same way. When you have finished massaging Stomach 28, slide your thumbs back to Liver 13. In this way, you make a circle on each side of the body. Repeat the acupressure of Liver 13 and the Stomach points three times.

Conception Vessel 8—Spirit Gate (Figures 1 and 2)

Place the ball of one hand on the navel. With light circling pressure, massage the point for two to three minutes.

> **Note**
>
> Moxibustion (see page 65) is especially beneficial on the navel, that is, Conception Vessel 8.

Kidney 15 to 21 (Figures 3 and 4)

Massage these points with your partner lying down. Place the tips of your thumbs on the Kidney 15 pair of points. Massage these points with steady pressure in synchrony with your partner's breathing, increasing the pressure when your partner exhales, and decreasing the pressure as he or she inhales, for four or five breathing cycles. Then massage the points using circling pressure for at least one minute per point.

When you have finished massaging Kidney 15, slide the tips of your thumbs up to Kidney 16 and massage this and the following points in the same way. When you have finished massaging Kidney 21, lift both your hands and place them again on Kidney 15. Massage these Kidney points five times in this way.

> **Caution**
>
> Note that Stomach 26, 27, and 28 and Kidney 15 and 16 must not be massaged during pregnancy!

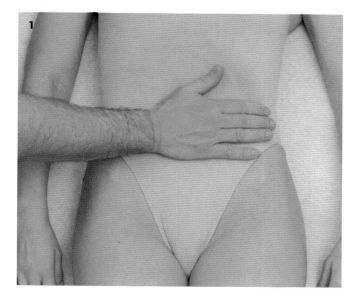

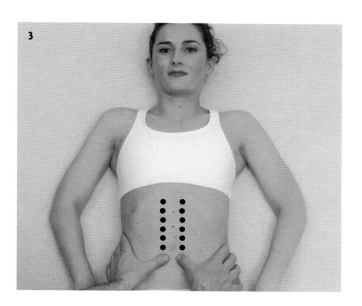

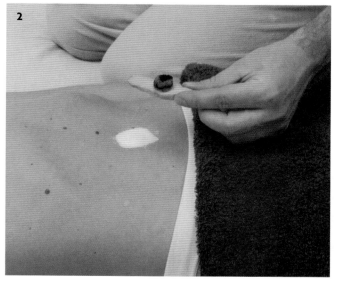

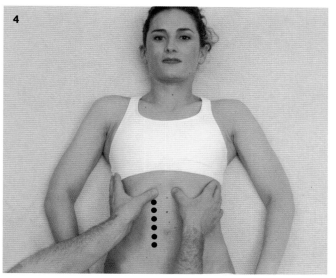

Conception Vessel 8 is located exactly at the navel and is massaged only with the ball of the hand.

Moxibustion of Conception Vessel 8 can be helpful for treating acute and chronic intestinal infections.

Left: Kidney 15 is located 2 cun below the level of the navel.

Right: Kidney 21 is the last point in this sequence.

Locating the Points on the Lower Abdomen

Several important points of the Gall Bladder and Spleen meridians are located in the area of the lower abdomen. These points are described in this section.

The Gall Bladder meridian runs from the head and shoulder down to the armpit and, from there, in a zigzag movement along the side of the body down to the hip and buttocks region. It then continues down the side of the leg, across the ankle, and along the top of the foot to a point at the outer edge of the toenail of the fourth toe. The Spleen meridian originates on the inside of the foot at the big toe and runs up along the leg, past the groin, and along the side of the abdomen and chest to the level of the shoulder joint. Here it turns and passes down to the armpit.

Gall Bladder 25—Capital Gate

This point is located at the lower edge of the free end of the twelfth rib. It is used to treat problems in the lumbar spine and the lower ribs. It is also used to treat ailments in the lower urinary tract and abdominal and intestinal area, including tension in the upper abdomen, flatulence, and intestinal infections.

Gall Bladder 28—Linking Path

This point is located slightly below the iliac crest. It is massaged to treat menstruation problems. This point should not be massaged during pregnancy.

Spleen 13—Bowel Abode

Spleen 13 is located 4 cun to the side of the body's middle axis and 4 cun below the level of the navel, slightly above the edge of the groin. This point regulates the activity of the intestines and Stomach and is used to treat tension and bloating in these areas. It should not be massaged during pregnancy.

Caution

Note that Gall Bladder 28 and Spleen 13 must not be massaged during pregnancy!

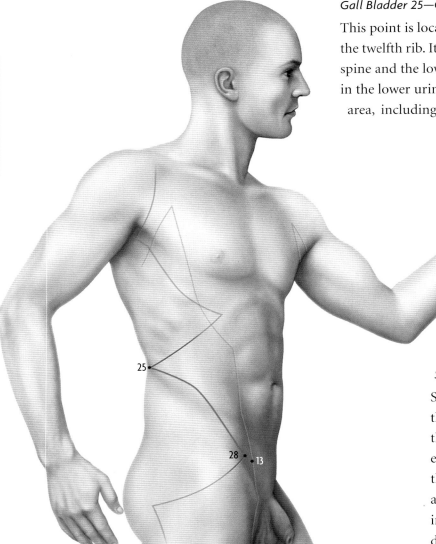

The Gall Bladder and Spleen meridians take very different paths along the body's sides and lower abdomen.

| Dark green | Gall Bladder meridian | Gall Bladder 25, 28 |
| Olive | Spleen meridian | Spleen 13 |

Massaging the Points on the Lower Abdomen

These points occur in pairs. Both points in each pair, one on each side of the body's middle axis, are massaged with the thumbs at the same time, with your partner lying relaxed on his or her back. Before you begin massaging the first point, Gall Bladder 25, note that these points are located in an area that can be very sensitive to the touch. Inform your partner about the location you will be massaging, and make sure to warm your hands before you begin.

Gall Bladder 25—Capital Gate (Figure 1)

The massage of this point proceeds in three stages: steady pressure, circling pressure, and gliding. Begin the massage with steady pressure in rhythm with your partner's breathing, slightly increasing the pressure when your partner exhales and decreasing it a little when he or she inhales. Then apply circling pressure for two to three minutes. Finally, glide both thumbs to Gall Bladder 28, making sure not to lose contact with your partner's skin as you slide your hands from point to point.

Gall Bladder 28 and Spleen 13 (Figures 2 and 3)

Gall Bladder 28 is massaged in the same manner as Gall Bladder 25. Begin the massage with steady pressure in rhythm with your partner's breathing, and then apply circling pressure for two to three minutes. Finally, slide your thumbs across the skin to Spleen 13, and massage this point in the same way. When you have finished, lift your hands and place the tips of your thumbs again on Gall Bladder 25, beginning a new massage cycle. Carry out five complete cycles.

To conclude, rub all three points for three to five minutes with a flattened hand in the direction in which their meridians flow. That is, use a downward stroke for the two Gall Bladder points and an upward stroke for the Spleen point.

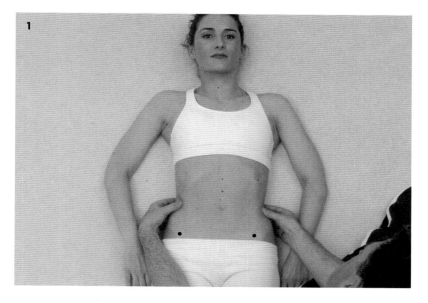

Be very careful when massaging Gall Bladder 25; this is a sensitive spot. The point is located on each side, slightly behind Gall Bladder 26, where the thumbs rest in this illustration. Massage the point with your index fingers.

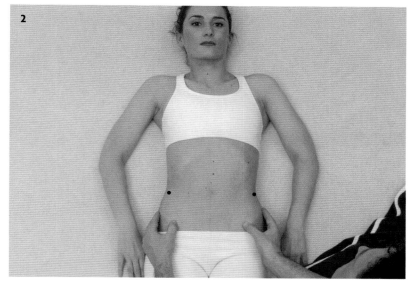

Here, both thumbs rest on Gall Bladder 28.

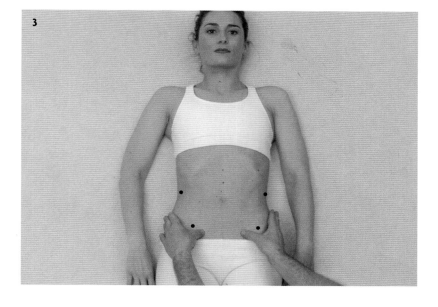

Spleen 13 is located 4 cun below the level of the navel and 4 cun to the side of the body's middle axis.

The Points of the Three Yang Meridians on the Upper Arms

Three meridians run along the outside and back of the upper arms: the Large Intestine, Triple Heater, and Small Intestine meridians. This section discusses the most effective points for acupressure of these meridians and their treatment possibilities.

Locating the Points on the Upper Arms: The Large Intestine Meridian

The Large Intestine meridian runs along the outside of the upper arm. When carried out as a sequence, massage of the points Large Intestine 11 to 15 stimulates the flow of energy in the Large Intestine meridian.

Note

For the upper arms, you can massage either yourself or a partner. In either case, you should massage first all the points on one arm, and then all the points on the other. You can also apply moxibustion to any of these points.

The Large Intestine meridian contains a number of important points on the outside of the upper arm that can be massaged to alleviate pain in that area.

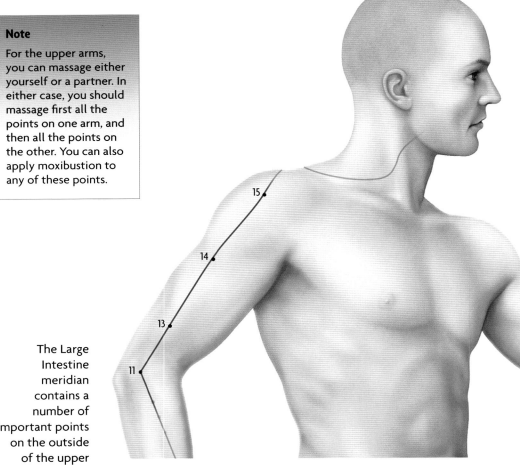

| Blue | Large Intestine meridian | Large Intestine 11, 13–15 |

Large Intestine 11—Pool at the Bend

This point is easiest to locate when the elbow is bent at a right angle. In this position, Large Intestine 11 is located between the outer edge of the elbow fold and the knobby protrusion of the elbow bone.

This point has a wide range of applications. It can be used to treat acute infections in the throat and neck area that are accompanied by fever and headaches, as well as pain in the elbow or lower arm, hypertension, and psychological and psychosomatic ailments. It also can be massaged to alleviate allergies.

Large Intestine 13—Arm Five Li

Because of its location, Large Intestine 13 is also known as Arm Five Li, or Five Lengths of the Hand. This point is located 3 cun above Large Intestine 11. It can be used to treat pain in the upper arm, as well as limited range of motion in the shoulder.

Large Intestine 14—Upper Arm

Large Intestine 14 is 7 cun above Large Intestine 11, on the outside of the upper arm. It can be used to treat pain in the bicep and shoulder muscles. This point can also be massaged to treat eye illnesses as well as lymph blockages in the neck, throat, and armpit area.

Large Intestine 15—Shoulder Bone

This point is easiest to locate when the arm is extended to the side, away from the body. In this position, Large Intestine 15 is between the front and middle part of the deltoid muscle that shapes the contour of the shoulder. Because of its location it is also called Shoulder Bone, though in fact it is located slightly in front of and below the actual bone. This point is used to treat problems in the shoulder joint, including limited range of motion, as well as itchy rashes.

Massaging the Points on the Upper Arms: The Large Intestine Meridian

Acupressure of the four points of the Large Intestine meridian on the upper arms is done in a sequence from the elbow to the shoulder. The massage proceeds from one point to the next with a gliding movement, thus connecting the four points. However, any of these points can also be massaged individually for its specific effects; in this case, the point should be massaged for two to three minutes.

Large Intestine 11 and Large Intestine 13 to 15 (Figures 1–4)

Begin with Large Intestine 11. With the tip of your index finger, apply first steady and then circling pressure for one to two minutes. Then glide your index finger along the skin to Large Intestine 13, and massage this point in the same manner. Repeat this procedure for Large Intestine 14 and 15. When you have finished massaging Large Intestine 15, start again at Large Intestine 11, and repeat the sequence five times.

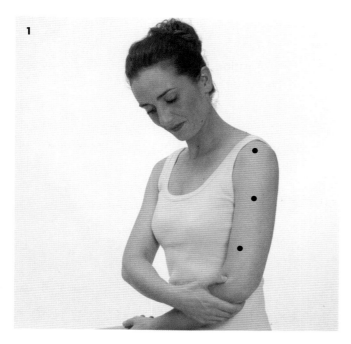

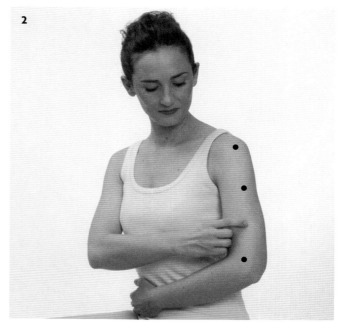

Left: Begin the sequence with Large Intestine 11.

Right: Follow the course of the meridian to Large Intestine 13 without losing contact with your partner's skin.

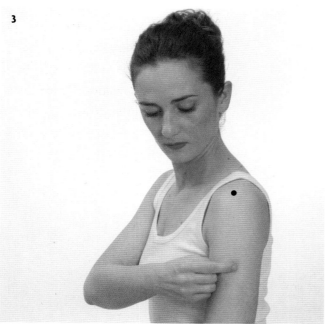

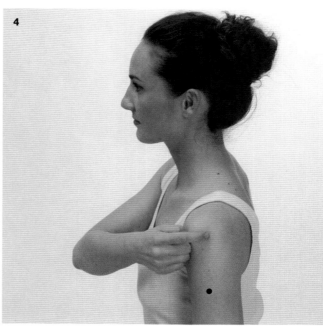

Left: After massaging Large Intestine 13, continue to Large Intestine 14.

Right: The sequence ends with the massage of Large Intestine 15.

Locating the Points on the Upper Arms: The Triple Heater Meridian

The upper arms also contain three important points of the Triple Heater meridian, which are described in this section. When massaged in sequence, these points stimulate the flow of energy in the Triple Heater meridian.

The Triple Heater meridian begins at the side of the nail of the ring finger and runs along the back of the hand and the outside of the lower arm to the elbow. From there it runs up along the outside of the upper arm in an almost straight line to the shoulder. There it continues along the side of the neck to just below the earlobe, where it curves around the back of the ear and runs forward to the temple.

Triple Heater 10—Celestial Well

This point is easiest to locate when the elbow is bent. In this position, Triple Heater 10 is located in the indentation behind the tip of the elbow. It can be massaged to treat pain in the shoulder, upper arm, and elbow joint or swelling caused by infection of the lymph passages in the throat, neck, or armpit.

Triple Heater 13—Upper Arm Convergence

Triple Heater 13 is located 3 cun below Triple Heater 14. It is used to treat pain in the shoulder, neck, and upper arm, as well as problems with the thyroid and infections of the lymph passages of the throat, neck, and armpit.

Triple Heater 14—Shoulder Bone Hole

Triple Heater 14, also called Shoulder Bone Hole, is easiest to locate when the arm is raised horizontally. In this location, it is in the indentation of the deltoid muscle. Since acupressure of this point stimulates the flow of energy in the Triple Heater meridian and generally increases the flexibility of the shoulder joint, you can massage it to treat pain that limits the range of motion of the shoulder joint.

Note

Triple Heater 10, 13, and 14 all have one thing in common: they offer the possibility of positively influencing the flow of qi (life energy). This energy can be organized and focused to alleviate pain.

The Triple Heater meridian contains twenty-three acupressure points. Points 10, 13, and 14 are treated most frequently.

| **Purple** | Triple Heater meridian | Triple Heater 10, 13, 14 |

Massaging the Points on the Upper Arms: The Triple Heater Meridian

Acupressure of these three points of the Triple Heater meridian is done in a sequence from the elbow to the shoulder, in keeping with the direction of the meridian. Note again that you should maintain contact with the skin while moving from one point to the next. This creates a treatment sequence connecting the three points that is repeated several times. Depending on the ailment you wish to treat, however, you can also massage individual points of this sequence, for two to three minutes each.

Triple Heater 10, 13, and 14 (Figures 1–3)

For this massage your partner should sit down, with his or her shoulders loose and relaxed, but not falling forward. Begin by treating Triple Heater 10, using the tip of your thumb to apply first steady pressure for thirty seconds and then circular pressure for one to two minutes. Then slide your thumb along the skin to Triple Heater 13, and massage it in the same way. Finally, slide your thumb along the meridian to Triple Heater 14, and massage it in the same way as well. Then lift your hand, reposition your thumb on Triple Heater 10, and begin again. Complete five repetitions of this sequence.

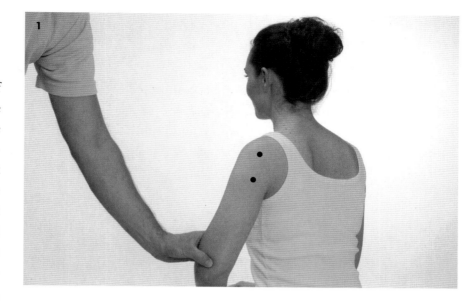

Begin the sequence by massaging Triple Heater 10.

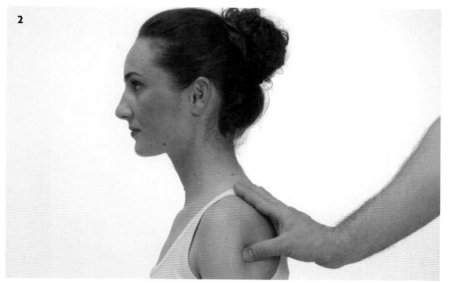

Continue along to Triple Heater 13.

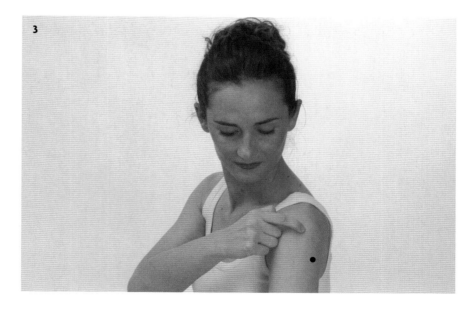

Because of its location, Triple Heater 14 is especially well suited for self-massage.

Locating the Points on the Upper Arms: The Small Intestine Meridian

The Small Intestine meridian is the third energy pathway that runs along the back of the upper arms and contains points important in acupressure.

This meridian begins on the pinkie finger and runs along the side of the hand up to the wrist, and from there along the back of the arm to the back of the shoulder. From there, it zigzags to the upper edge of the shoulder blade and up to the side of the neck. From here, it continues past the joint of the lower jaw to the cheekbone before ending at the ear. When carried out as a sequence, the massage of the three Small Intestine points found on the upper arm stimulates the flow of energy in the Small Intestine meridian.

Small Intestine 8—Small Sea

Small Sea is located between the tip of the elbow and the bony protrusion of the ulna. Since the point has a general pain- and cramp-relieving effect, it is massaged in the case of pain in the arms, shoulder, or lower jaw. The point also has a strong calming effect that has even been described as sedating, and thus it is frequently massaged in the case of psychological and psychosomatic illnesses. The point is also used to treat flus and colds accompanied by fever.

Small Intestine 9—True Shoulder

Small Intestine 9, also known as True Shoulder, is easiest to locate when the arm is hanging down loosely. In this position, it is located 1 cun above the top of the armpit on the back of the body. Acupressure of this point is useful in treating pain in the shoulder joint and upper arm. This point can also be massaged to treat problems in lymph flow in the neck, throat, and armpit area.

Small Intestine 10—Upper Arm Shu

This point is also easiest to locate when the arm hangs down loosely. In this position, it is located above the armpit on the back of the body in an indentation below the upper edge of the shoulder blade. Small Intestine 10 has the same treatment applications as Small Intestine 9.

Note

When you massage the points on one arm as a sequence, make sure that your thumb or index finger maintains contact with the skin of the arm as you proceed, gently gliding your fingertip across the skin from point to point.

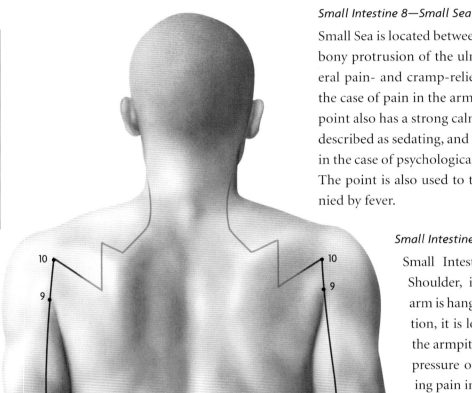

The Small Intestine meridian makes several sharp turns on the back of the shoulders before rising up along the sides of the neck.

| **Red** | Small Intestine meridian | Small Intestine 8–10 |

Massaging the Points on the Upper Arms: The Small Intestine Meridian

Acupressure of the points of the Small Intestine meridian begins at the elbow and moves up toward the shoulder. Once again, note that you should maintain contact with the skin when moving from one point to the next, thus creating a treatment sequence connecting the three points. However, depending on the ailments you are aiming to relieve, you can also massage individual points of this sequence, for at least two to three minutes each. Small Intestine 8 and 9 are well suited for self-massage; they can be massaged not with your thumb but with the tip of your index finger, beginning with Small Intestine 8.

Small Intestine 8 to 10 (Figures 1–3)

Carry out this massage with your partner sitting down. Begin by using the tip of your thumb to apply steady pressure to Small Intestine 8 for one to two minutes. Then apply circling pressure for the same amount of time. Now glide your thumb across the skin to Small Intestine 9, and massage it in the same way. Then follow the meridian with your thumb to Small Intestine 10, and massage it in the same way. Perform this sequence a total of five times, each time beginning at Small Intestine 8.

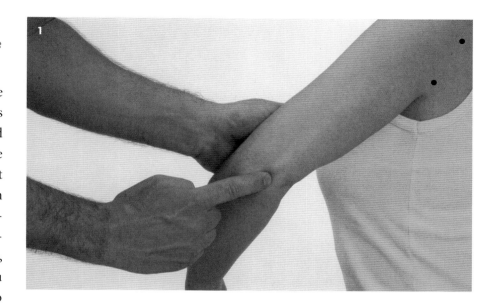

Small Intestine 8 is located in an indentation immediately adjacent to the elbow.

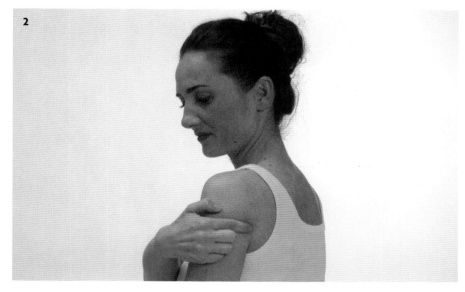

Maintain contact with the skin as your finger moves from one point to the next.

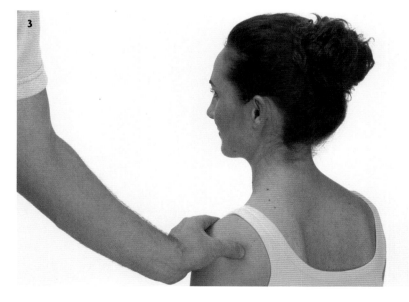

Small Intestine 10 is located directly below the upper edge of the shoulder blade.

The Points of the Three Yin Meridians on the Upper Arms

Three yin meridians run from outside to inside on the inside and front of the upper arms: the Lung, Pericardium, and Heart meridians.

Locating the Points on the Upper Arms: The Lung Meridian

The Lung meridian begins in the upper chest between the first and second ribs. It then runs out to the arm and down the inside of the upper arm to the elbow. From here it continues along the inside of the lower arm to the thumb. Massaged as a sequence, the Lung points of the upper arm stimulate the flow of energy in the Lung meridian. Follow this massage with acupressure of the points of the Pericardium and Heart meridians.

Lung 3—Celestial Storehouse

Lung 3, called Celestial Storehouse in traditional Chinese medicine,

is located 3 cun below the fold of the armpit at the outer edge of the biceps muscle. It is massaged especially to treat illnesses of the respiratory passages. Because of its effects in stopping bleeding, it is also effective for treating nosebleeds.

Lung 4—Guarding White

Lung 4 is located 5 cun above the elbow at the edge of the biceps muscle. Massage of this point is helpful in treating illnesses of the respiratory passages as well as chest pains.

Lung 5—Cubit Marsh

This point is located on the inside (thumb side) of the elbow, next to the easy-to-feel tendon of the biceps muscle. In traditional Chinese medicine this point is said to have the ability to reduce lung heat, expel mucus, and strengthen the respiratory passages. It is thus used to treat illnesses of the respiratory passages that are accompanied by a lot of phlegm or very thick phlegm. It can also be helpful in

The Lung meridian is one of the three yin pathways running along the inside of the upper arms.

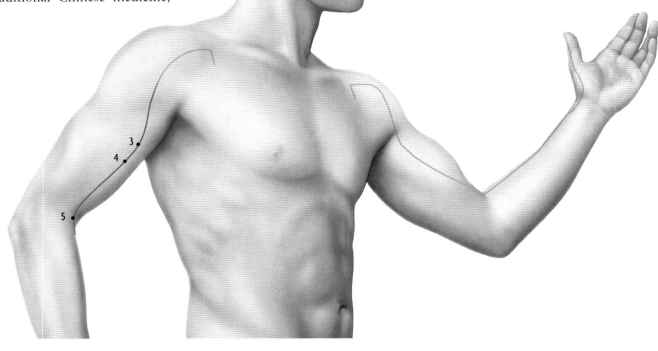

| Blue | Lung meridian | Lung 3–5 |

treating any type of shortness of breath or infection of the upper and lower respiratory passages. Acupressure of this point is also helpful in treating pain in the elbow.

Massaging the Points on the Upper Arms: The Lung Meridian

Acupressure of these Lung points should begin at the shoulder and move down toward the elbow. Again, note that your finger should glide as it moves from point to point, never losing contact with the skin. This creates a treatment sequence connecting the three points. Of course, depending on the aim of your treatment, you can also massage individual points for a duration of at least two to three minutes. These three points are also well suited for self-massage; as you would for a partner, for self-massage you should use your thumb and begin your massage at Lung 3.

Lung 3 to 5 (Figures 1–3)

The massage is given with your partner sitting down. Apply first steady and then circling pressure on Lung 3 for one to two minutes. Then slide your thumb over the skin to Lung 4 and massage this point in the same way. Repeat this process for Lung 5. Go through this sequence five times, beginning each time at Lung 3.

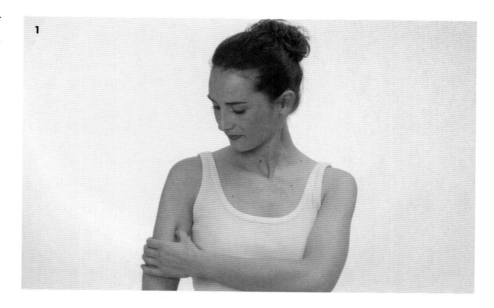

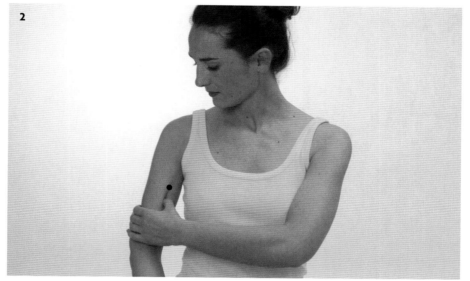

Lung 3 is located 3 cun below the armpit, at the outer edge of the biceps muscle.

Move your thumb 1 cun down from Lung 3 to reach Lung 4.

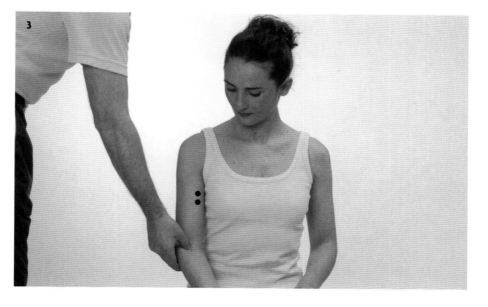

Lung 5 is located in an indentation in the inside fold of the elbow.

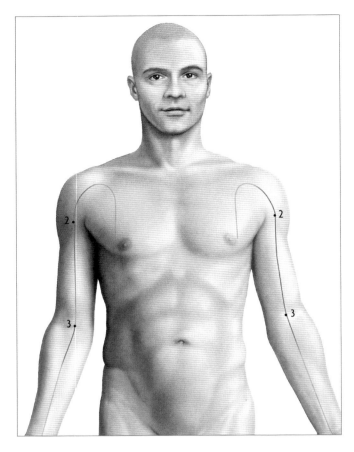

The Pericardium meridian runs from the chest along the front of the shoulders and the insides of the arms down to the hands.

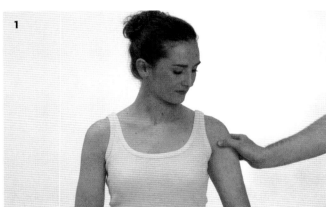

Pericardium 2 is located 2 cun from the top of the armpit.

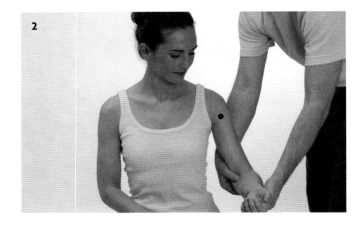

Pericardium 3 is located in the middle of the elbow fold.

Locating the Points on the Upper Arms: The Pericardium Meridian

The second yin meridian on the inside of the upper arm is the Pericardium meridian. It has two points in this region that are important in acupressure. Massaging the two points together stimulates the flow of energy in the Pericardium meridian.

Pericardium 2—Celestial Spring

This point is located 2 cun to the side of the armpit fold on the front of the arm. It is used to treat acute and chronic bronchitis as well as pain caused by a constriction of the coronary vessels.

Pericardium 3—Marsh at the Bend

Pericardium 3 is located in the middle of the elbow fold, on the inner side of the easy-to-feel tendon of the biceps muscle. This point is helpful in treating painful coronary problems. It can also be massaged to alleviate illnesses of the upper abdomen, such as stomachaches and acute infections of the stomach's mucous membrane accompanied by nausea and vomiting. This point is also used to treat anxiety, panic, and fever.

Massaging the Points on the Upper Arms: The Pericardium Meridian

The two points of the Pericardium meridian can be massaged in a sequence, from the upper arm down to the elbow. They can be linked in this sequence by gliding your hand along the skin as you move from Pericardium 2 to 3. You can also massage each point individually for its specific effects. In this case, the point should be treated for two to three minutes.

Pericardium 2 and 3 (Figures 1 and 2)

Carry out the massage with your partner sitting down. Begin with acupressure on Pericardium 2. With the tip of your thumb, apply first steady and then circling pressure for one to two minutes each. Then slide your thumb along the meridian to Pericardium 3, making sure to maintain contact with the skin as you move. Massage this point in the same way. Repeat this sequence a total of five times, beginning each time at Pericardium 2.

Locating the Points on the Upper Arms:
The Heart Meridian

The Heart meridian runs along the inside of the arm. When you massage its points on the upper arm in a sequence, you stimulate the flow of energy in this meridian.

Heart 1—Highest Spring

This point is located in the middle of the armpit. It is used to treat so-called functional ailments of the heart; these are ailments that do not have a clear organic cause. It is also helpful in the treatment of paralysis and circulation problems in the arms.

Heart 2—Cyan Spirit

This point is located 3 cun above the elbow, on the inside of the upper arm. It is massaged to relax the tendons and muscles and alleviate pain in the upper arms.

Heart 3—Lesser Sea (Yin Pathway)

When the elbow is bent, Heart 3 is located midway between the end of the elbow fold and the noticeable protrusion of the upper arm bone. It is used to treat motion problems and skin sensitivity in the arm, especially in the elbow. It is also used to treat chest pains, as well as sleeping problems and psychological difficulties.

Massaging the Points on the Upper Arms:
The Heart Meridian

These points are massaged from the armpit to the elbow, with your hand sliding between the points to create a sequence. Each point can also be massaged individually for its specific effects; in this case, the point should be massaged for two to three minutes.

Heart 1 to 3 (Figures 1 and 2)

With the tip of your thumb, apply first steady and then circling pressure on Heart 1 for thirty seconds. Then slide your thumb to Heart 2 and massage this point in the same way, followed by Heart 3. Repeat this sequence a total of five times, beginning each time at Heart 1.

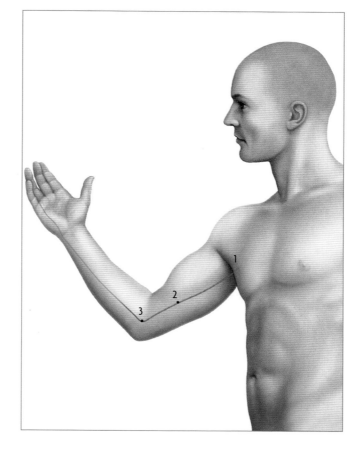

The Heart meridian begins in the armpit and runs along the inside of the arm down to the pinkie finger.

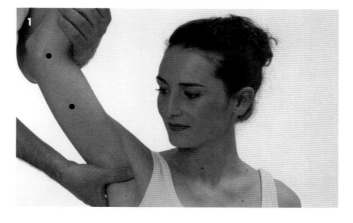

Massage Heart 1 at the armpit using the tip of your thumb.

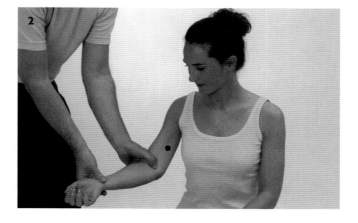

Use one hand to support the lower arm at the wrist as you use the thumb of your other hand to massage Heart 3.

The Points of the Three Yang Meridians on the Lower Arms

The three yang meridians described for the upper arms—the Large Intestine, Triple Heater, and Small Intestine meridians—continue on the lower arms.

Locating the Points on the Lower Arms: The Large Intestine Meridian

Massage of the points described in this section is useful in treating pain and range of motion problems in the hands, lower arms, elbows, upper arms, shoulders, and

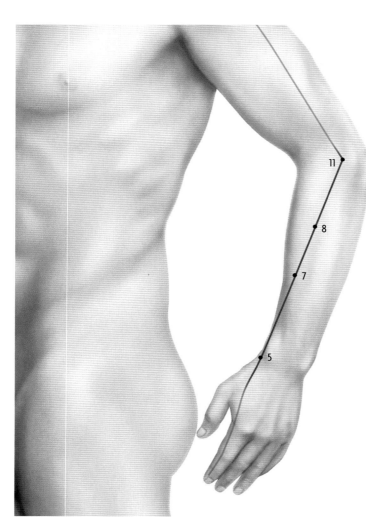

The Large Intestine meridian runs from the hand across the outside of the lower arm to the upper arm, continuing to the shoulder, neck, and face.

| Blue | Large Intestine meridian | Large Intestine 5, 7, 8, 11 |

neck. Massaging the points as a sequence stimulates the flow of energy in the Large Intestine meridian.

Large Intestine 5—Yang Ravine

Extending your thumb away from your hand creates an indentation between the tendons on the thumb side of the wrist. Between these tendons is Large Intestine 5, also known as Yang Ravine. It is used to treat pain in the wrist, acute infections in the head, eye, and mouth, and ear ailments such as ringing in the ear and hardness of hearing.

Large Intestine 7—Warm Dwelling

When your elbow is slightly bent, Large Intestine 7, known traditionally as Warm Dwelling, is located 5 cun up from the wrist fold on the outside of the lower arm. This point can be used to treat ailments in the throat-nose-mouth area such as sore throat and infections of the mucous membranes of the mouth or nose. Massage of Large Intestine 7 is also useful in treating nosebleeds.

Large Intestine 8—Lower Ridge

When your elbow is slightly bent, Large Intestine 8 is located 4 cun below the fold in the elbow on the outside of the arm. The most important applications for Large Intestine 8 are in treatments for pain in the elbow joint and lower arm as well as headaches, dizziness, and drowsiness.

Large Intestine 11—Pool at the Bend

When your elbow is slightly bent, Large Intestine 11, known traditionally as Pool at the Bend, is located midway between the end of the elbow fold and the protruding bone of the elbow, on the outside of the arm. This point is used to treat pain in the elbow and lower arm, as well as acute infections in the throat and head that are accompanied by fever and headaches. This point can also be used to alleviate itchiness caused by allergies; for this reason it is also called the anti-allergy point.

Massaging the Points on the Lower Arms: The Large Intestine Meridian

Acupressure on the four points of the Large Intestine meridian proceeds up from the wrist to the elbow. As you move from one point to the next, your finger should not leave the skin; instead, your finger should simply glide over the skin, forming a massage sequence that connects the four points. Of course, depending on the ailment being treated, you can also massage any of these points individually for its specific effects; in this case, massage the point for at least two to three minutes. The points are well suited for self-treatment; just as you would with a partner, use the tip of your thumb and begin the massage with the fifth point of the meridian.

Large Intestine 5, 7, 8, and 11 (Figures 1–3)

Begin by massaging Large Intestine 5 with the tip of your thumb, applying first steady and then circling pressure for one to two minutes. Making sure to maintain contact with the skin, slide the tip of your thumb across the skin to Large Intestine 7, and massage this point in the same way. Repeat this process for Large Intestine 8 and 11. When you have finished massaging Large Intestine 11, repeat the sequence, beginning at Large Intestine 5, for a total of five repetitions.

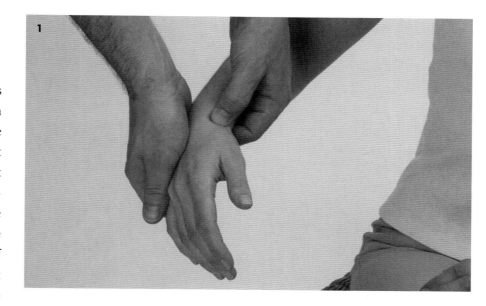

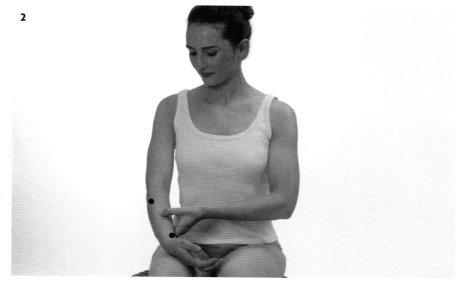

Massage Large Intestine 5 using the tip of your thumb on the indentation of the outside of the wrist.

Large Intestine 8 is located 4 cun below Large Intestine 11.

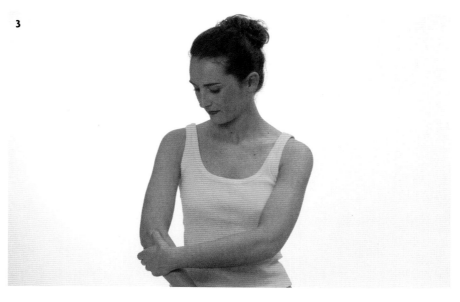

Bend your elbow at a right angle to find Large Intestine 11, located next to the outside edge of the elbow.

Locating the Points on the Lower Arms: The Triple Heater Meridian

Acupressure of the points of the Triple Heater meridian on the lower arms is useful in treating pain and range of motion problems in the hands, lower arms, elbows, upper arms, shoulders, and neck. Massaging the points as a sequence stimulates the flow of energy in the Triple Heater meridian.

Triple Heater 4—Yang Pool

This point is located on the back of the wrist in the center of the fold in the skin. It is used to treat pain in the wrist, shoulder, and back.

Triple Heater 5—Outer Pass

This point is located 2 cun up from the wrist in the noticeable gap between the radius and ulna. It is used to treat pain and range of motion problems in the hand, shoulder, and back. It can also be used to treat headaches as well as illnesses of the upper respiratory passages that are accompanied by fever. This point has also proven effective in treating acute eye and ear infections.

The Triple Heater meridian runs along the backs of the hands and the outside of the lower arms up to the shoulders, neck, and head.

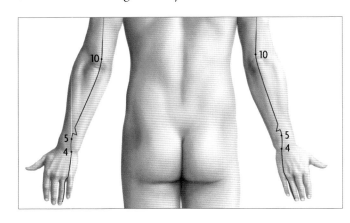

Triple Heater 10—Celestial Well

When your elbow is bent, Triple Heater 10, known as Celestial Well in traditional Chinese medicine, is located 1 cun up from the tip of the elbow, in an indentation found there. This point is helpful in the treatment of pain in the elbow joint, upper arm, and shoulder as well as swelling of the lymph nodes in the throat, neck, and armpit.

Massaging the Points on the Lower Arms: The Triple Heater Meridian

Massage the three points of the Triple Heater meridian from the wrist to the elbow on the outside of the upper arm. Move from point to point with a sliding movement, never breaking contact with the skin, to connect the points in a massage sequence. You can also massage any of these points individually for its specific effects; in this case, massage the point for at least two to three minutes.

Triple Heater 4, 5, and 10 (Figures 1 and 2)

For this massage your partner should sit down. Begin with Triple Heater 4, using the tip of your thumb to apply first steady and then circling pressure for one to two minutes. Making sure to maintain contact with your partner's skin, move the tip of your thumb across the skin to Triple Heater 5, and massage this point in the same way. Then move your thumb along the meridian to the Triple Heater 10, and massage this point in the same way. After you have massaged Triple Heater 10, repeat the sequence, beginning at Triple Heater 4, for a total of five repetitions.

Left: Triple Heater 4 is massaged in the middle of the back of the wrist.

Right: Finish your massage with Triple Heater 10.

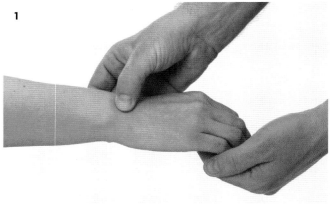

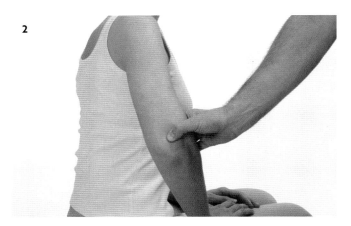

Locating the Points on the Lower Arms: The Small Intestine Meridian

Acupressure of the Small Intestine meridian on the lower arms is effective in treating pain and range of motion problems of the hands, lower arms, elbows, upper arms, shoulders, and neck. When carried out as a sequence, massage of these points stimulates the flow of energy in the Small Intestine meridian.

Small Intestine 5—Yang Valley

Small Intestine 5 is on the back and outside (toward the pinkie finger) of the wrist. It is used to treat pain in the wrist, as well as feverish infections and headaches.

Small Intestine 7—Branch of the Main Pathway

This point is located 5 cun up from the wrist on the outside of the lower arm. Because of its generally calming effects, the point is used to treat psychosomatic and psychological problems. It is also used to treat pain in the lower arm.

Small Intestine 8—Small Sea

This point, referred to in traditional Chinese medicine as Small Sea, is located between the tip of the elbow and the protrusion of the ulna. Because this point has a relaxing and pain-inhibiting effect, it is used to treat pain in the arm, shoulder, and lower jaw. Small Intestine 8 can also be massaged to treat psychosomatic and psychological ailments as well as feverish infections such as the flu.

Massaging the Points on the Lower Arm: The Small Intestine Meridian

Massage the three points of the Small Intestine meridian from the wrist to the elbow. Move from point to point with a sliding movement, never breaking contact with the skin, to connect the points in a massage sequence. Depending on the ailment being treated, you can also massage any of these points individually for its specific effects; in this case, massage the point for at least two to three minutes.

Small Intestine 5, 7, and 8 (Figures 1 and 2)

For this massage your partner should sit down. Begin with Small Intestine 5, using the tip of your thumb to apply first steady and then circling pressure for one to two minutes. Making sure to maintain contact with your partner's skin, move the tip of your thumb across the skin to Small Intestine 7, and massage this point in the same way. Then move your thumb along the meridian to Small Intestine 8, and massage this point in the same way. After you have massaged Small Intestine 8, repeat the sequence, beginning at Small Intestine 5, for a total of five repetitions.

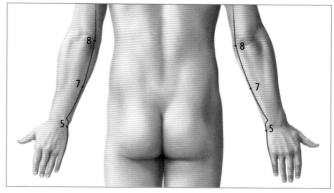

The Small Intestine meridian runs from the pinkie finger along the back of the lower arm.

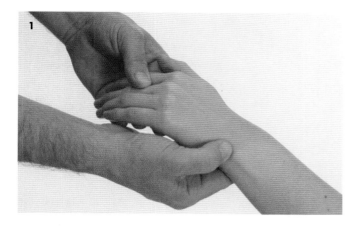

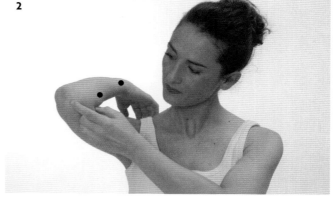

Left: Begin the sequence by massaging Small Intestine 5.

Right: Follow the course of the meridian to Small Intestine 8.

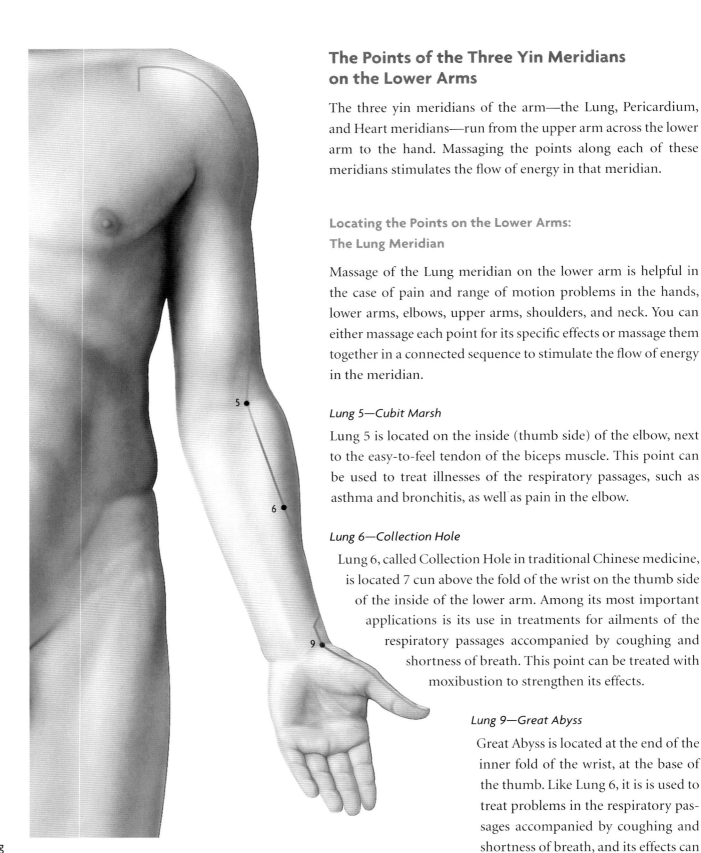

The Points of the Three Yin Meridians on the Lower Arms

The three yin meridians of the arm—the Lung, Pericardium, and Heart meridians—run from the upper arm across the lower arm to the hand. Massaging the points along each of these meridians stimulates the flow of energy in that meridian.

Locating the Points on the Lower Arms: The Lung Meridian

Massage of the Lung meridian on the lower arm is helpful in the case of pain and range of motion problems in the hands, lower arms, elbows, upper arms, shoulders, and neck. You can either massage each point for its specific effects or massage them together in a connected sequence to stimulate the flow of energy in the meridian.

Lung 5—Cubit Marsh

Lung 5 is located on the inside (thumb side) of the elbow, next to the easy-to-feel tendon of the biceps muscle. This point can be used to treat illnesses of the respiratory passages, such as asthma and bronchitis, as well as pain in the elbow.

Lung 6—Collection Hole

Lung 6, called Collection Hole in traditional Chinese medicine, is located 7 cun above the fold of the wrist on the thumb side of the inside of the lower arm. Among its most important applications is its use in treatments for ailments of the respiratory passages accompanied by coughing and shortness of breath. This point can be treated with moxibustion to strengthen its effects.

Lung 9—Great Abyss

Great Abyss is located at the end of the inner fold of the wrist, at the base of the thumb. Like Lung 6, it is is used to treat problems in the respiratory passages accompanied by coughing and shortness of breath, and its effects can be enhanced through moxibustion.

The Lung meridian runs along the inside of the upper and lower arm.

Blue	Lung meridian	Lung 5, 6, 9

Massaging the Points on the Lower Arms: The Lung Meridian

Acupressure of the three points of the Lung meridian on the lower arms is carried out from top to bottom, beginning at the elbow with Lung 5 and ending at Lung 9 at the wrist. You can massage the points along the Lung meridian as a sequence, moving your hand from point to point in a gliding movement. You can also massage any of these points individually for its specific effects; in this case, massage the point for two to three minutes.

Lung 5, 6, and 9 (Figures 1–3)

For this massage have your partner sit down. Begin with Lung 5, using the tip of your thumb to apply first steady and then circling pressure for thirty seconds. Making sure to maintain contact with the skin, slide the tip of your thumb across the skin to Lung 6, and massage this point in the same way. Then move your thumb along the meridian to Lung 9, and massage it in the same way. When you have finished massaging this point, repeat the sequence, beginning at Lung 5, for a total of five repetitions.

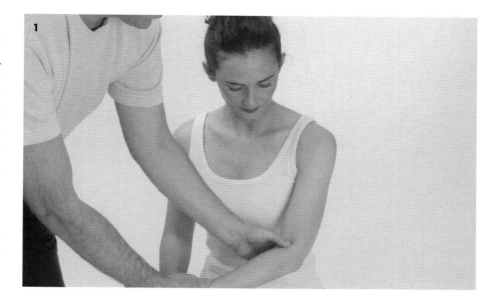

Massage Lung 5 with your thumb on the inside of the elbow.

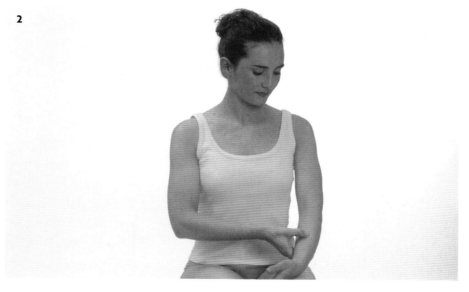

Lung 6 is located 7 cun above the wrist.

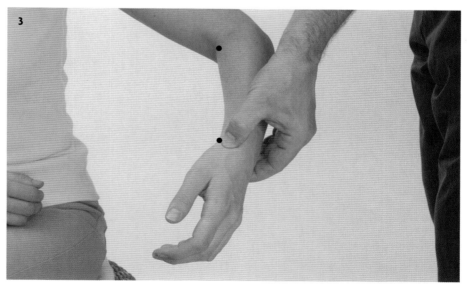

Massage Lung 9 with your thumb on the thumb side of the wrist.

Locating the Points on the Lower Arms: The Pericardium Meridian

The Pericardium meridian runs along the lower arm from the inside of the elbow across the palm to the tip of the middle finger. Its points are frequently massaged to treat pain in the chest area as well as abdominal pains, but it can also be used to treat anxiety.

Pericardium 3—Marsh at the Bend

This point is located exactly in the middle of the elbow fold, next to the easy-to-feel tendon of the biceps muscle. It is used to treat stomachaches, nausea, and vomiting, as well as pains in the chest area.

Pericardium 6—Inner Pass

This point is located 2 cun up from the inside fold of the wrist, on a line connecting Pericardium 3 and 7. It has a range of applications and is used primarily to treat stomachaches, vomiting, and nausea, as well as pain and range of motion problems in the lower arm. Massage of this point can be used as a complement to medical treat-

ment in the case of feelings of constriction and pain in the chest area.

Pericardium 7—Great Mound

When your wrist is slightly bent, Pericardium 7 is located in the middle of the inside fold of the wrist. Because of its calming and relaxing effect, this point is used to treat psychological and psychosomatic problems. It can also be used to alleviate pain in the chest.

Massaging the Points on the Lower Arms: The Pericardium Meridian

Massage of the points on the Pericardium meridian proceeds from the elbow down to the wrist on the inside of the lower arm. You can connect these points in a sequence by gliding your hand from one point to the next as you proceed. You can also massage any of these points individually for its specific effects; in this case massage the point for two to three minutes.

Pericardium 3, 6, and 7 (Figures 1 and 2)

This massage is carried out with your partner sitting down. Begin with Pericardium 3, using the tip of your thumb to apply first steady and then circling pressure for thirty seconds. Making sure to maintain contact with the skin, move the tip of your thumb across the skin to Pericardium 6, and massage this point in the same way. Then move your thumb along the meridian to Pericardium 7, and massage this point in the same way. When you have finished, repeat the sequence, beginning at Pericardium 3, for a total of five repetitions.

The Pericardium meridian runs along the inside of the upper and lower arms.

Left: Begin the massage on the inside of the elbow at Pericardium 3.

Right: Massage Pericardium 7 on the inside of the wrist.

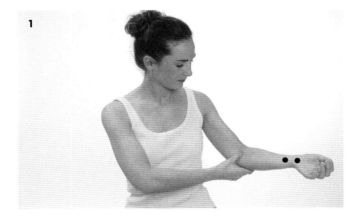

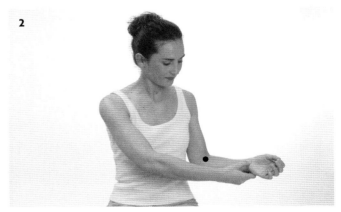

Locating the Points on the Lower Arms: The Heart Meridian

The Heart meridian runs from the elbow (on the side of the pinkie finger) down the inside of the lower arm and across the palm to the pinkie finger. Its points are massaged to treat pain in the chest area as well as psychological and psychosomatic problems and nervousness.

Heart 3—Lesser Sea (Yin Pathway)

When the elbow is bent, Heart 3, known as Lesser Sea or Yin Pathway in traditional Chinese medicine, is located midway between the end of the elbow fold and the noticeable protrusion of the upper arm bone. This point is used to treat pain, range of motion, and sensitivity problems in the arm and elbow. It is also used to treat pain in the chest, such as that caused by a constriction of the coronary vessels, as well as sleeping problems and psychological symptoms such as confusion or depression.

Heart 7—Spirit Gate

Find the end of the inside fold of the wrist on the pinkie side; move 0.5 cun toward the side of the thumb and you have located Heart 7. Because of the calming effects this point has on the heart, it is used to treat pain in the heart region, as well as in the case of so-called functional heart ailments. In addition, because of its calming effects on the psyche, this point can be used to alleviate anxiety.

Massaging the Points on the Lower Arms: The Heart Meridian

Massage the two points of the Heart meridian on the inside of the lower arm from the elbow to the wrist. You have the choice between two types of acupressure: you can connect the individual points in the massage through a gliding movement, or you can massage each point individually for its specific effects. In the latter case, massage each point for two to three minutes.

Heart 3 and 7 (Figures 1 and 2)

The massage is carried out with your partner sitting down. Begin with Heart 3, using the tip of your thumb to apply first steady and then circling pressure for one to two minutes. Making sure to maintain contact with your partner's skin, move the tip of your thumb across the skin to Heart 7, and massage it in the same way. When you have finished, repeat the sequence, beginning at Heart 3, for a total of five repetitions. In addition to pressure massage, you can also use moxibustion on Heart 7 with a moxa pin or a moxa cigar.

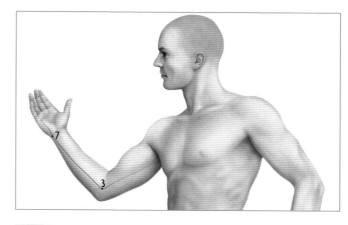

The Heart meridian begins in the armpit and runs along the inside of the arm to the palm and pinkie finger.

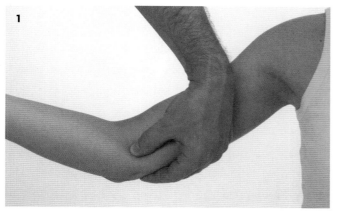

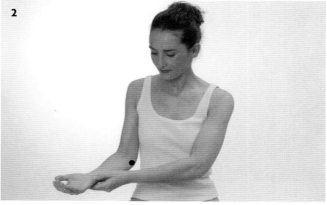

Left: Take the inside of the upper arm into your hand to massage Heart 3.

Right: Heart 7 is well suited for self-massage.

The Points on the Hands

On the two hands, or to be more precise, their fingers, three energy pathways originate: the Large and Small Intestine meridians and the Triple Heater meridian. All three meridians run from top to bottom along the body when the hands are overhead, meaning they are yang meridians (see page 33).

In addition, three energy pathways end in the hand: the Lung, Heart, and Pericardium meridians. Since all three of these meridians run from bottom to top along the body, they are yin meridians (see page 33).

Locating the Points on the Hands

This section describes the very effective points of these meridians on the hands. On the Large Intestine meridian you will massage the points Large Intestine 1 and 4, on the Small Intestine meridian the point Small Intes-

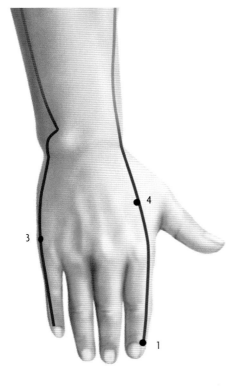

Caution

Large Intestine 4 has the ability to cause contractions and as such must not be massaged during pregnancy!

The Small Intestine meridian and Large Intestine meridian run along the back of the hand.

Blue	Large Intestine meridian	Large Intestine 1, 4
Red	Small Intestine meridian	Small Intestine 3

tine 3, on the Pericardium meridian the point Pericardium 8, and on the Lung meridian the points Lung 7, 10, and 11. Some of these points can be treated not only with the standard pressure application but also with warmth using moxibustion. However, use only the specific aids of traditional Chinese medicine for this purpose to avoid injury. When treating your own hand you can use the moxa pin or cigar. You will be able to relax and enjoy the treatment better, however, if a partner carries out the traditional warmth treatment for you; for this it is best to use loose mugwort in a moxa box.

Large Intestine 1—Metal Yang

The starting point of the Large Intestine meridian, Large Intestine 1, known as Metal Yang in traditional Chinese medicine, is located at the lower edge of the nail of the index finger, on the side closer to the thumb. Traditional Chinese medicine knows this as a point that dissolves heat and removes infections. In addition, it expands the senses and clears the power of the mind. The point is used to treat acute infections in the mouth and throat, such as gum infections, sore throats, and tonsillitis. This point can also be massaged as a complementary therapy in the case of fainting.

Large Intestine 4—Valley of Union

This point is easiest to locate when you make an O with your thumb and index finger, pressing the tips of the two fingers firmly against each other. This causes a small bulge of muscle to rise just above the web of skin between the index finger and thumb, on the back of the hand; this bulge marks the site of Large Intestine 4. This is the most effective point for relieving acute pain. In addition, it can be used to treat ailments of the lower arm and hand, feverish colds, and infections in the mouth and throat. Because Large Intestine 4 may cause contractions, it must not be massaged during pregnancy.

Small Intestine 3—Back Ravine

To locate this point, make a loose fist. Below the pinkie finger, at the level of the middle of the palm and over the pinkie's metacarpal bone, will be a fold of skin. Small

Intestine 3 is located at the outside edge of that fold. This point is effective for treating pain in the arm and back. It can be especially helpful in the case of pain in the cervical spine and in the lower back. Another use of this point is to treat eye problems such as cornea infections and sties. Because of its balancing effects this point can also be used to treat psychosomatic and psychological problems.

Pericardium 8—Palace of Toil

Pericardium 8, known in traditional Chinese medicine as Palace of Toil, is located on the palm of the hand at the place where, with a closed fist, the tip of the middle finger touches the inside of the palm. Pericardium 8 has psychologically balancing effects and is thus often used to treat psychological and psychosomatic problems. Other uses are in the treatment of pain in the mouth cavity, for which acupressure of this point can reduce swelling and prevent infection. Pericardium 8 can also be massaged to stop nosebleeds. Finally, it can help alleviate pain in the chest area.

Lung 7—Broken Sequence

Lung 7, known in traditional Chinese medicine as Broken Sequence, is located 1.5 cun above the fold of the wrist on the thumb side of the inner arm. Traditional Chinese medicine ascribes to this point the ability to influence and spread Lung qi. For this reason, Lung 7 is used especially to treat colds and problems in the respiratory passages such as coughing and shortness of breath. Moreover, the point can be used to treat pain or paralysis in the lower arm and the hand. You can also treat this point with moxibustion using a moxa pin, herb, or cigar.

Lung 10—Fish Border

Known as Fish Border in traditional Chinese medicine, this point is located at the outer edge of the ball of the thumb. According to Chinese medicine it cleanses the lungs and calms coughs. It is used to treat a variety of problems of the respiratory passages. It can be treated with pressure as well as moxibustion.

Lung 11—Lesser Shang

Lung 11, also known as Lesser Shang, is located on the outer edge of the nail of the thumb. According to Chinese medicine this point cleanses the lungs and soothes the throat. It has excellent effects for painful swelling in the throat area and is effective in treating coughing and shortness of breath. Beyond this, it also helps to keep your senses and awareness clear. Massage this point in cases of impaired consciousness accompanied by an increase of the body temperature, as in cases of heat exhaustion or heat stroke.

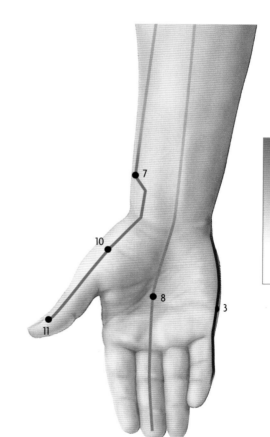

Note

Lung 11 is frequently very painful to the touch. Pressure should be applied only gradually, beginning with light pressure that is increased slowly but steadily.

Red	Small Intestine meridian	Small Intestine 3
Purple	Pericardium meridian	Pericardium 8
Blue	Lung meridian	Lung 7, 10, 11

The Pericardium and Lung meridians run along the palm of the hand; the third point of the Small Intestine meridian can be seen at the edge of the palm.

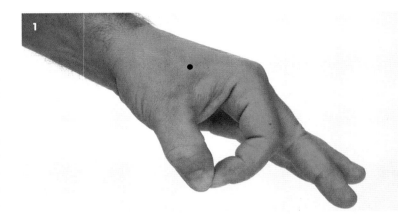

To locate Large Intestine 4, press the tips of your thumb and index finger against each other. The point is located in the small muscle bulge that forms just above the web of skin between the thumb and index finger.

To massage Large Intestine 4, take the base of the thumb between your thumb and index finger.

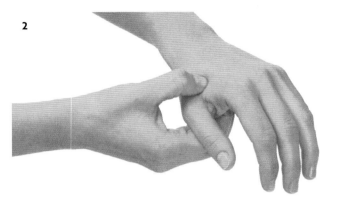

Pericardium 8 is located at the spot at which the middle finger touches the palm in a loose fist.

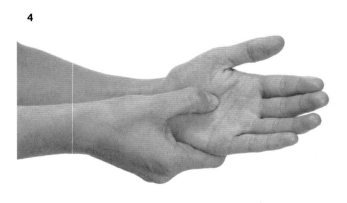

Massage Pericardium 8 using the tweezers grip.

Massaging the Points on the Hands

Acupressure of the points on the hands requires a great deal of empathy from the person giving the massage. As you practice acupressure on these points, pay attention to your partner's facial expression to make sure you register any discomfort early on.

Large Intestine 1—Metal Yang

You can massage Large Intestine 1 with your partner either lying down or sitting up. Locate the point at the edge of the nail of the index finger. With the tip of your thumb, apply steady pressure for two to three minutes.

> **Note**
> Large Intestine 1 is usually very sensitive, meaning that pressure should be applied only gradually.

Large Intestine 4—Valley of Union (Figures 1 and 2)

Massage this point using your thumb and index finger as tweezers: the thumb rests on Large Intestine 4, with the tip of your index finger providing the stabilizing base. First apply steady pressure in synchrony with your partner's breathing, slightly increasing the pressure as your partner exhales and decreasing the pressure as he or she inhales. After ten to fifteen breathing cycles, switch to a circling massage of the point.

> **Caution**
> Large Intestine 4 must not be massaged during pregnancy!

Pericardium 8—Palace of Toil (Figures 3 and 4)

You can massage Pericardium 8, or Palace of Toil, with your partner either sitting up or lying down. Massage this point using your thumb and middle finger as tweezers. In this case the tip of the middle finger provides the balancing base for the thumb, which applies pressure to the point. Apply first steady pressure and then circling pressure for a total of two to four minutes.

Small Intestine 3—Back Ravine (Figure 1)

You can massage Small Intestine 3 with your partner either sitting up or lying down. Using your thumb or index finger, apply first steady and then circling pressure. Since this point tends to be very painful when corresponding ailments are present, you should begin with very light pressure. In addition to pressure, you can apply moxibustion to this point, using one of the specific aids described on page 65.

Lung 11—Lesser Shang (Figure 2)

Massage Lung 11 with your partner either sitting up or lying down. Locate the point on the edge of the nail using the tip of your thumb. Then apply steady pressure for two to three minutes. If you want, you can apply moxibustion in addition to pressure massage to this point.

Lung 10—Fish Border (Figure 3)

Massage Lung 10 with your partner either sitting up or lying down. If you are massaging yourself, it is better to do so sitting up. Locate the point using the tip of your thumb on the ball of the wrist. Apply first steady and then circling pressure for two to three minutes. Your partner will find this massage more comfortable if you support his or her wrist with your free hand.

Lung 7—Broken Sequence (Figure 4)

Massage this point with your partner either sitting up or lying down. If you are massaging yourself, you will be more comfortable sitting up and placing your arm on your thigh. Apply first steady pressure and then circling pressure for two to three minutes.

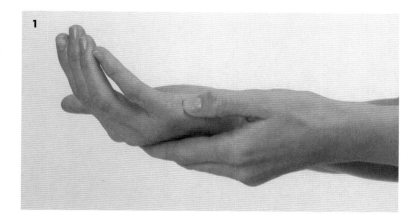

Massage Small Intestine 3 at the end of the fold of skin on the palm at the base of the pinkie.

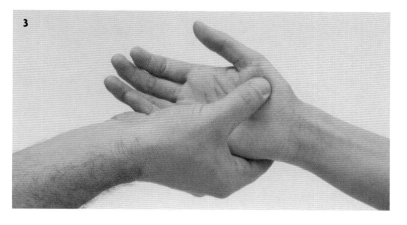

Lung 11 is located next to the outside edge of the thumbnail.

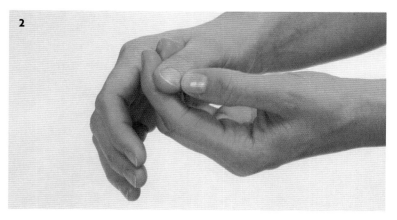

Massage Lung 10 on the outside edge of the ball of the thumb.

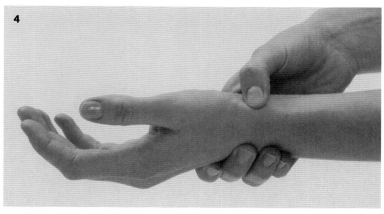

Lung 7 is located 1.5 cun above the wrist on the thumb side of the lower arm.

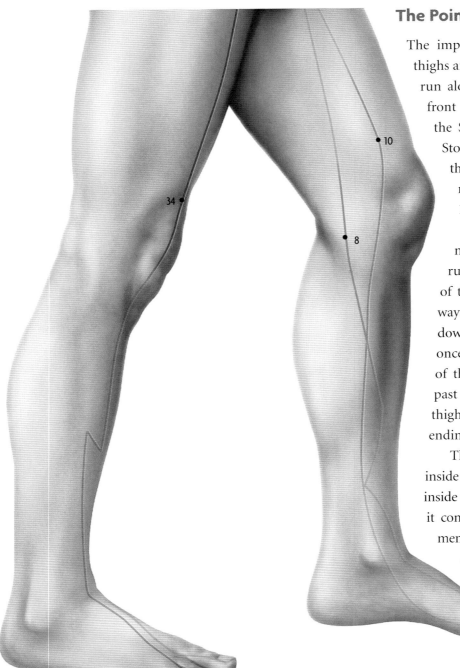

The Points on the Thighs

The important acupressure points on the thighs are located on several meridians that run along this part of the body. On the front and inside of the thighs these are the Stomach meridian, with the point Stomach 34; the Spleen meridian, with the point Spleen 10, and the Liver meridian, with the points Liver 8, 10, and 11.

The Stomach meridian originates in the face under the eye and runs almost vertically down to the top of the collarbone before moving sideways across the chest and then running down to the upper abdomen, where it once again returns closer to the center of the body. From there it runs down past the groin and down the front of the thigh to the calf and the top of the foot, ending on the second toe.

The Spleen meridian begins on the inside of the foot and runs up along the inside of the leg to the groin. From there it continues along the side of the abdomen and chest to the shoulder, where it changes directions and runs down again to the armpit.

The Liver meridian begins in the big toe and runs along the top of the foot and up the inside of the leg. In this area it runs into the Spleen meridian at several points. The Liver meridian also runs through the groin and up the side of the abdomen until ending just below the sixth rib.

On the back of the thighs are the points of the Urinary Bladder meridian, of which Urinary Bladder 37 and 40 are especially important for acu-

The Stomach, Spleen, and Liver meridians run over the front and inside of the thighs.

Khaki	Stomach meridian	Stomach 34
Olive	Spleen meridian	Spleen 10
Light green	Liver meridian	Liver 8

pressure. The Urinary Bladder meridian originates on the inside edge of the eyes and runs over the head to the nape, where it splits into two branches that run down along the body almost parallel to the spine. These branches run over the buttocks and backs of the thighs before reuniting at the backs of the knees. The meridian continues along the back of the leg down to the outside of the ankle and ends at the outside of the small toe.

On the outside of the thighs are the points Gall Bladder 30 and 31, two of the most frequently treated points on the Gall Bladder meridian. This meridian begins at the outer edge of the eye and continues in a zigzag line around the ear. From the mastoid process it makes a large arc across the side of the head to the forehead and then runs back along to the side of the neck. From there it runs in a zigzag line across the shoulder and down along the side of the body and the outside of the leg to top of the foot, ending at the fourth toe.

Locating the Points on the Thighs: The Front

The points on the front of the thighs are massaged to treat pain and range of motion problems in the legs, as well as stomachaches and menstrual problems.

Stomach 34—Beam Hill

Stomach 34 is traditionally known as Beam Hill. When the knee is bent, this point is located 2 cun above the outer and upper edge of the kneecap. It is used to treat stomachaches as well as range of motion problems, swelling, and pain in the knees.

Spleen 10—Sea of Blood

When the knee is bent, this point is located 2 cun above the upper inner edge of the kneecap. Spleen 10, also called Sea of Blood, is used to treat pain in the knee and on the inside of the thigh as well as gynecological problems such as

those occurring with menstruation. Massage of Spleen 10 is also useful in the treatment allergies; it can be used very effectively to treat skin rashes and eczema caused by allergies.

Liver 8—Spring at the Bend

This point is located on the inside of the thigh at the level of the knee; when the knee is bent, you will find it in the middle of the end of the knee fold in an indentation between two tendons. Massage of this point has positive effects on pain and range of motion problems in the knee, sexual problems in men, and gynecological conditions.

Massaging the Points on the Thighs: The Front

Stomach 34, Spleen 10, and Liver 8 are all important acupressure points on the front of the thighs. When treating the points Spleen 10 and Liver 8, ask your partner to take a comfortable position, either lying down or—as illustrated here—sitting up.

1 Stomach 34—Beam Hill (Figure 1)

Massage Beam Hill with your partner sitting up; if you are massaging yourself, you should sit up as well. Massage the point using first steady pressure and then circling pressure for a total of two to three minutes. You can also apply moxibustion (see page 65) to this point.

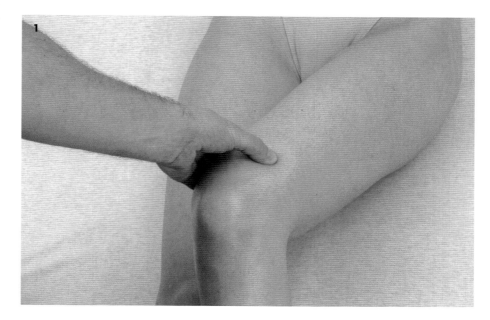

For massage of Stomach 34, the leg should be slightly bent at the knee.

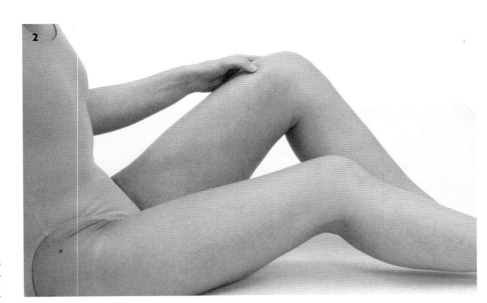

Spleen 10 is well suited for self-massage.

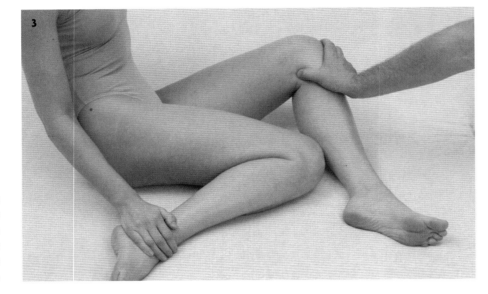

Liver 8, on the inside of the knee, is easiest to massage when the knee is slightly bent.

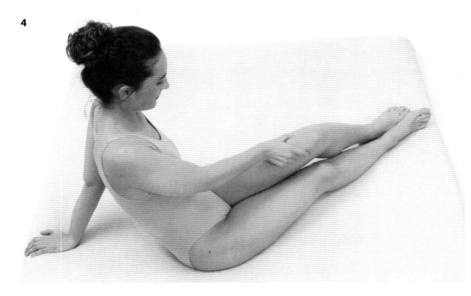

To treat problems in the knee, you can massage the two points Stomach 34 and Spleen 10 at the same time.

Spleen 10—Sea of Blood (Figure 2)

Treat Sea of Blood with the tip of your thumb, applying first steady and then circling pressure for a total of two to three minutes. If you wish, you can also use moxibustion on this point.

Liver 8—Spring at the Bend (Figure 3)

Treat Liver 8 with the tip of your thumb, applying first steady and then circling pressure for a total of two to three minutes. If you wish, you can also use moxibustion on this point.

Treating Stomach 34 and Spleen 10 Simultaneously (Figure 4)

If you have some experience with acupressure, it is possible to massage two points at the same time. The two points Spleen 10 and Stomach 34, discussed above, are especially well suited for this. To massage them simultaneously, take the knee between your thumb and index finger with the tweezers grip, placing the top of the thumb on Stomach 34 and the index finger on Spleen 10. Apply first steady and then circling pressure. In this case too you can use moxibustion on these points.

Locating the Points on the Thighs: The Back

These points are massaged to treat problems in the back, legs, or abdomen.

Urinary Bladder 37—Gate of Abundance

This point is located on the back of the thigh, 6 cun below the lower buttock fold. It is used to treat pain in the back and groin.

Urinary Bladder 40—Bend Middle

Urinary Bladder 40 is found in the middle of the back of the knee. It is massaged to treat range of motion problems and cramps in the legs as well as acute and chronic gastrointestinal conditions.

Massaging the Points on the Thighs: The Back

The two points on the back of the each thigh are best massaged with your partner lying on his or her stomach.

Urinary Bladder 37—Gate of Abundance (Figures 1 and 2)

Massage this point for two to three minutes using the tip of your thumb, applying first steady and then circling pressure. You can also massage this point using the ball of your hand, again using first steady and then circling pressure.

Urinary Bladder 40—Bend Middle (Figure 3)

Massage this point using the tip of your thumb for two to three minutes, applying first steady and then circling pressure.

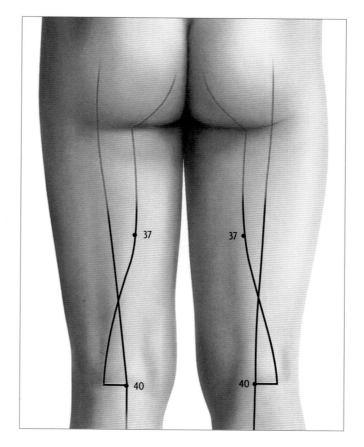

The two branches of the Urinary Bladder meridian merge at the knee.

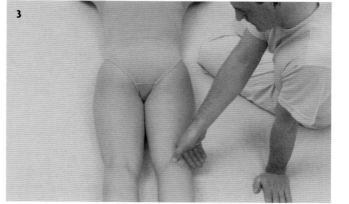

Urinary Bladder 37 is massaged 6 cun below the lower edge of the buttock.

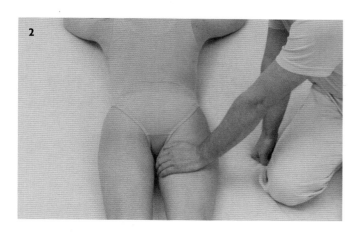

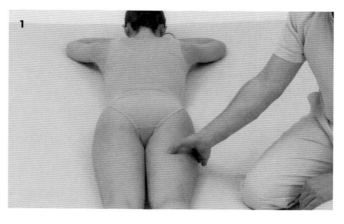

Left: You can massage Urinary Bladder 37 with either your fingertips or the ball of your hand.

Right: Urinary Bladder 40 is located in the middle of the back of the knee.

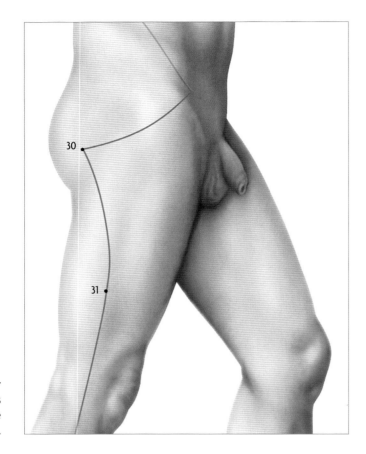

The Gall Bladder meridian runs along the outside of the leg.

Locating the Points on the Thighs: The Outside

You can use the points Gall Bladder 30 and 31 to treat pain in the back and legs.

Gall Bladder 30—Jumping Round

It is easiest to locate this point with your partner on his or her side and his or her hip joint bent. Imagine a line running from the bottom of the sacrum (at the top of the seam between the buttocks) to the greater trochanter (a prominence at the top of the femur). If you divide the line into three equal parts, Gall Bladder 30 is located at the spot that divides the middle from the outer third. It is used to treat pain in the lower back, pain along the course of the sciatic nerve, and range of motion problems in the legs.

Gall Bladder 31—Wind Market

This point is located 7 cun up from the knee on the outside of the thigh. It is massaged in the case of pain or paralysis in the legs.

Massaging the Points on the Thighs: The Outside

Massage these points with your partner lying comfortably on his or her side.

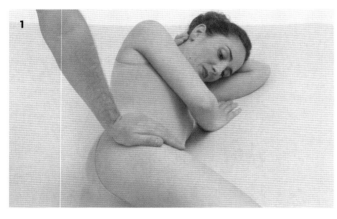

Place the ball of your hand on the side of the buttocks and apply first steady and then circling pressure on Gall Bladder 30.

Gall Bladder 30—Jumping Round (Figures 1 and 2)

Have your partner bend his or her leg at the hip to help you locate the point, as just described. Massage the point with the ball of your hand or the tip of your elbow, applying first steady and then circling pressure for two to three minutes.

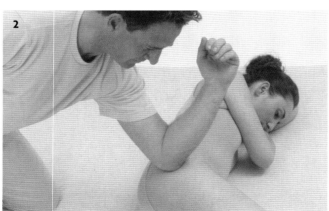

Left: You can also massage Gall Bladder 30 with your elbow instead of the ball of your hand.

Right: Massage Gall Bladder 31 using the tip of your thumb or the ball of your hand.

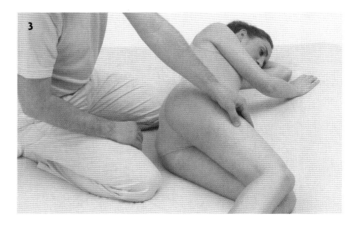

Gall Bladder 31—Wind Market (Figure 3)

Using the tip of your thumb or ball of your hand, apply first steady pressure and then circling pressure.

Locating the Points on the Thighs: The Inside

Two important points of the Liver meridian are located on the inside of the thighs, below the groin.

Liver 10—Foot Five Li (Five Lengths to the Foot)

Liver 10, known as Foot Five Li in traditional Chinese medicine, is located 3 cun below the upper edge of the pubic bone on the inside of the thigh. It is used to treat prostate infections and anuria.

Liver 11—Yin Corner

Liver 11 is located 2 cun below the upper edge of the pubic bone on the inside of the thigh. Massaging this point can regulate menstruation and increase the chances of conception in the case of fertility problems; this point is used in the treatment of female reproductive disturbances.

Massaging the Points on the Thighs: The Inside

To massage the points on the inside of the thighs, have your partner lie on his or her back. If you are massaging yourself, it is better to sit up.

Liver 10—Foot Five Li (Five Lengths to the Foot) (Figure 1)

Locate the point and massage it with the tip of your thumb, applying first steady and then circling pressure for a total of two to three minutes.

Liver 11—Yin Corner (Figure 2)

Massage this point with the tip of your thumb, applying first steady and then circling pressure for a total of two to three minutes.

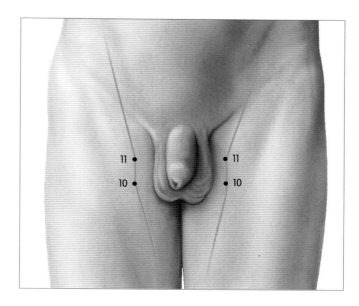

The Liver meridian runs along the inside of the thighs to the groin.

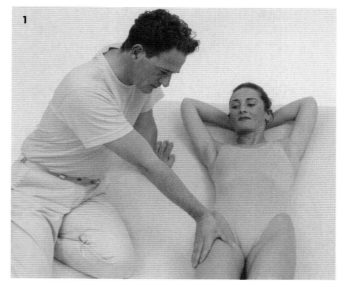

Liver 10 is massaged 3 cun below the upper edge of the pubic bone.

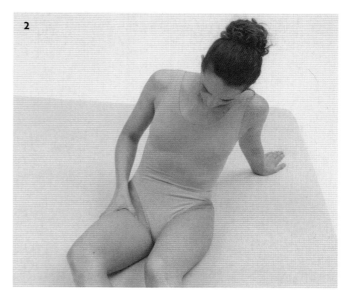

Liver 11 is 1 cun up from Liver 10.

The Points on the Calves

The most important acupressure points on the front of the calves belong to the Stomach meridian—Stomach 36, 38, and 40. On the back of the calves is the Urinary Bladder meridian, of which the points Urinary Bladder 56 and 60 are the most widely used. On the outside of the calves is the Gall Bladder meridian, of which Gall Bladder 34 and 39 are the most widely used. Finally, on the inside of the calves are the points Kidney 7 and Spleen 6 and 9.

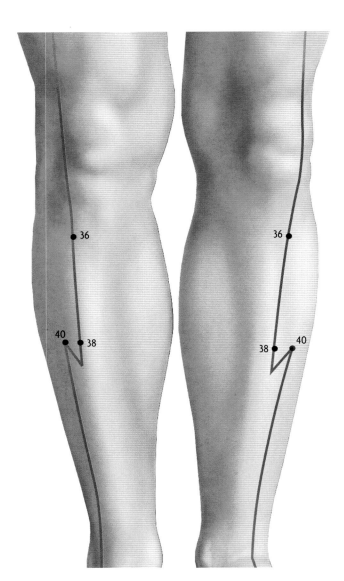

The Stomach meridian runs along the front of the calves down to the tops of the feet.

| **Khaki** | Stomach meridian | Stomach 36, 38, 40 |

Locating the Points on the Calves: The Front

Stomach 36, 38, and 40 can be treated with both massage and moxibustion to alleviate a variety of problems.

Stomach 36—Leg Three Li (Three Lengths to the Foot)

To locate Stomach 36, first find the protrusion of the shinbone just below the knee. Stomach 36 is at the level at which the protrusion turns into the front edge of the shinbone, 1 cun toward the outside of the leg. This is one of the most important points of the body. Traditional Chinese medicine sees it as a point that harmonizes the intestines and regulates qi. It can strengthen both body and mind and can balance cold and dampness. Massaging this point strengthens especially the Stomach and Spleen and can stimulate the immune system and prevent illnesses. This point is also used to treat problems with digestion and range of motion and diminished sensation or numbness in the leg.

Stomach 38—Ribbon Opening

This point is located 8 cun below the outer indentation of the knee. It can be used to treat pain in the calf, stomachaches, and pain that limits range of motion of the shoulder.

Stomach 40—Beautiful Bulge

Stomach 40 is located at the same height as Stomach 38, but 1.5 cun further toward the outside of the leg. This point is used to treat problems in the respiratory passages, such as asthma and bronchitis, as well as psychological and psychosomatic problems. Because of its ability to cause the expulsion of mucus, it can be used to treat illnesses accompanied by heavy phlegm.

Massaging the Points on the Calves: The Front

These points are usually massaged with your partner lying on his or her back. If you are massaging the three points as a sequence, the duration of pressure on each point in the sequence is one to two minutes. As you move from point to point, make sure you do not lose contact with your partner's skin. If you are massaging a single point individually, the duration of pressure increases to two to three minutes.

Stomach 36—Leg Three Li (Three Lengths to the Foot) (Figure 1)

To massage Stomach 36, use your thumb to apply first steady pressure and then circling pressure.

Stomach 38—Ribbon Opening (Figure 2)

Massage Stomach 38 using the tip of your thumb, applying first steady and then circling pressure.

Stomach 40—Beautiful Bulge (Figure3)

Massage Stomach 40 with the tip of your thumb, using first steady and then circling pressure. The massage takes two to three minutes.

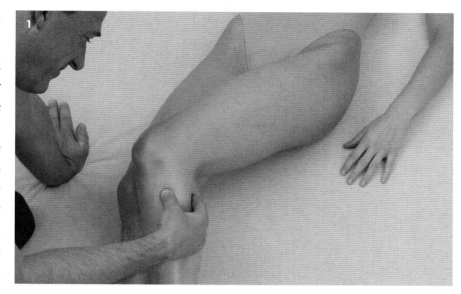

Stomach 36 is massaged 1 cun to the side of the front edge of the shinbone.

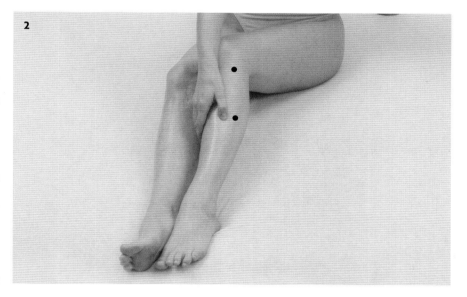

Stomach 38 is 8 cun below the indentation of the knee.

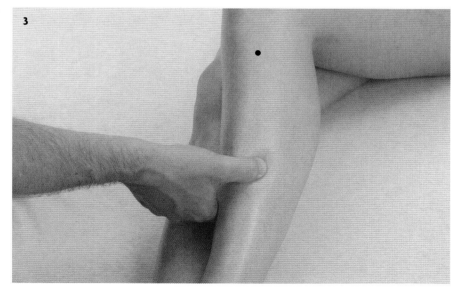

Stomach 40 is located 1.5 cun toward the outside of the calf from Stomach 38.

Locating the Points on the Calves: The Back

The Urinary Bladder meridian runs on the back of the calves. The points Urinary Bladder 56 and 60 are useful especially in treating local ailments in the calves and heels. Urinary Bladder 60 is also used to treat back and neck pain.

Urinary Bladder 56—Sinew Support

Urinary Bladder 56 is located 5 cun below the back of the knee, between the two heads of the calf muscle, which has an important function in bending the knee and rolling the foot. Traditional Chinese medicine sees this point as being able to relax the tendons and alleviate pain. For this reason, Urinary Bladder 56 is often used in cases of calf cramps and pain in the calf. It is also sometimes used to treat hemorrhoids.

Urinary Bladder 60—Kunlun Mountains

Urinary Bladder 60 is located midway between the highest rise of the outside ankle and the Achilles tendon. Traditional Chinese medicine holds that this point can relax both tendons and muscles, alleviate pain, and clear heat. It is thus used to treat pain in the heel and the lower back as well as the neck. Since Urinary Bladder 60 can have effects on contractions, it should not be massaged during pregnancy.

Note

Please note that Urinary Bladder 60 must not be massaged during pregnancy since it can cause the onset of contractions!

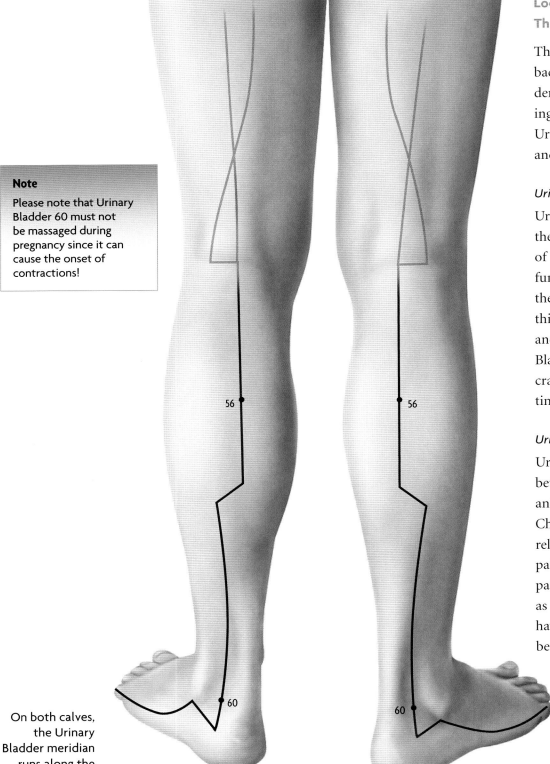

On both calves, the Urinary Bladder meridian runs along the back of the calf to the heel and along the outside of the foot to the small toe.

Black	Urinary Bladder meridian	Urinary Bladder 56, 60

Massaging the Points on the Calves: The Back

Acupressure of the two points of the Urinary Bladder meridian on the back of the calves is done one after the other. Begin with Urinary Bladder 56 below the knee, and then move to Urinary Bladder 60. You can treat the points as a sequence, connecting the two points with a gliding movement of your hand. Alternatively, you can massage the points separately according to the ailment you are seeking to address, in which case the duration of massage for the individual point should be two to three minutes.

Urinary Bladder 56—Sinew Support (Figures 1 and 2)

The massage is carried out with your partner lying down on his or her stomach. You can massage this point using either the tip of your thumb or the ball of your hand. Either way, apply first steady and then circling pressure for a total of two to three minutes.

Urinary Bladder 60—Kunlun Mountains (Figure 3)

Use the tweezers grip to massage Kunlun Mountains, placing your thumb on the point and using your index finger below the heel to create a balancing point for your thumb. Apply first steady pressure and then circling pressure to the point for one to two minutes each.

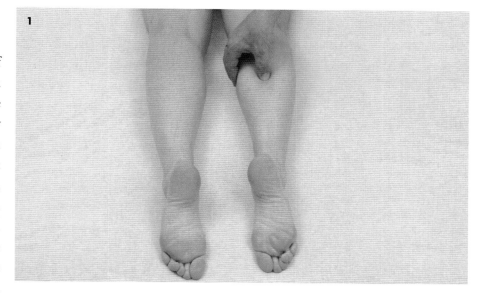

1

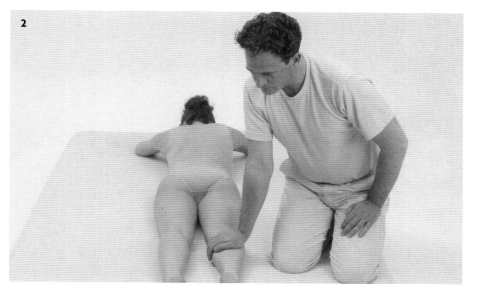

Urinary Bladder 56 is located 5 cun below the fold of the knee between the two heads of the calf muscle.

2

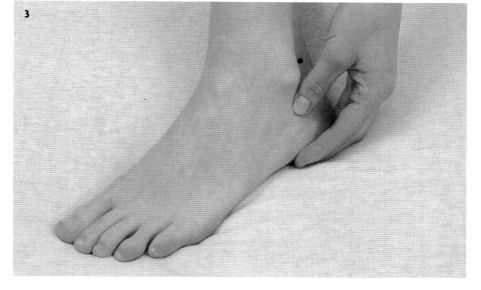

When massaging a point using the ball of your hand, try to exert pressure only from the hand and not from the arm.

3

Massage Urinary Bladder 60 (see point marked on illustration) midway between the highest rise of the outside ankle and the Achilles tendon.

Locating the Points on the Calves: The Outside

The Gall Bladder meridian runs on the outside of the calves. Gall Bladder 34 and 39 are used to treat gallbladder problems or pain in the knees or cervical spine.

Gall Bladder 34—Mound Spring

Gall Bladder 34, known traditionally as Mound Spring, is located in a small depression in front of and slightly below the head of the fibula. This point can be massaged to treat pain in the knee, gallbladder ailments, or side-specific paralysis.

Gall Bladder 39—Suspended Bell

Gall Bladder 39, known traditionally as Suspended Bell, is located 3 cun above the highest rise of the outside of the ankle at the front of the fibula. This point can be massaged to treat problems in the cervical spine, pain or lack of strength in the calf, and side-specific paralysis.

Massaging the Points on the Calves: The Outside

Massage Gall Bladder 34 and 39 with your partner lying down. If you are massaging yourself, you will find it easier to reach these points if you sit up. Note that both points can be treated not just with pressure but also with warmth, meaning moxibustion (see page 65).

Gall Bladder 34—Mound Spring (Figure 1)

Massage this point on the outside of the calf using the tip of your thumb. Apply first steady and then circling pressure for two to three minutes.

Gall Bladder 39—Suspended Bell (Figure 2)

Massage this point in the same manner as Gall Bladder 34, using the tip of your thumb for two to three minutes.

Left: The Gall Bladder meridian runs along the outside of the calf to the fourth toe.

Top right: Gall Bladder 34 is massaged just below the head of the fibula.

Bottom right: Gall Bladder 39 is 3 cun above the outside of the ankle.

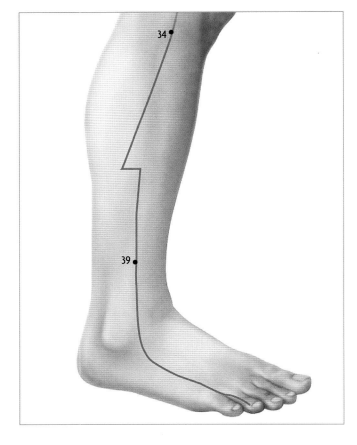

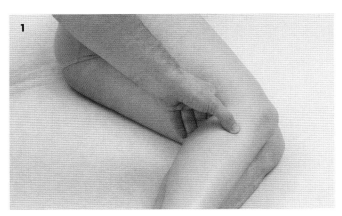

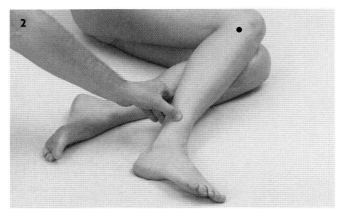

Locating the Points on the Calves: The Inside

The Kidney and Spleen meridians run on the inside of the calves. Their treatment areas are presented here.

Kidney 7—Recover Flow

Kidney 7 is located 2 cun above the highest rise of the inside of the ankle, just inside the Achilles tendon. This point is used to treat insufficient or excessive sweat production as well as edema.

Spleen 6—Three Yin Intersection

Spleen 6 is located 3 cun above the highest rise of the inside ankle at the back edge of the shinbone. It has regulating effects for gynecological issues and also can be massaged to treat sexual dysfunctions in men and bladder problems.

Spleen 9—Yin Mound Spring

This point is located at the back edge of the shinbone, just below the knee. It is used to treat pain in the knee as well as bladder problems, intestinal infections, or a tendency to edema.

Massaging the Points on the Calves: The Inside

Massage these points with your partner lying down on his or her back. If you want to massage the three points on yourself, it is easier to do so while sitting up.

Kidney 7—Recover Flow

Have your partner bend his or her leg slightly outward. Massage this point using your thumb, applying first steady and then circling pressure for two to three minutes.

Spleen 6—Three Yin Intersection (Figure 1)

Your partner remains lying down with his or her leg bent outward. Apply first steady and then circling pressure for two to three minutes using your thumb.

Spleen 9—Yin Mound Spring (Figure 2)

Again, your partner remains lying down with his or her leg turned slightly outward. Massage this point with your thumb, applying first steady and then circling pressure for two to three minutes.

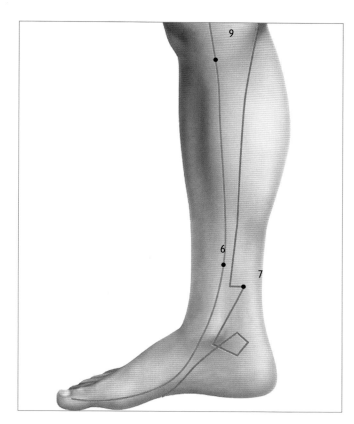

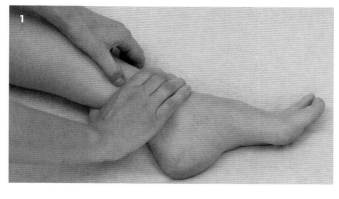

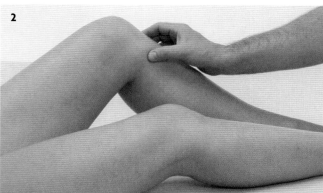

Left: The Kidney (gray) and Spleen (olive) meridians run along the inside of the calf.

Top right: Spleen 6 is located 3 cun above the inside of the ankle.

Bottom right: Spleen 9 is massaged with the leg turned slightly outward.

The Points on the Feet

Useful points on the top of the foot are Stomach 41 and 44 and Liver 3. On the outside of the foot the points Urinary Bladder 67 and Gall Bladder 41 have special importance. On the inside of the foot are the Kidney and Spleen meridians, of which the points Kidney 3 and 6 and Spleen 3 are especially helpful.

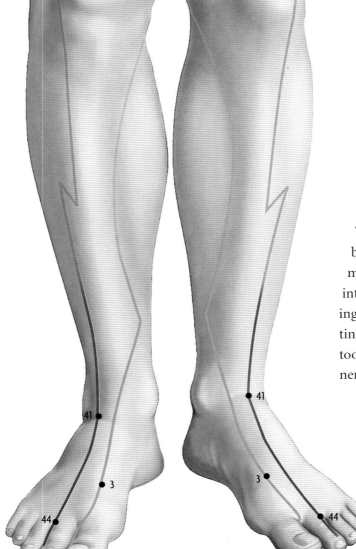

Locating the Points on the Feet: The Top of the Feet

These points can be sensitive to pressure in the case of a wide variety of ailments. They have effects ranging from relieving pain in the foot to alleviating toothaches. A detailed description of their treatment possibilities is presented here.

Stomach 41—Ravine Divide

Stomach 41, known in traditional Chinese medicine as Ravine Divide, is located in an indentation in the middle of the front horizontal fold of the upper ankle. According to Chinese medicine, this point strengthens qi and the Spleen and has calming effects on body and mind. The point can be used to treat a wide range of ailments, including constipation, headaches accompanied by dizziness or drowsiness, impaired consciousness or loss of consciousness, and high fever.

Stomach 44—Inner Court

This point is located at the edge of the web of skin between the second and third toes. It too has harmonizing effects on qi, as well as on the stomach and intestines. Moreover, it has the ability to reduce swelling. Stomach 44 is used to treat infections in the intestines, throat, nose, mouth, tonsils, or gums, as well as toothaches, nosebleed, headaches, and paralysis of facial nerves.

Liver 3—Great Surge

Liver 3 is located on the top of the foot in the indentation between the first and second metatarsals. Because of its harmonizing effects it is especially helpful for treating menstruation problems, constipation, and urination problems. Moreover, it is used to treat pain in the feet and legs.

The Stomach and Liver meridians run along the top of the feet.

Khaki	Stomach meridian	Stomach 41, 44
Light green	Liver meridian	Liver 3

Massaging the Points on the Feet: The Top of the Feet

If you are massaging a partner, he or she should lie down. If you are massaging yourself, it is more comfortable to reach these points sitting up.

Stomach 41—Ravine Divide (Figure 1)

Using your thumb, apply first steady and then circling pressure to the point. If you want, you can use not just pressure but also moxibustion on this point.

Stomach 44—Inner Court (Figure 2)

Grasp the "webbing" between the second and third toes between the tips of your thumb and index finger, using the tweezers grip, and massage the point using first steady and then circling pressure. You can also use moxibustion on this point.

Liver 3—Great Surge (Figure 3)

Massage this point for two to three minutes using the tip of your thumb, applying first steady and then circling pressure. You can also use moxibustion on this point.

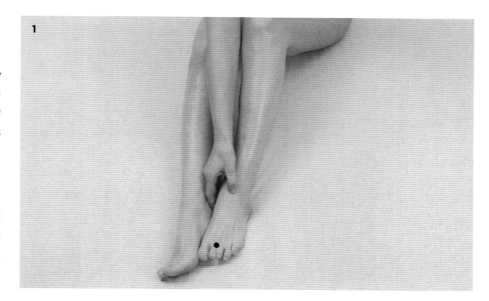

Stomach 41 is massaged in the front fold of the ankle.

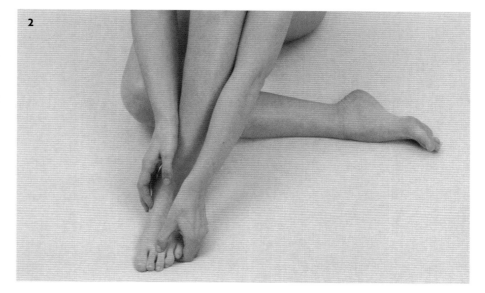

Stomach 44 is located at the beginning of the space between the second and third toes.

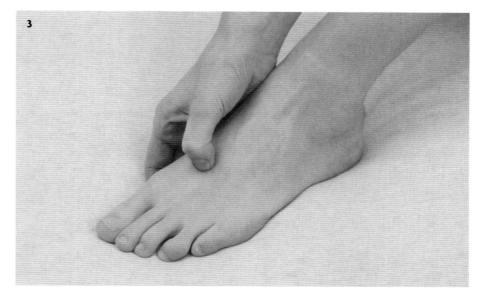

Liver 3 is located on the top of the foot in the indentation between the first and second metatarsals.

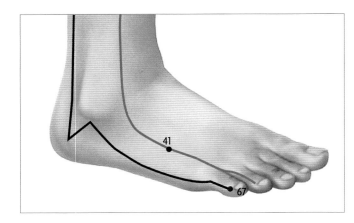

The Gall Bladder meridian (dark green) and Urinary Bladder meridian (black) run along the outside edge of the foot.

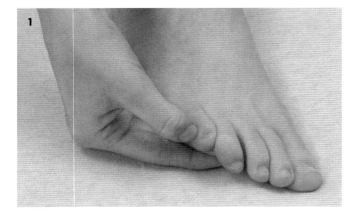

1

Urinary Bladder 67 is massaged next to the nail of the small toe.

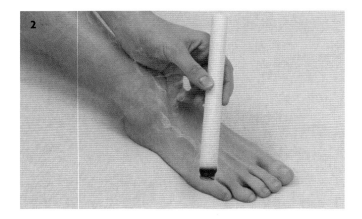

2

You can use moxibustion, for example with a moxa cigar, on Urinary Bladder 67.

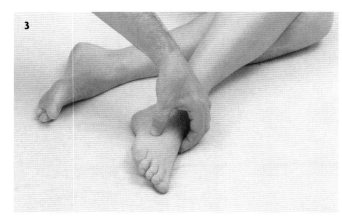

3

Gall Bladder 41 is best massaged using the tweezers grip.

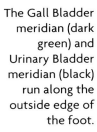

Locating the Points on the Feet: The Outside

In the case of headache or pain in a foot, check point Gall Bladder 41 to see whether it is sensitive to pressure, and if it is, massage it. Since Urinary Bladder 67 can promote contractions, you must not massage this point during pregnancy.

Urinary Bladder 67—Reaching Yin

This point is located next to the bottom outer edge of the nail of the small toe. It is used to treat headaches, infections of the mucous membranes of the nose, and nosebleeds. This point has exceptional qualities in promoting healthy childbirth, being able to promote correct positioning of the fetus, contractions, and the expulsion of the placenta after childbirth. Please note that extreme care must be taken in the massage of this point on a pregnant woman; such massage should be undertaken only by licensed therapists.

Gall Bladder 41—Foot Overlooking Tears

Gall Bladder 41 is located on the top of the foot at the corner of the fourth and fifth metatarsals. It is used to treat pain in the feet, problems in the groin and abdomen, side-specific paralysis, and side-specific headaches.

Massaging the Points on the Feet: The Outside

To massage these points on a partner, have him or her lie down, with his or her leg turned slightly inward so that you can easily reach the outside of the foot. On yourself, you can massage these points only while sitting up.

Urinary Bladder 67—Reaching Yin (Figures 1 and 2)

Massage this point using the tip of your thumb for two to three minutes, applying first steady and then circling pressure.

Gall Bladder 41—Foot Overlooking Tears (Figure 3)

Massage this point using the tip of your thumb for two to three minutes, applying first steady and then circling pressure.

Locating the Points on the Feet: The Inside

Both the Kidney and the Spleen meridians run along the inside of the feet.

Kidney 3—Great Ravine

This point is located in the indentation between the highest point of the inside ankle and the Achilles tendon. It is used to treat range of motion problems in the legs, sexual problems in men, infections in the throat and mouth, and hypertension.

Kidney 6—Shining Sea

This point is located in the indentation below the inside ankle. It is used to treat gynecological problems, chronic infections of the mouth, and fatigue.

Spleen 3—Supreme White (Venus)

Spleen 3 is located on the inside of the foot next to and a little below the first base joint of the toe (at the ball of the foot). This point is used to treat acute or chronic gastrointestinal infections as well as digestive problems.

Massaging the Points on the Feet: The Inside

To massage these points, have your partner lie down with his or her leg turned slightly outward so that you can easily reach the inside of the foot. If you are massaging yourself, these points are easiest to reach when you sit up.

Kidney 3—Great Ravine (Figure 1)

Apply first steady and then circling pressure for two to three minutes with the tip of your thumb.

Kidney 6—Shining Sea (Figure 2)

Using the tip of your thumb, apply first steady and then circling pressure for two to three minutes.

Spleen 3—Supreme White (Venus) (Figure 3)

Massage Spleen 3 using the tip of your thumb, applying first steady and then circling pressure for a total of two to three minutes.

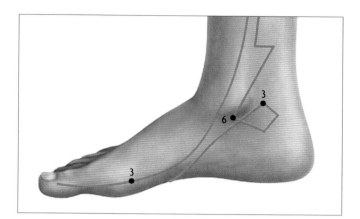

The Kidney meridian (light gray) and Spleen meridian (olive) run along the inside of the foot.

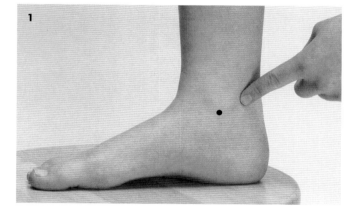

Kidney 3 (at finger) is massaged between the inside of the ankle and the Achilles heel.

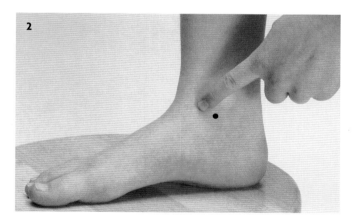

Kidney 6 is located in the indentation below the inside of the ankle.

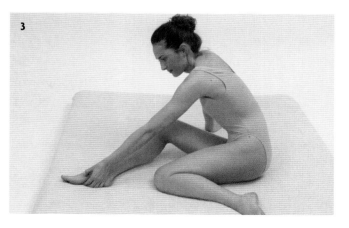

Use the tweezers grip to massage Spleen 3, located on the side of the foot.

Targeting Ailments with Acupressure

This section contains comprehensive information about some treatment possibilities using acupressure. Some common ailments and their possible treatments are described; you'll also find information about what you can do to ensure the success of the massage and how acupressure can support and complement medical treatment.

> **Note**
>
> Acupressure can be a complementary treatment method for chronic ailments, but its use should be discussed with a qualified health care practitioner before acupressure massage is begun.

Sleep Problems, Headaches, Fatigue

Sleep difficulties, headaches, and fatigue have become everyday illnesses. Using acupressure—if necessary in concert with medical treatment—you can successfully address these ailments.

Sleep Problems

Many of us suffer from some kind of sleep problem at least occasionally, if not chronically. A healthy, sufficiently long sleep is necessary for the whole body and especially for the central nervous system, and lack of sleep quickly leads to decreased attention span, decreased mental performance, irritation, depression, and nervousness. Young adults on average need seven to eight hours' sleep per night, while five to six hours is enough for older people. (This difference is important to consider, especially when you are dealing with older people who complain of sleep problems.)

Clinically, modern medicine differentiates between those who have difficulty falling asleep and those who have difficulty staying asleep. Difficulty falling asleep means that sufferers often lie awake for a long time after going to bed, while people who have difficulty staying asleep fall asleep normally but wake up several times during the night or wake up too early in the morning.

A third type of sleep issue that can reduce the depth and quality of night sleep without necessarily leading to waking is parasomnia, a sleep disorder that includes recurring nightmares, sleepwalking, and bed wetting. This type of sleep problem is especially common among children.

Sleep problems have a range of different causes. These include pain, such as may result from an illness or injury, as well as illnesses of the nervous system, such as depression, which are frequently accompanied by sleep difficulties.

In today's hectic times, many people who have to work at night, who work changing shifts, or who face constantly increasing pressure at work find it impossible to maintain a healthy sleep-wake rhythm. "Uppers" such as caffeinated drinks, drugs, and medication also disrupt our sleep patterns. Often, sufferers experience these symptoms over long periods of time, much as with a chronic illness. In such a situation, a vicious circle can ensue: the sufferers go to bed and from the outset do not expect to be able to fall asleep or stay asleep; their negative expectation becomes a part of the problem.

To break this cycle, it is important not simply to treat sleeping problems with sleeping pills, but rather to treat them in a way that allows sufferers to change their behavior. Examples of effective, quick, and easily learned techniques that allow sufferers to experience conscious relaxation include autogenic training and progressive muscle relaxation. (See glossary on page 232 for more information.)

What You Can Do

During the daytime you should make sure to get enough exercise, since only this can lead to a healthy fatigue in the evening. Do not drink stimulating drinks such as coffee or caffeinated soft drinks after lunch. Ensure a pleasant sleeping environment: Your bedroom should be dark and quiet. The best room temperature is between 60 and 65 degrees Fahrenheit. Treat yourself to a warm footbath before going to bed. In addition, you can drink warm milk or an herbal tea. Especially good choices for bedtime tea are melissa, hops, and lavender. If despite these measures you are not able to fall asleep, do not lie awake in the dark for longer than thirty minutes. If you cannot fall asleep in that time, it is better to read a book for a little while until you feel tired. Under no circumstances should you bring problems from your day to bed with you. To avoid this, carry out a relaxation exercise before going to bed, for example autogenic training or progressive muscle relaxation.

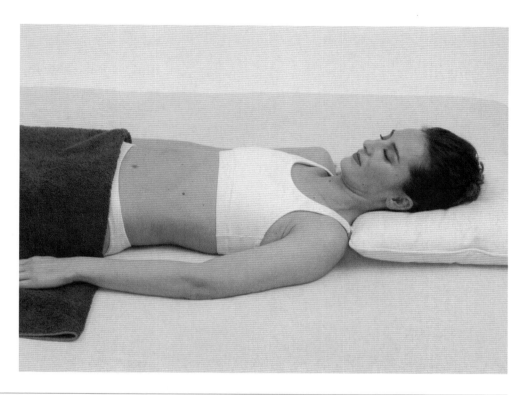

Progressive muscle relaxation can help you learn to consciously relax one body part after another.

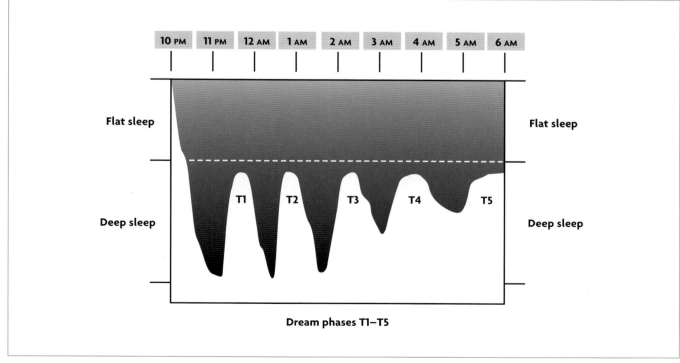

10 PM | 11 PM | 12 AM | 1 AM | 2 AM | 3 AM | 4 AM | 5 AM | 6 AM

Flat sleep

Flat sleep

T1   T2   T3   T4   T5

Deep sleep

Deep sleep

Dream phases T1–T5

During the night we undergo several phases with different depths of sleep.

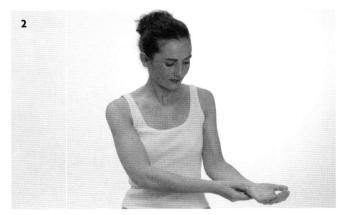

Heart 7 is located on the outside edge of the fold of the wrist.

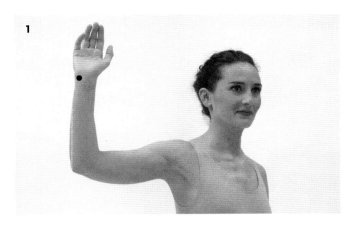

Massage Heart 7 using your thumb with steady and circling pressure.

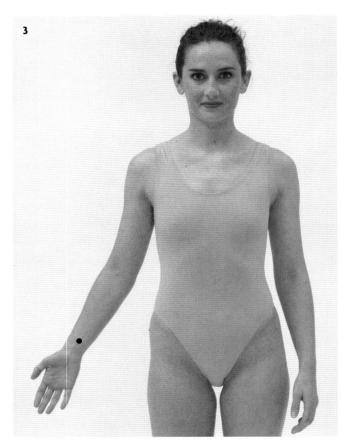

Left: Pericardium 6 is located 2 cun above the fold of the wrist.

Right: Massage Pericardium 6 using your thumb for two to three minutes with steady and circling pressure.

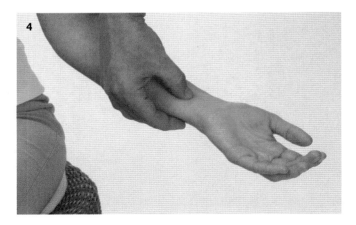

How Can Acupressure Help?

Stress is a frequent cause of sleep problems. Acupressure of the following points has calming effects and can help the body relax. A regular massage can help promote falling and staying asleep.

Heart 7—Spirit Gate (Figures 1 and 2)

How to locate the point: Heart 7 or Spirit Gate is located on the inside of the arm, on the outer edge of the inside fold of the wrist.

How to apply pressure to the point: Before massaging the point, warm your hands by rubbing your palms against each other or running warm water over your hands and lower arms. Then place your thumb on the point on one arm and massage it using first steady and then circling pressure for one to two minutes each first clockwise and then counterclockwise. Then massage the point on the other arm.

Pericardium 6—Inner Pass (Figures 3 and 4)

How to locate the point: Inner Pass is located 2 cun above the inside of the wrist, between the tendons in the middle of the inside of the arm.

How to apply pressure to the point: Place your thumb or index finger on this point and massage it for one to two minutes first with steady pressure and then with circular pressure, first clockwise and then counterclockwise. Then treat the point on the other arm in the same way.

Heart 3—Lesser Sea (Yin Pathway) (Figures 1 and 2)

How to locate the point: When the elbow is bent, you will find this point midway between the end of the elbow fold and the protrusion of the upper arm bone.

How to apply pressure to the point: Apply first steady pressure and then circling pressure, first clockwise and then counterclockwise. Repeat on the other arm. The massage should last for two to three minutes per arm.

Liver 3—Great Surge (Figures 3 and 4)

How to locate the point: Liver 3 or Great Surge is located on the top of the foot in an indentation between the first and second metatarsals.

How to apply pressure to the point: First warm the top of the foot and calf by gently rubbing the skin. Then press Liver 3 as hard as you can with the tip of your thumb or index finger. This can be painful. The pressure should be strong but bearable for about one minute. Then massage the point for another minute using small circling movements and less pressure, first clockwise and then counterclockwise. After treating this point for two to three minutes, treat the point on the other foot. You can also use moxibustion on this point, choosing between the three forms of the moxa herb: the moxa cigar, the moxa pin, or loose mugwort in a moxa box. The duration of the warmth treatment should be two to three minutes.

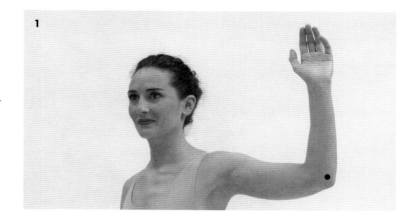

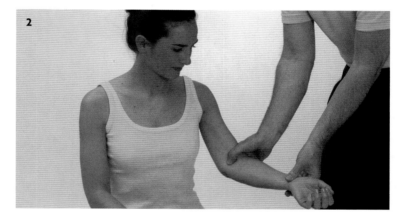

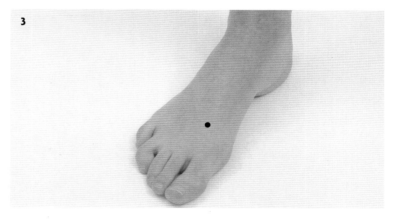

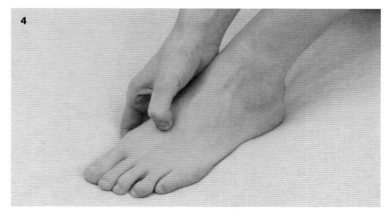

Heart 3 is located between the noticeable protrusion of the upper arm bone and the fold of the elbow.

Massage the point with first steady and then circular pressure.

Liver 3 is located on the top of the foot, in an indentation between the first and second metatarsals.

Massage the point using your thumb and applying steady and circling pressure.

Headaches and Migraines

Almost every person suffers from a headache at some point. However, among roughly a third of the population, headaches are so frequent or so severe that they require medical treatment. Headaches can be a symptom of many ailments, including muscle tension, infection, or a tumor. They can also be a side effect of certain types of medication, including medication to treat coronary problems or blood thinners that may be prescribed after a stroke. In addition, prolonged and regular use of pain medication can cause headaches. Among susceptible persons, even everyday occurrences such as low air pressure, changes in weather, or irregular meals can cause headaches. Other factors that can cause headaches include lack of sleep, continued stress, and physical tension. Oftentimes, several of these factors are present at once.

However, a headache is not just an indication of illness but can be an illness in itself. Examples of this include tension headaches, migraines, and cluster headaches. Of these types of headaches, the tension headache is the most frequent. This tends to be a slight pain occurring on both sides of the head that affects more than half the population. The reason for this is usually a combination of psychological strain and tension of the neck muscles. An imbalance of neurotransmitters in the brain can also contribute to tension headaches.

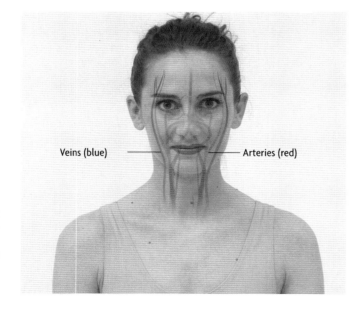

Veins (blue) — — Arteries (red)

Headaches can be caused by the contraction and relaxation of blood vessels in the head area.

Migraines are headaches that occur sporadically and can last up to several days, accompanied by symptoms such as nausea, vomiting, and sensitivity to light as well as problems with vision and sense of smell. Doctors believe that migraines are caused by circulation problems in the brain that lead to cramps and then dilations of the blood vessels.

The cluster headache is marked by very strong pain located on one side of the head. The illness is relatively rare and is observed predominantly among men. So far, the cause for cluster headaches has not been identified.

What You Can Do

Your health care provider may be able to prescribe medication depending on the intensity, frequency, and duration of headache attacks. But you yourself can contribute to the alleviation of pain and the success and sustainability of the therapy. Observe which factors cause the headaches. In what situations does the pain occur? Are changes in the weather, occurrence or resolution of stress, lack of sleep, or consumption of certain foods linked to the occurrence of headaches? Try to record the external circumstances that accompany the pain in a "headache diary." This will help you identify the causes of the headaches and avoid situations that can cause headaches. Make sure to get enough sleep and exercise and to have regular meals. It may also be helpful to learn certain relaxation techniques such as autogenic training or progressive muscle relaxation to enable you to better withstand stress. You should consume alcohol and nicotine at only very low levels, if at all, since their consumption too can cause headaches. Also pay attention to your posture, particularly in situations of psychological tension, to avoid developing muscle tensions.

How Can Acupressure Help?

Acupressure is extremely effective in alleviating headaches. The treatment possibilities for acupressure in this area are as varied as the causes for headaches.

Gall Bladder 20—Wind Pool (Figures 1 and 2)

How to locate the point: Wind Pool is located at the base of the back of the head, on both sides of the middle axis next to the muscles that can be felt there.

How to apply pressure to the point: Place both thumbs on the points to the left and right of the middle axis of the head. Massage the points using first steady pressure and then circling pressure, in clockwise and then counterclockwise movements, for one to two minutes each. If you wish, you can also apply a traditional warmth treatment to this point using the specific moxibustion aids (see page 65).

> **Caution**
> If headaches persist or severe headaches occur suddenly and without discernible cause, you should consult a qualified health care practitioner.

Gall Bladder 21—Shoulder Well (Figures 3 and 4)

How to locate the point: With your partner leaning his or her head slightly forward, locate the dorsal process of the seventh cervical vertebra. Using your other hand, locate the highest elevation of the shoulder. Shoulder Well is located midway between these two points.

How to apply pressure to the point: The point is massaged using the tip of the thumb with first steady and then circling pressure for one to two minutes each. Afterward knead and rub the surrounding muscles for the same amount of time. This may be uncomfortable for your partner, since there frequently is painful muscle tension in this area. You can also treat this point with heat using moxibustion; the warmth treatment should last two to three minutes per point.

> **Caution**
> Gall Bladder 21 must not be massaged during pregnancy!

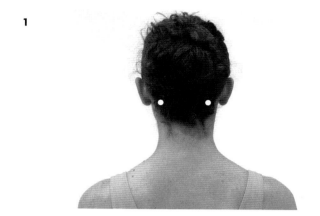

1

Gall Bladder 20 is located at the base of the back of the head.

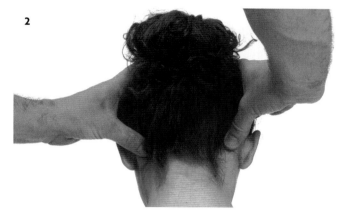

2

Massage both Gall Bladder 20 points at the same time using the tips of your thumbs.

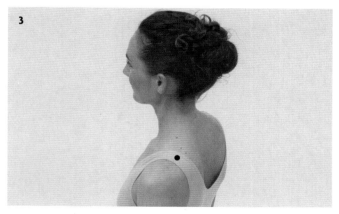

3

Gall Bladder 21 is located midway between the seventh cervical vertebra and the highest rise of the shoulder.

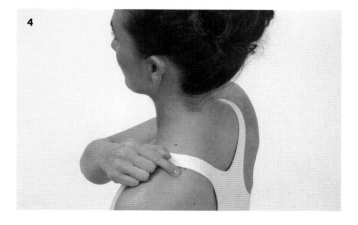

4

Use steady and circling pressure on this point.

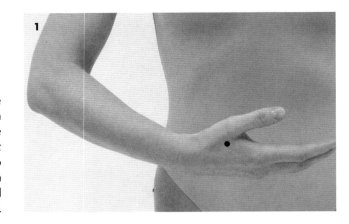

Large Intestine 4 is located on the small bulge of muscle just above the web of skin between the thumb and the index finger.

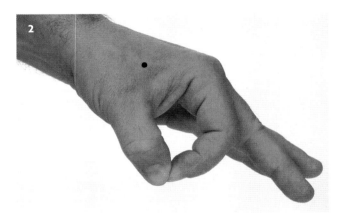

To locate the point, make an O with your thumb and index finger.

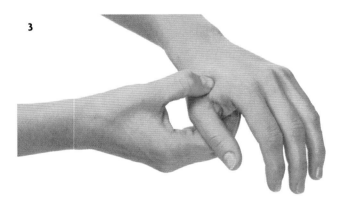

Massage the point using the tip of your thumb and index finger in the tweezers grip.

Left: Small Intestine 3 is located at the end of the skin fold over the base joint of the pinkie.

Right: Massage the point using steady and circling pressure.

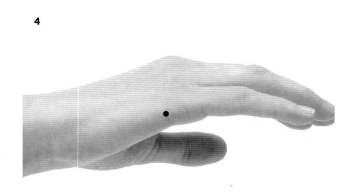

Large Intestine 4—Valley of Union (Figures 1–3)

How to locate the point: This point is easiest to locate when you make an O with your thumb and index finger, pressing the tips of the two fingers firmly against each other. This causes a small bulge of muscle to rise just above the web of skin between the index finger and thumb, on the back of the hand; this bulge marks the site of Large Intestine 4.

How to apply pressure to the point: Take one hand in a tweezers grip between your thumb and index finger, with your thumb resting on Large Intestine 4 and the tip of the index finger on the other side of the hand as a balancing point. First apply steady pressure in rhythm with your partner's breathing: increase the pressure while your partner exhales and slightly decrease the pressure while he or she inhales. After ten to fifteen breathing cycles, switch to massaging the point with circling pressure. Then massage Large Intestine 4 on the other hand. If you want, you can also apply moxibustion to this point.

> **Caution**
>
> Please note that Large Intestine 4 must not be massaged during pregnancy!

Small Intestine 3—Back Ravine (Figures 4 and 5)

How to locate the point: When the hand is folded loosely into a fist, this point is located at the edge of the hand, at the end of the skin fold over the pinkie finger's metacarpal bone.

How to apply pressure to the point: Small Intestine 3 can be treated with your partner either sitting up or lying down. If you are massaging yourself, it is easier to do so

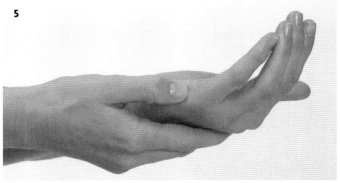

sitting up. Using the tip of your index finger or thumb, apply first steady and then circling pressure. Since this point tends to be very painful in the case of its respective ailments, you should always begin the massage using only light pressure.

Stomach 36—Leg Three Li (Three Lengths to the Foot) (Figures 1 and 2)

How to locate the point: Locate the triangular protrusion of the shin below the knee. Stomach 36 is at the level at which the protrusion turns into the front edge of the shinbone, 1 cun toward the outside of the leg.

How to apply pressure to the point: Begin by applying steady pressure on the point using the tip of your thumb. Then apply circling pressure, first clockwise and then counterclockwise. The treatment of the point should take a total of two to three minutes, after which you should switch to the point on the other leg. If you wish, you can also apply a traditional heat treatment to this point. Use one of the specific aids for moxibustion for this purpose: the moxa cigar, moxa pin, or loose mugwort in a moxa box. The duration of moxibustion should be two to three minutes per point. If your partner experiences an unpleasant heat sensation before the end of this time period, reduce the duration of the warmth treatment.

Urinary Bladder 60—Kunlun Mountains (Figures 3 and 4)

How to locate the point: Kunlun Mountains is located between the highest rise of the outside ankle and the Achilles tendon.

How to apply pressure to the point: Place the tip of your thumb on Urinary Bladder 60, and support the rest of the foot by placing the other fingers of the same hand under the heel. Apply first steady and then circling pressure for two to three minutes, then switch to Urinary Bladder 60 on the other foot. You can also apply moxibustion to this point. Depending on the heat sensitivity of your partner, such a treatment can last up to two to three minutes on each point. Adjust the duration of this treatment based on the wishes of your partner.

> **Caution**
> Please note that Urinary Bladder 60 must not be massaged—or have moxibustion applied to it—during pregnancy!

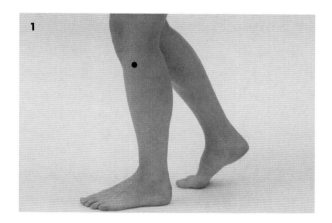

Stomach 36 is located below and to the side of the knee.

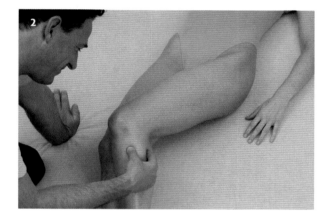

Use your thumb to massage Stomach 36, applying first steady and then circling pressure.

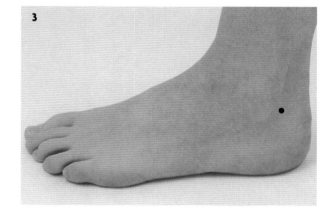

Kunlun Mountains is located between the highest rise on the outside of the ankle and the Achilles tendon.

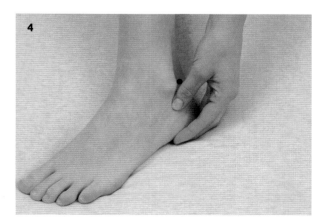

Massage the point with your thumb, applying steady and circling pressure just behind the ankle bone.

Fatigue

Every one of us has some experience with feelings of fatigue that occur from time to time. We know fatigue to be an alarm signal from the body after excessive physical or mental exertion, as well as an accompanying symptom of frequent illnesses such as infections, and a consequence of psychological illnesses such as depression. It can also be a symptom of severe illnesses such as cancer.

Fatigue can also be a side effect of certain medications and of combinations of medications, including those used to treat cardiovascular problems and allergies as well as sleep disorders. Another factor contributing to fatigue is continuous exposure to toxins and heavy metals in our surroundings, at work and at home.

Among an increasing share of the population, however, fatigue is occurring so frequently and severely and with such a long duration that physicians refer to it as an illness in itself, the so-called chronic fatigue syndrome ("burnout syndrome"). Among sufferers, this syndrome can lead to a serious decrease in the quality of life and ability to perform, up to the point where even small demands of everyday life can no longer be taken care of.

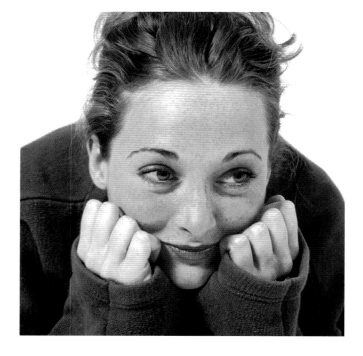

States of fatigue are reactions of the body to physical or psychological strain that should be taken seriously.

Many people suffering from chronic fatigue syndrome have an imbalance in the chemical substances of their brain, although organic causes do not exist in all sufferers. For some patients, links to long and excessive strain, for example stress at the workplace, is present, although this is not true for all. In the end, the causes for chronic fatigue syndrome have not yet been comprehensively identified.

What You Can Do

To help your health care provider identify the best course of treatment, you can think about the following: When did you start noticing a decrease in your ability to handle pressure? What were your life circumstances at that point in time? Could certain events be causes for the onset, for example professional or personal stress of a long duration, increased stress and worry, a family crisis, prolonged illness, sleeping problems, medication, renovations at home, or a move? How have your symptoms progressed—did they slowly worsen, have they remained steady, or do they occur sporadically?

Be sure to get enough sleep and exercise and to eat regular meals. A balanced sleep-waking rhythm is important for the regeneration of both body and mind. Without it, fatigue is an alarm signal from your body that you should be taking very seriously. Your diet can also increase the resilience of your body. Avoid fatty foods and cold foods such as ice cream and cold drinks. Reduce the consumption of alcohol and nicotine so as not to place unnecessary stress on your body. Also reduce your consumption of coffee. Although coffee is commonly believed to be a stimulating drink, in the long run, like a drug, it weighs the body down and suppresses natural regeneration phases. Instead, drink milder green tea as a "waking drink" or stimulating herbal teas such as lemongrass or lemon verbena.

If you must face stressful situations increasingly often, it may also be useful to learn specific relaxation techniques such as autogenic training or progressive muscle relaxation.

How Can Acupressure Help?

Acute fatigue can be positively influenced through acupressure. If, however, you are suffering from frequent or even constant exhaustion, you should not confine yourself to acupressure but should also consult with a qualified health care practitioner to identify the causes and work to address them.

Stomach 36—Leg Three Li (Three Lengths to the Foot) (Figures 1 and 2)

How to locate the point: Locate the triangular protrusion of the shinbone below the knee. Stomach 36 is at the level at which the protrusion turns into the front edge of the shinbone, 1 cun toward the outside of the leg.

How to apply pressure to the point: Begin by applying steady pressure to the point using the tip of your thumb. Then apply circling pressure, first clockwise and then counterclockwise. The treatment of this point should take about two to three minutes altogether. Then massage the point on the other leg in the same manner.

Pericardium 6—Inner Pass (Figures 3 and 4)

How to locate the point: This point is located 2 cun above the inside fold of the wrist, between the tendons in the middle of the inside of the arm.

How to apply pressure to the point: Place the tip of your thumb or index finger on the point and massage it for two to three minutes with steady and then circling pressure, first clockwise and then counterclockwise. Then massage the point on the other arm in the same manner.

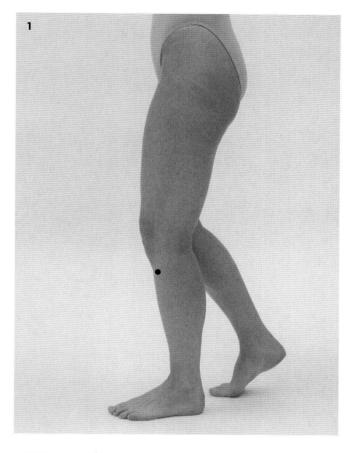

Stomach 36 is located to the side of and below the knee.

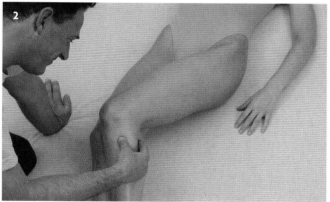

Use the tip of your thumb to massage Stomach 36.

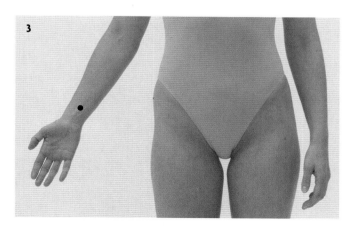

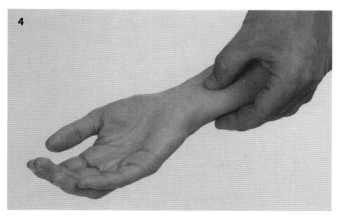

Left: Pericardium 6 is located on the inside of the lower arm.

Right: Pericardium 6 is massaged using the tweezers grip.

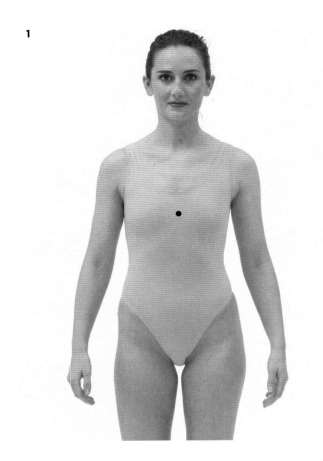

1

Conception Vessel 17—Chest Center (Figures 1 and 2)

How to locate the point: Chest Center is located on the sternum at the level of the nipples, on the middle axis of the body. The point can also be located by counting the ribs, beginning from the collarbone: it is on the middle of the chest at the level of the gap between the fourth and fifth ribs.

How to apply pressure to the point: Massage Conception Vessel 17 with the tip of your index finger, applying first steady and then circling pressure for one to two minutes each. It is possible that the treatment of this point will resolve psychological tensions; in fact, your partner may begin to cry, which for him or her will likely cause a feeling of relief.

Spleen 6—Three Yin Intersection (Figures 3 and 4)

How to locate the point: Three Yin Intersection is located one hand width, or 3 cun, above the highest point of the inside ankle on the back edge of the shinbone. This point is usually very sensitive to pressure.

How to apply pressure to the point: First warm the feet by rubbing them. Then massage the point with your thumb, applying steady and then circling pressure, first clockwise and then counterclockwise, for one to two minutes each. Then massage the point on the other leg in the same way.

> **Caution**
> Spleen 6 can cause early contractions and thus must not be massaged during pregnancy!

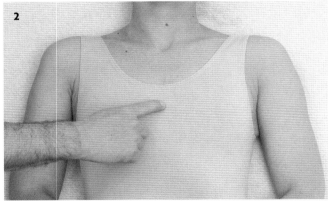

2

Massage
Conception
Vessel 17
carefully, using
the tip of your
index finger.

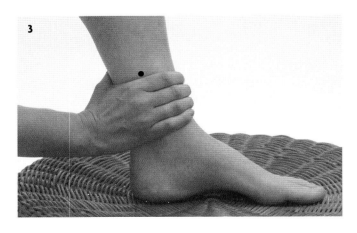

3

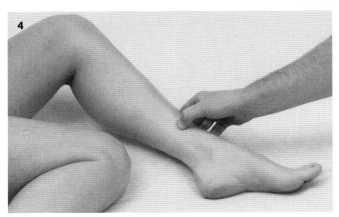

4

Left: Spleen 6
is located one
hand-width
above the inside
of the ankle.

Right: Massage
the point using
steady and
circling pressure
with the tip of
your thumb.

Acupressure to Treat Sleeping Problems, Headaches, and Fatigue

Sleeping Problems

Heart 7 is located on the inside of the wrist. Massage the point using steady and then circling pressure, first clockwise and then counterclockwise.

Pericardium 6 is 2 cun above the wrist, between the two tendons in the middle of the inside of the arm. Massage the point on both arms using steady pressure and then circling pressure, first clockwise and then counterclockwise.

Heart 3 is located between the inside of the elbow and the protrusion of the upper arm bone. It is easiest to locate with the arm slightly bent. Massage the point using your thumb, applying first steady and then circling pressure for two to three minutes.

Liver 3 is located on the top of the foot in an indentation between the first and second metatarsal bones. Press the point as strongly as possible and then massage it gently with circular pressure, first clockwise and then counterclockwise, on both feet.

Headaches and Migraines

Gall Bladder 20 is located at the base of the back of the head, on either side of the body's middle axis and between the muscles of the neck. Massage the two points simultaneously using your thumbs, applying first steady and then circling pressure.

Gall Bladder 21 is located midway between the seventh cervical vertebra and the highest rise of the shoulder. Press it with steady and circling pressure and then knead the surrounding muscles.

Large Intestine 4 is located on the small muscle bulge that forms between your thumb and index finger when you press your thumb against your hand. Massage it on both hands with the tweezers grip, applying first steady and then circling pressure.

When the hand is folded loosely into a fist, Small Intestine 3 is located at the end of the skin fold beneath the pinkie metacarpal. Massage it with steady and circling pressure on both hands, but be careful since these points are frequently sensitive to pressure.

Below the knee you can feel the triangular protrusion of the shinbone. From here, point Stomach 36 is located 1 cun toward the outside of the leg. Massage it on both legs using first steady and then circling pressure.

Urinary Bladder 60 is located between the highest rise of the outside of the ankle and the Achilles tendon. Massage it on both legs using first steady and then circling pressure for one to two minutes.

Fatigue

Below the knee you can feel the triangular protrusion of the shinbone. From here, point Stomach 36 is located 1 cun toward the outside of the leg. Massage it on both legs using first steady and then circling pressure.

Pericardium 6 is 2 cun above the wrist, between the tendons on the inside of the arm. Massage it on both arms using first steady and then circling pressure.

Conception Vessel 17 is located at the level of the gap between the fourth and fifth ribs, directly on the body's middle axis. Massage it using first steady and then circling pressure for one to two minutes.

Spleen 6 is located one hand width above the highest rise of the inside of the ankle, on the back edge of the shinbone. Since this point is usually very sensitive to pressure, massage it on both legs carefully, using steady and then circling pressure, first clockwise and then counterclockwise.

Breathing Problems

The upper respiratory passages—nose, mouth, and trachea—are in constant contact with causes of illnesses such as viruses or bacteria, which we ingest in the air we breathe. For this reason many infectious diseases begin with symptoms in the respiratory passages, such as a stuffy or runny nose, sore throat, and cough.

Bronchitis and Bronchial Asthma

Bronchitis, an infection of the bronchi, is characterized by an initially dry cough that becomes productive after a few days, meaning the sufferer can cough up phlegm. Bronchitis is frequently accompanied by a light fever, headache, or pain behind the sternum during a coughing fit. If acute bronchitis does not heal within two weeks, it is wise to consult with your health care provider, because if bacteria attack the already weakened mucous membranes in the lungs, pneumonia could ensue.

Chronic bronchitis refers to a bronchial infection that is almost steady, occurring for at least three months during two consecutive years. The most frequent cause of chronic bronchitis is smoking. Oftentimes, harmful substances from the environment such as dust and

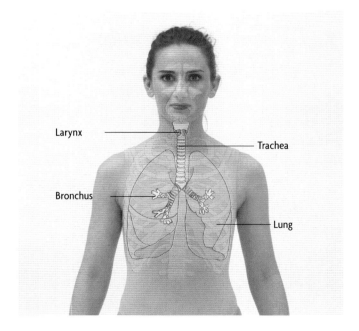

The larynx, trachea, lungs, and bronchi are all part of the respiratory passages.

Larynx

Trachea

Bronchus

Lung

exhaust fumes can also contribute to chronic bronchitis. Chronic bronchitis has become a common illness. It is treated primarily by prescribing medication to loosen the phlegm, making it easier to cough out the secretions. If the presence of bacteria is confirmed, treatment with antibiotics may be necessary.

Another illness that damages the mucous membranes of the bronchi is bronchial asthma. Damage of the mucous membranes in this case is accompanied by the increased production of phlegm and a sporadic constriction of the bronchi, leading sufferers to repeatedly suffer from shortness of breath. Causes of asthma are manifold, ranging from physical exertion and infections of the respiratory passages to allergies. About half of all asthma patients are children under the age of ten. Medical treatment is absolutely necessary for asthma.

In treating asthma, medication is divided into "as needed" medication, to be taken to end an asthma attack, and constant medication, to be taken regularly to reduce the frequency of attacks. Medication usually serves to reduce infections and to temporarily dilate the respiratory passages.

What You Can Do

If you are suffering from bronchitis, drink a lot of fluids to loosen the phlegm. Plant-based substances such as menthol, eucalyptus, and thyme encourage the expulsion of loosened phlegm and are especially good for children. Massage with various preparations of essential oils can support treatment to stop infection and loosen phlegm. For asthma sufferers it is very important to avoid products that cause allergic reactions. Of course, to avoid such products asthmatics would need to know that they were allergic to them. Finally, acupressure and special breathing techniques can help sufferers to regain more control over their breathing.

How Can Acupressure Help?

To treat problems with the respiratory passages, acupressure of certain points can alleviate coughing, calm the irritated bronchial mucous membranes, lower fever, and loosen tense respiratory muscles.

In addition, the massage of individual points such as Stomach 36 stimulates the immune system and thus strengthens the body's ability to fend off infections. Other points that can be used to treat breathing problems are located on the Lung meridian.

Lung 1—Central Treasury (Figures 1 and 2)

How to locate the point: Central Treasury is located 6 cun to the side of the middle axis, in a small indentation 1 cun beneath the collarbone. It can be especially sensitive in cases of ailments of the respiratory passages. Thus, be sure to begin the massage using gentle pressure.

How to apply pressure to the point: Apply steady pressure in sync with your partner's breathing for one minute, slightly increasing pressure as your partner exhales and decreasing pressure as he or she inhales. Then apply moderately strong circular pressure with your index finger, first clockwise and then counterclockwise. Massage the point for two to three minutes altogether, then switch to the point on the other side of the body.

Lung 9—Great Abyss (Figures 3 and 4)

How to locate the point: Great Abyss is located on the end of the inner fold of the wrist, at the base of the thumb.

How to apply pressure to the point: Apply steady pressure to Lung 9 for one to two minutes. Then apply circling pressure, first clockwise and then counterclockwise. Massage the point on the other wrist in the same way.

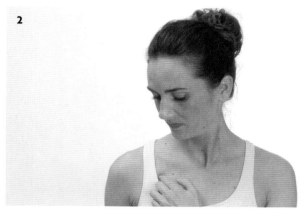

Lung 1 is located 6 cun to the side of the middle axis and 1 cun beneath the collarbone.

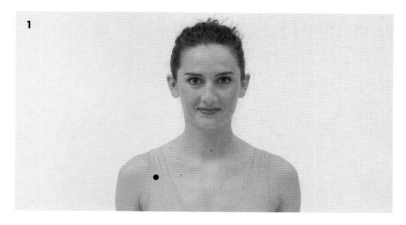

Lung 1 is well suited for self-massage because of its location.

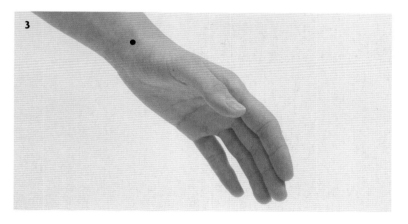

Lung 9 is located on the thumb side of the inside fold of the wrist.

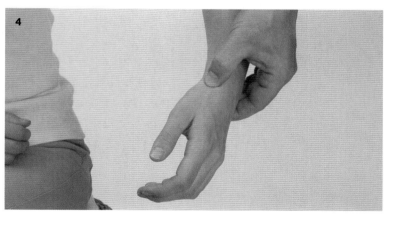

Massage the point using steady and circling pressure with the tweezers grip.

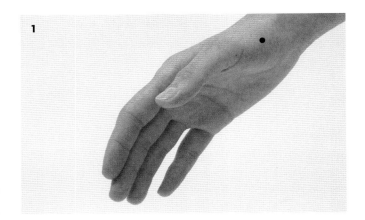

Lung 10 is located below the base joint of the thumb.

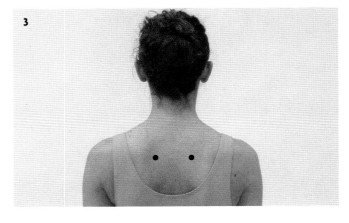

Massage the point using the tweezers grip with steady and circling pressure.

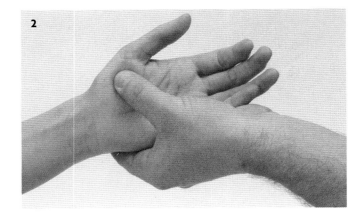

The two points of Urinary Bladder 13 are located on each side of the body's middle axis.

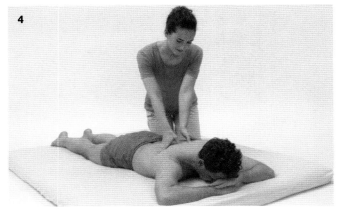

Left: Let your partner massage you.

Right: You can also massage these points using tennis balls.

Lung 10—Fish Border (Figures 1 and 2)

How to locate the point: This point is located at the midpoint of the bone that runs along the fleshy mound below the thumb, at the point where the skin from the back of the hand and the palm meet. Chinese medicine refers to this area as the "border between red and white skin."

How to apply pressure to the point: Place the tip of your thumb on the point and apply first steady and then circling pressure for a total of two to three minutes. Massage the point on the other side in the same way.

Urinary Bladder 13—Lung Shu (Figures 3–5)

The point Urinary Bladder 13, despite being located on the Urinary bladder meridian, also has a particular influence on the Lung.

How to locate the point: Locate the seventh cervical vertebra; this is the one that protrudes the most when you bend your head slightly forward. From here, count down three vertebrae and then locate the gap between the third and fourth vertebrae. Lung Shu is at the level of this gap, 1.5 cun to either side of the spine.

How to apply pressure to the point: Massage both of the Urinary Bladder 13 points using first steady and then circling pressure. The massage should last two to three minutes altogether. Another possibility for self-massage of this point is to use two tennis balls. Place one under each of the two points, and lie on the balls for two to three minutes.

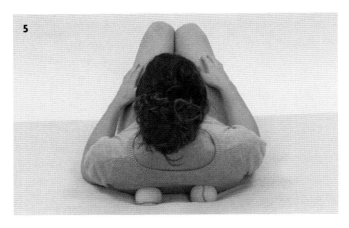

Yintang—Hall of Seal (Figures 1 and 2)

This point can be included in the massage if the frontal sinus is affected at the same time.

How to locate the point: The extra point Yintang is located on the middle axis of the face exactly between the two eyebrows.

How to apply pressure to the point: First apply steady pressure to the point. Since Yintang is located in a very sensitive part of the head, begin by applying light pressure and let yourself be guided by your partner's sensitivity to pressure. Then massage the point for one to two minutes with small circling movements, first clockwise and then counterclockwise.

Gall Bladder 20—Wind Pool (Figures 3 and 4)

How to locate the point: Gall Bladder 20 or Wind Pool is located at the base of the back of the head, on both sides of the middle axis next to the muscles that can be felt there.

How to apply pressure to the point: Massage Gall Bladder 20 on both sides at the same time, using the tips of your thumbs and applying steady pressure and then circling pressure, first clockwise and then counterclockwise, for one to two minutes each. In addition to regular pressure massage you can also apply a heat treatment to this point using the specific aids of moxibustion. However, since the two points are located at the beginning of the hairline on the back of the head, care should be taken when applying moxibustion.

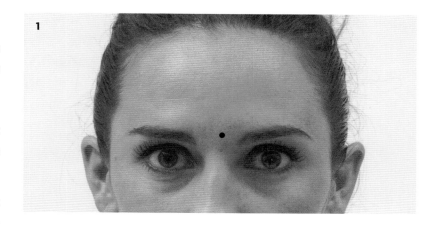

Extra point Yintang is located exactly between the eyebrows.

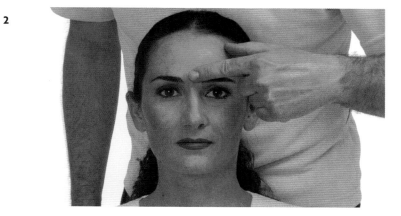

Massage the point using the tip of your index finger and applying steady and circling pressure.

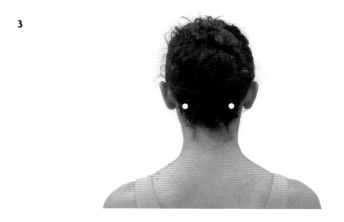

At the base of the back of the head are the two points of Gall Bladder 20.

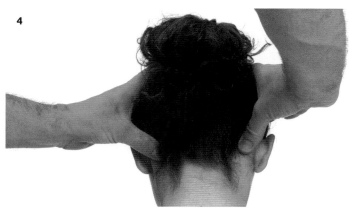

Massage both points simultaneously using your thumbs.

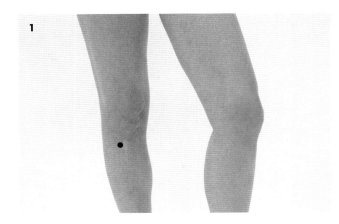

Stomach 36 is located below the knee on the side of the leg.

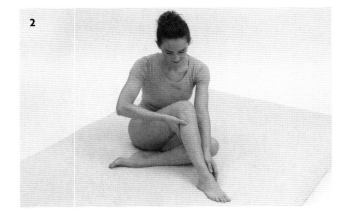

Because of its location, Stomach 36 is well suited for self-massage.

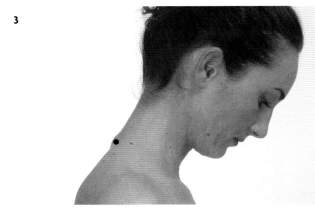

Bend your head forward to find Governor Vessel 14, located just below the dorsal process of the lowest cervical vertebra.

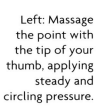

Left: Massage the point with the tip of your thumb, applying steady and circling pressure.

Right: Then rub across the point with the palm of your hand.

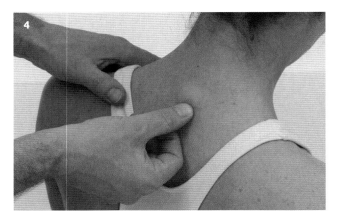

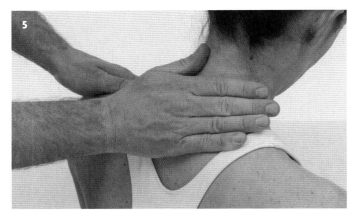

Stomach 36—Leg Three Li (Three Lengths to the Foot) (Figures 1 and 2)

How to locate the point: Locate the triangular protrusion of the shinbone below the knee. Stomach 36 is at the level at which the protrusion turns into the front edge of the shinbone, 1 cun toward the outside of the legs.

How to apply pressure to the point: Begin by applying strong and steady pressure to the point using the tip of your thumb or your index or middle finger. Then apply circling pressure, first clockwise and then counterclockwise, for one minute in each direction. Conclude by loosely rubbing the outside of the calf with your palm for about two minutes, applying only light pressure. Then switch to the other leg and repeat the massage on the point there.

Governor Vessel 14—Great Hammer (Figures 3–5)

How to locate the point: Governor Vessel 14 is located on the spine between the lowest cervical vertebra and the uppermost thoracic vertebra. Place your fingertips between the shoulders on the cervical vertebrae and bend your head slightly forward to facilitate locating the points. The dorsal process of the lowest cervical vertebra will protrude slightly more in this position, and in the gap below this dorsal process is the Governor Vessel 14.

How to apply pressure to the point: Begin by applying steady pressure to the point using the tip of your thumb. Then apply circling pressure, first clockwise and then counterclockwise, for one minute in each direction. Then use your palm to rub the skin around Governor Vessel 14 for about three minutes.

Sinus Ailments

The paranasal sinuses (properly known as the frontal, maxillary, ethmoidal, and sphenoidal sinuses) are air-filled cavities in the cranial bones that connect to the nasal cavity via small openings. They are lined with the same mucous membranes found in the nose.

During the course of an infection, for example a cold, the mucous membranes in the paranasal sinuses can swell up and produce an increased amount of secretions. This can lead to an infection of the paranasal sinuses called sinusitis.

Since the sinus openings into the nasal cavity are constricted because of the swollen mucous membranes, secretions cannot flow easily and the openings become clogged up. This creates a blunt pressure pain in the middle of the forehead, above the cheekbones and the eye area, which can sometimes be perceived as a pulsing pain. Strong headaches and fever can accompany this inflammation.

What You Can Do

To improve the ability of secretions to flow out in the case of a paranasal sinus infection, the swelling of the mucous membranes has to be reduced. Helpful treatments to reduce the swellling include over-the-counter nose drops, warmth applications using an infrared lamp, and steam inhalations, particularly when the steam is mixed with decongestant essential oils. One alternative to nose drops, which over time can damage the nose's mucous membranes, is to rinse the nose with salt solutions. Plant-based preparations (most often tinctures taken orally) made of verbena, gentian root, sorrel, elder petals, and primrose petals are effective in reducing swellings and infections and can also be given to children.

Traditional Chinese medicine sees functional relations between the mucous membranes of the sinuses and the intestines. Frequently recurring infections of the sinuses can thus indicate problems in the intestines. If you suspect that such a relation may be true in your case, it is best to consult a therapist schooled in traditional Chinese medicine. It is possible that an intestinal cleansing, accompanied by changes in your diet, may help alleviate your problems.

How Can Acupressure Help?

In the cases of sinus infections, acupressure works on several levels. For one, the infection can be influenced using points such as Large Intestine 4. The headaches that often accompany these infections can be alleviated through the massage of selected acupressure points. Moreover, the massage of points such as Large Intestine 20 can contribute to the thinning of mucus, enabling it to flow better and thus reducing the dull pressure pain in the eye area. However, keep in mind that you should consult a physician in the case of continued sinus problems.

Caution

Acute feverish infections in the frontal and maxillary sinuses are very serious and must be treated by a physician.

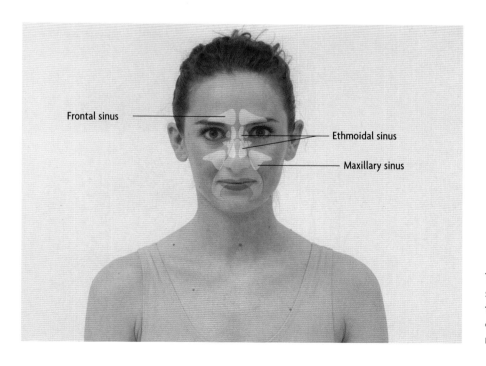

Frontal sinus — Ethmoidal sinus — Maxillary sinus

The paranasal sinuses include the frontal, ethmoidal, and maxillary sinuses.

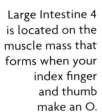

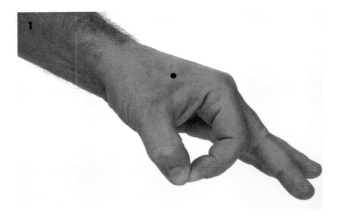

Large Intestine 4 is located on the muscle mass that forms when your index finger and thumb make an O.

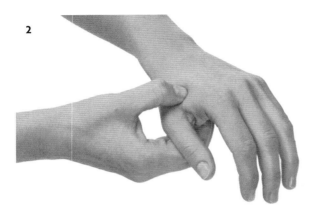

Massage the point using the tweezers grip . . .

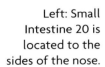

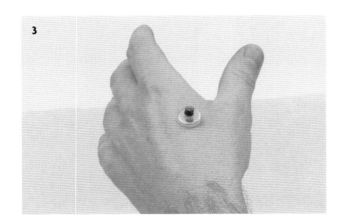

. . . and then carry out a moxibustion on it.

Left: Small Intestine 20 is located to the sides of the nose.

Right: Massage the two points one after the other or simultaneously.

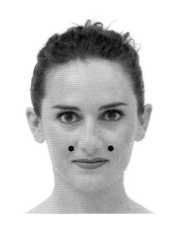

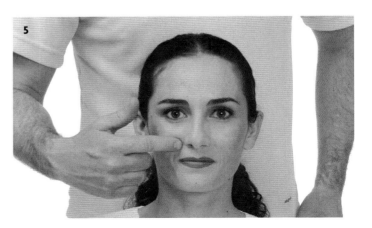

Large Intestine 4—Valley of Union (Figures 1–3)

How to locate the point: This point is easiest to locate when you make an O with your thumb and index finger, pressing the tips of the two fingers firmly against each other. This causes a small bulge of muscle to rise just above the web of skin between the index finger and thumb, on the back of the hand; this bulge marks the site of Large Intestine 4.

How to apply pressure to the point: First rub the thumb side of the hand for one to two minutes, until the skin is warm. Then use your thumb to apply steady pressure to Large Intestine 4 for about two minutes. Follow this with small circling movements on the point, using moderately strong pressure. Then massage the point on the other hand in the same way. If you want, you can also apply moxibustion to the points on the two hands. For this, you can either use a moxa pin (as illustrated in the photo) or a moxa cigar.

> **Caution**
> Do not massage Large Intestine 4 during pregnancy.

Large Intestine 20—Welcome Fragrance (Figures 4 and 5)

How to locate the point: Large Intestine 20 is located on both sides of the nose, at the beginning of the fold in the skin that runs from the nose to the edge of the mouth.

How to apply pressure to the point: You can treat the two Large Intestine 20 points (one on each side of the nose) either at the same time or one after the other, using the tips of your index fingers. Since this is a rather sensitive spot, be sure to find the appropriate amount of pressure. Massage the point with steady pressure and then circling pressure, first clockwise and then counterclockwise, for about one minute.

Yintang—Hall of Seal (Figures 1 and 2)

How to locate the point: Hall of Seal is located exactly between the eyebrows (see the black point in illustration 1).

How to apply pressure to the point: Using your index finger, apply steady pressure to the point for about one minute, and then massage it for another minute using circling pressure, first clockwise, then counterclockwise.

Urinary Bladder 2—Bamboo Gathering (Figures 1 and 3)

How to locate the point: Urinary Bladder 2 is located on the inside edge of the eyebrows (see the white points in illustration 1).

How to apply pressure to the point: Place the tips of your index fingers on each of the Urinary Bladder 2 points. Apply steady and then circling pressure for one to two minutes each. Then move your index fingers slightly further out from the midline (at most 1 cm) before returning back to the point.

Urinary Bladder 10—Celestial Pillar (Figures 4 and 5)

How to locate the point: Urinary Bladder 10 is located 1.5 cun to the side of the middle axis, in an indentation just under the bony edge of the back of the head.

How to apply pressure to the point: Massage the two points of Urinary Bladder 10 either simultaneously or one after the other. Apply steady and circling pressure on the points for one to two minutes each.

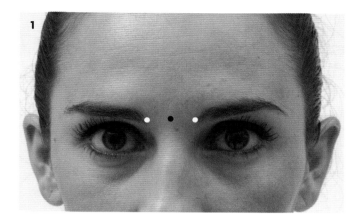

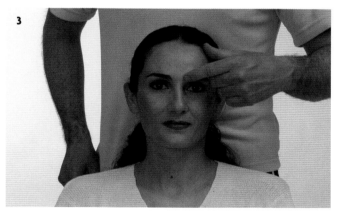

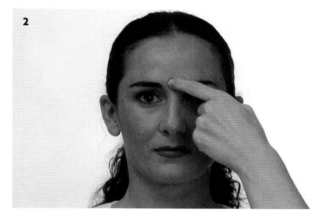

The extra point Yintang is located between the eyebrows, while the points of Urinary Bladder 2 are located at the inside edge of the eyebrows.

Hall of Seals is well suited for self-massage.

Use your index finger to massage Urinary Bladder 2.

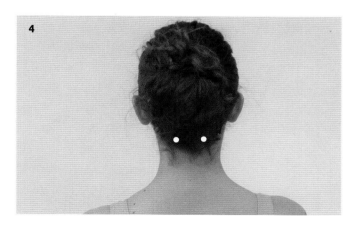

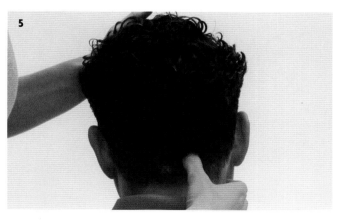

Left: Urinary Bladder 10 is located at the bony edge on the back of the head.

Right: Massage Urinary Bladder 10 using the tip of your thumb.

Colds and the Flu

Colds and flus occur most frequently during the wet and cold winter months. Aside from weakness in an individual's immune system, external factors such as cold, wetness, and draft play an important role in supporting an infection. First indications of a cold are usually a scratch in the throat or itch in the nose. This is followed by a runny or stuffy nose, cough, headaches, and joint pains. If a fever accompanies these symptoms, we refer to the infection as a flu. This infection is not the same as true influenza, a viral infection that recurs in epidemics and can have life-threatening consequences.

Note

Strengthen your immune system early, before the onset of the wet and cold seasons, through measures such as:

- Enjoying sauna sessions
- Switching between hot and cold water during the shower
- Eating a diet rich in vitamins and minerals

Plant-based substances such as echinacea also strengthen the immune system and can even be taken at the onset of a cold.

What You Can Do

In the case of a normal cold free of complications, you do not necessarily need to take any medication at all. As the old saying goes, a cold treated with medicine lasts one week—and without medicine seven days. Nonetheless, you can alleviate the symptoms of a cold by using nose drops or a spray to reduce the swelling of the mucous membranes twice a day. Note that you should discontinue use of this after one week at the most, since you otherwise run the danger of damaging the nose's mucous membranes. An alternative to nose drops with fewer side effects are steam inhalations with essential oils such as eucalyptus and melissa. For a dry cough, substances that encourage the thinning and expulsion of mucus are the first choice. Among plant-based preparations, thyme has an excellent mucus-releasing effect.

It is very important that you drink plenty of liquids during a cold, so that secretions can remain fluid. Moreover, especially for children, warm chest wraps and herbal teas can alleviate symptoms. If the cold is accompanied by a feeling of fatigue or increased sensitivity to cold, the patient should stay in bed. If fever occurs, you should consult a physician after at most two days.

How Can Acupressure Help?

Acupressure reduces the symptoms of a cold, such as headache, fever, and cough. At the same time, acupressure can boost the immune system via points such as Stomach 36. To counter a cold or flu and to positively influence recovery, the following points can be massaged: Yintang, Large Intestine 4 and 20, Governor Vessel 14, and Lung 7 and 9. Moreover, you can rub the skin over

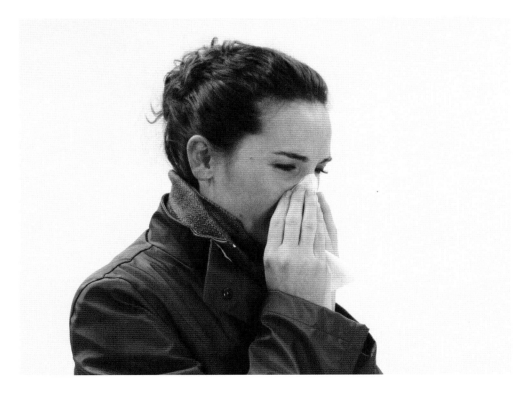

Especially in the cold and wet times of the year, you run the risk of catching a cold.

the forehead. If you yourself are suffering from a cold, you should ask your partner to carry out the massage so that you can relax.

Yintang—Hall of Seal (Figures 1 and 2)

How to locate the point: The extra point Yintang is located exactly between the eyebrows.

How to apply pressure to the point: With the tip of your index finger, apply steady pressure to Yintang for one to two minutes. Since the point is located in a very sensitive area of the head, you should begin by applying light pressure, adjusting your pressure based on your partner's sensitivities. Follow this by applying circling pressure, first clockwise and then counterclockwise, for one to two minutes. If you are experienced with moxibustion, you can apply a warmth treatment to the extra point. Use only the specific aids of moxibustion (see page 65) on this sensitive point.

Large Intestine 20—Welcome Fragrance (Figures 3 and 4)

How to locate the point: This point is located on both sides of the nose, at the beginning of the fold in the skin that runs from the nose to the edge of the mouth.

How to apply pressure to the point: You can massage the two Large Intestine 20 points at the same time or one after the other. Make sure to find the right amount of pressure to use on this sensitive point, adjusting your pressure based on your partner's sensitivities. Begin massaging Large Intestine 20 with steady pressure for one to two minutes. Then apply circling pressure for one to two minutes, first clockwise and then counterclockwise.

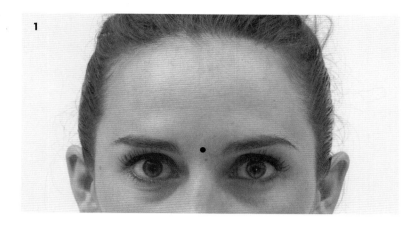

The extra point Yintang is located exactly between the eyebrows.

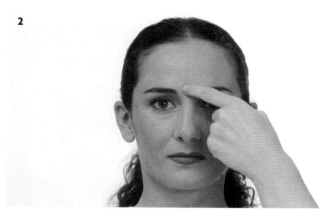

Because of its location, this point is well suited for self-massage.

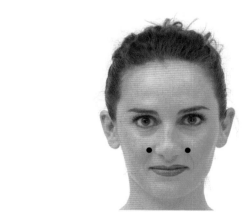

Large Intestine 20 is located next to the nose.

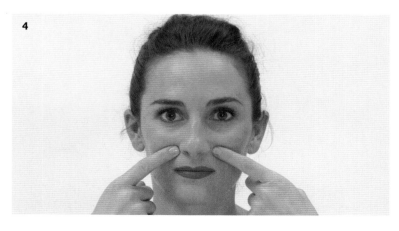

You can massage both points simultaneously using the tips of your index fingers.

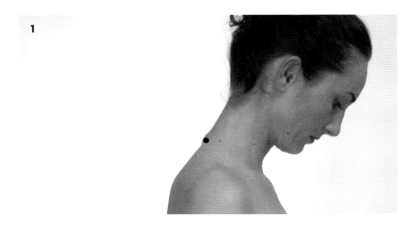

Bend your head forward . . .

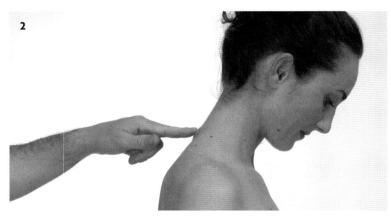

. . . and locate Governor Vessel 14 just below the dorsal process of the lowest cervical vertebra.

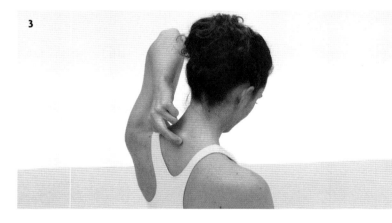

You can massage Governor Vessel 14 on yourself, placing your index and middle fingers on top of each other.

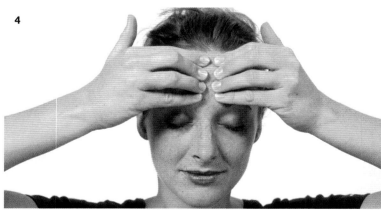

Rub your fingertips along your forehead from the middle axis to the temples.

Governor Vessel 14—Great Hammer (Figures 1–3)

How to locate the point: Governor Vessel 14 is located on the spine, between the lowest cervical vertebra and the topmost thoracic vertebra. Place your fingertips between the shoulders on the spine and have your partner bend his or her head slightly forward to help in locating this point. With the head bent forward, the dorsal process of the lower cervical vertebra will protrude slightly; Great Hammer is just below this dorsal process.

How to apply pressure to the point: Begin acupressure of Governor Vessel 14 using steady pressure, followed by circling pressure, first clockwise and then counterclockwise, for one minute each. Then use your palm to strongly rub the skin surrounding Governor Vessel 14 for about three minutes. If you are massaging a partner, you can also apply moxibustion to this point. Use only the specific aids of moxibustion on this part of the body.

Rubbing the Skin above the Forehead (Figure 4)

Because colds and flus are often accompanied by pain in the forehead area, it is often useful to massage the forehead to relieve these ailments. However, in doing so, be sure to let yourself be guided by the sensitivity of your partner, since the forehead is often very sensitive to pressure in these cases.

Place your fingertips across from each other on the forehead on the left and right sides of the middle axis, above the eyebrows. From there, with light and pleasant pressure, stroke the skin out toward the temples. Then return your fingertips to the middle axis of the head, but start at a slightly higher point than before, and again move your fingers to stroke the skin toward the temples. In this way, move up from the eyebrows to the hairline above the forehead. Depending on your partner's sensitivity, the duration of the massage should be two to three minutes.

Lung 7—Broken Sequence (Figure 1)

How to locate the point: The seventh point of the Lung meridian is located on the inside of the lower arm, 1.5 cun above the inside fold of the wrist, in a small indentation on the side of the thumb.

How to apply pressure to the point: Place the tip of your thumb on Lung 7. Apply strong, steady pressure for two to three minutes, adjusting your pressure as needed based on your partner's preferences. Then apply circling pressure to the point for one to two minutes, first clockwise and then counterclockwise. Now switch to the other hand to massage Lung 7 there in the same way. Aside from traditional pressure application, you can also apply a warmth treatment to these points, using the aids for moxibustion made from mugwort (see page 65).

Lung 9—Great Abyss (Figures 2 and 3)

How to locate the point: The ninth point of the Lung meridian is located on the inside of the wrist crease, on the thumb side of the wrist.

How to apply pressure to the point: Massage this point in the same manner described for Lung 7 above. Using the tip of your thumb or index finger, apply steady pressure on the point. Then apply circling pressure, first clockwise and then counterclockwise. Finally, massage Lung 9 on the other hand in the same manner. You can apply moxibustion on this point too, using either a moxa cigar, a moxa pin, or loose mugwort in a moxa box.

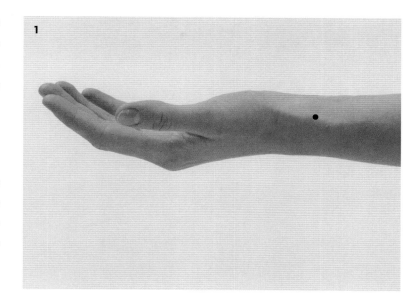

Lung 7 is located in the small indentation on the thumb side of the lower arm.

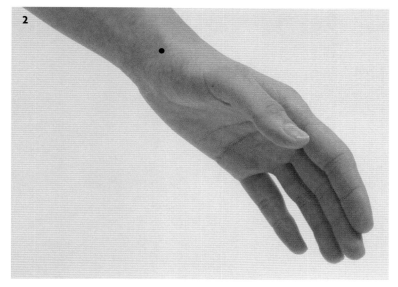

Lung 9 is located 1.5 cun toward the hand from Lung 7.

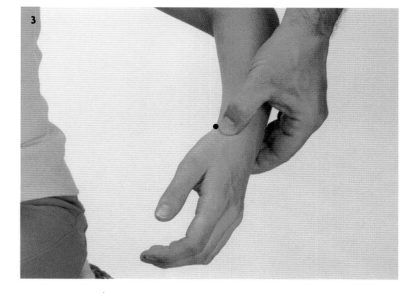

Use the tip of your thumb to massage this point.

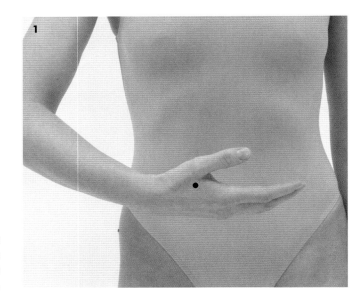

Locate Large Intestine 4 on the muscle bulge . . .

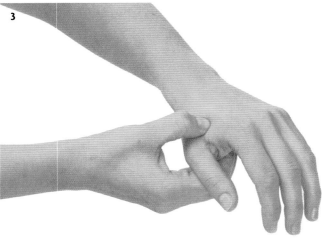

. . . that forms when the thumb and index finger form an O.

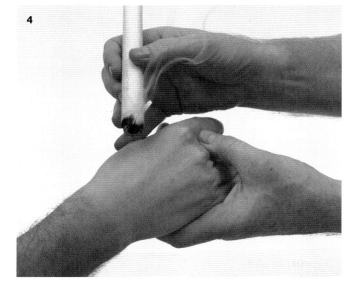

Left: Massage the point using the tweezers grip.

Right: You can also apply moxibustion to this point.

Large Intestine 4—Valley of Union (Figures 1–4)

How to locate the point: This point is easiest to locate when you make an O with your thumb and index finger, pressing the tips of the two fingers firmly against each other. This causes a small bulge of muscle to rise just above the web of skin between the index finger and thumb, on the back of the hand; this bulge marks the site of Large Intestine 4.

How to apply pressure to the point: Before massaging this point, warm the hand by rubbing it from its base to the index finger for one to two minutes. The skin may turn slightly red as it warms from the rubbing; this is no cause for worry. With the tip of your thumb, apply relatively strong steady pressure for two minutes. Then apply circling pressure for one to two minutes. Then treat the point on the other hand in the same way: first rub the hand and then massage Valley of Union. If you wish, you can also apply a traditional Chinese warmth treatment to these points. Use only the specific aids for moxibustion, meaning the mugwort in the form of a cigar or pin or loose in the moxa box.

Caution
Do not massage Large Intestine 4 during pregnancy!

Acupressure to Treat Breathing Problems

Bronchitis and Bronchial Asthma

Lung 1 is located 6 cun to the side of the body's middle axis near the shoulder. Massage it on both sides using first steady and then circling pressure for two to three minutes.

Lung 9 is located on the inside of the wrist, on the crease below the ball of the thumb. Massage it on both hands using first steady and then circling pressure.

Lung 10 is located below the base of the thumb joint. Massage it on both hands using first steady and then circling pressure for two to three minutes.

Urinary Bladder 13 is located 1.5 cun to the side of the middle axis, at the level of the gap between the third and fourth vertebrae. Massage it on either side with your thumbs or with tennis balls for about two minutes.

The extra point Yintang is located exactly between the eyebrows. Massage it using first steady and then circling pressure.

Gall Bladder 20 is located at the base of the back of the head, next to the large neck muscles. Massage it on both sides using first steady and then circling pressure with your thumbs.

Stomach 36 is located 3 cun below the indentation of the knee on the outside of the knee. Massage it on both legs using first steady and then circling pressure; follow up by rubbing it with your palm.

Governor Vessel 14 is located between the lowest cervical vertebra and uppermost thoracic vertebra. Massage it using first steady and then circling pressure; follow up by rubbing it.

Sinus Problems

Large Intestine 4 is located on the muscle bulge that forms between the thumb and index finger when they form an O. Massage it using first steady and then circling pressure on both hands.

Large Intestine 20 is located next to the nose. Massage it on both sides using first steady and then circling pressure.

The extra point Yintang is exactly between the eyebrows. Massage it using steady and then circling pressure, first clockwise and then counterclockwise.

Urinary Bladder 2 is located at the inside edge of the eyebrows. Massage it on both sides using first steady and then circling pressure.

Urinary Bladder 10 is located below the base of the back of the head. Massage it on both sides using first steady and then circling pressure.

Colds and the Flu

The extra point Yintang is located exactly between the eyebrows. Massage it using first steady and then circling pressure for two to three minutes.

Large Intestine 20 is located on both sides of the nose. Massage it on both sides using first steady and then circling pressure.

Governor Vessel 14 is located between the lowest cervical vertebra and the uppermost thoracic vertebra. Massage it using first steady and then circling pressure; follow up by rubbing it.

Place your fingertips along the middle axis of the forehead, above the eyebrows. From here, stroke outward with light pressure to the temples. Repeat as you work your way up to the hairline.

Lung 7 is located on the thumb side of the arm, 1.5 cun up from the wrist. Massage it on both arms using steady and then circling pressure, first clockwise, then counterclockwise.

Lung 9 is located on the inside crease of the wrist, below the ball of the thumb. Massage it using first steady and then circling pressure.

Large Intestine 4 is located on the muscle bulge that forms between the thumb and index finger when they form an O. Massage it on both hands using first steady and then circling pressure.

Problems in the Urogenital System

The urogenital system includes the urinary tract, the kidneys, the ureter, the bladder, the urethra, and the reproductive organs. Common health issues in this area include painful, recurring urinary tract infections and, among women, menstruation problems. Acupressure is suitable as a gentle, supportive complementary therapy in the treatment of these conditions.

Menstrual Problems and Premenstrual Syndrome

Menstrual problems are relatively common and can in most cases be positively influenced by herbal treatments. These problems include pain during menstruation and abnormally profuse, abnormally long, or sporadic menstrual flow. Causes include hormonal irregularities or

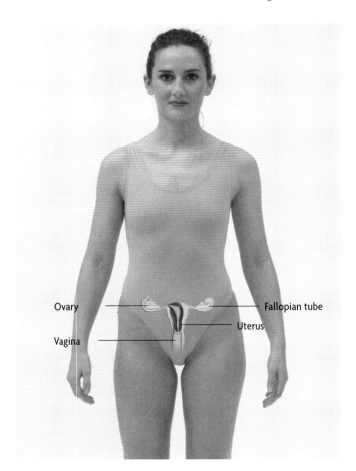

Ovary
Fallopian tube
Uterus
Vagina

Changes in the structure of the mucous membranes of the uterus lead to menstruation of different strengths.

organic changes such as benign tumors or infections in the uterus. Emotional states often vary with hormonal levels and can cause difficulties during the menstrual cycle.

The complete lack of menstruation is referred to as amenorrhea. This condition is normal in times of change, such as during puberty or menopause, after childbirth, or just after you have stopped taking birth control pills. The most common reason for the lack of menstruation is pregnancy. But amenorrhea can also be an indication of problems with metabolism, such as diabetes or a thyroid ailment, or a functional problem of the reproductive organs.

Another very common menstrual complaint is premenstrual syndrome (PMS). This syndrome is characterized by a collection of different symptoms and affects many women two to ten days before menstruation. Sufferers complain of headaches, difficulty sleeping, food cravings, constipation, depression, anxiety, and nervousness as well as water retention in the chest that often causes a pulling pain. Usually these problems disappear with the onset of menstruation.

What You Can Do

If you experience a problem with your menstruation, keep a menstruation calendar that records the timing, duration, and strength of your menstural flow, and show this to your physician. If no organic changes can be identified as the cause, try taking plant-based preparations to restore balance in the hormonal system. Preparations made from borage, lady's mantle, monk's pepper tree, valerian, and silverweed are especially well suited for this, as they have a balancing effect on hormones and overall relaxing effects.

Baths and footbaths are also helpful for well-being and relaxation. For this, begin with lukewarm water in a suitable vessel, and gradually add hot water during the bath until you have reached a pleasant temperature. A balanced diet that is not too high in fats and salt is also important. Finally, try to take more time for yourself and to pay attention to your own needs.

How Can Acupressure Help?

Acupressure on the points discussed below can reduce pain during menstruation and contribute to physical and psychological relaxation. Acupressure can also help normalize menstruation. For these purposes the points Stomach 28 to 30, Stomach 36, and Spleen 6 are frequently used. Also helpful is massage of the abdomen and the sacrum region. This massage is especially pleasurable and relaxing when given by a partner, although self-treatment is also possible.

Massaging the Abdomen

Lie down on your back in a comfortable position. To make sure that your abdomen is relaxed, place a rolled-up blanket or small pillow under your knees. Place your fingertips next to each other just below the base of the arch of the rib cage, exactly on the body's middle axis. Apply pressure while exhaling, maintain steady pressure for one to two minutes, and release pressure while inhaling. In this manner, massage the abdomen point by point, from top to bottom. This massage reaches important points of the Conception Vessel and thus has positive influence on menstrual problems. The two illustrations show the location of the points Conception Vessel 6, 7, 9, and 10 on the body's middle axis. The point Conception Vessel 8 is directly on the navel. It must not be massaged but can be treated with moxibustion (see page 65).

> **Caution**
>
> Do not carry out this massage during pregnancy, since it can cause the onset of contractions!

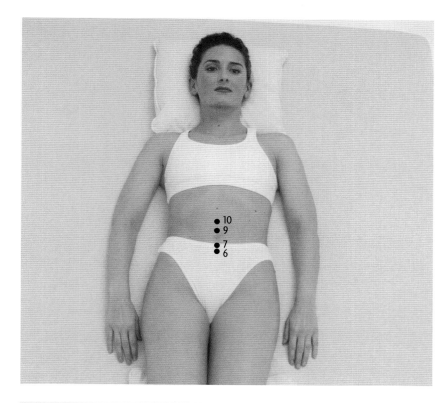

Locate the points on the body's middle axis below the arch of the rib cage.

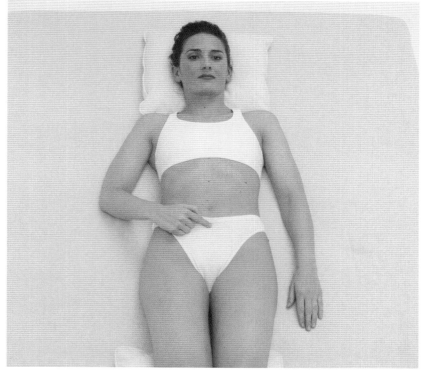

Massage the points from top to bottom.

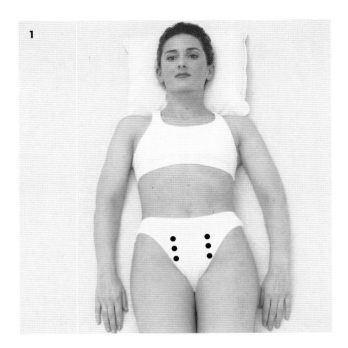

Stomach 28 to 30 are located on both sides of the body's middle axis.

Stomach 28 to 30 (Figures 1 and 2)

These three points are very effective for treating menstruation problems. Since they also have effects on the uterus, these points must not be massaged during pregnancy.

How to locate the points: Stomach 28 to 30 are located 2 cun from the middle axis of the body on either side. They are arranged one on top of the other: Stomach 28 is located 3 cun below the navel, Stomach 29 is 4 cun below the navel, and Stomach 30 is 5 cun below the navel.

How to apply pressure to the points: Press the three points on both sides one after the other with your fingertips. Apply first steady and then circling pressure for one to two minutes each.

> **Caution**
> These three points should not be massaged during pregnancy!

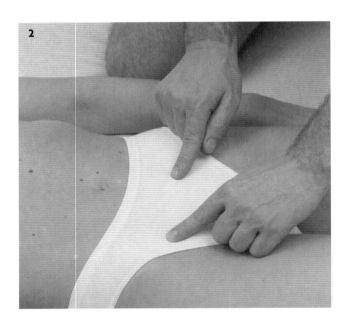

Massage the points on both sides of the middle axis simultaneously.

Rubbing the Sacrum (Figures 3 and 4)

Rubbing the sacrum region provides relief especially for problems in the abdomen, and especially if the massage is given by a partner. The sacrum region encompasses the points Urinary Bladder 27 to 35 (see page 92), which are very helpful in treating problems in the lower body. This rubbing massage will include and activate these points. If you are massaging yourself, lie down on your side; if you are massaging a partner, have her lie on her stomach. Rub the palm of your hand across the sacrum for four to five minutes. Make sure that your palm maintains constant contact with the skin in order to create a pleasurable sensation of warmth.

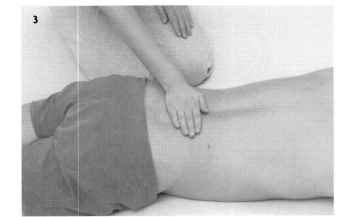

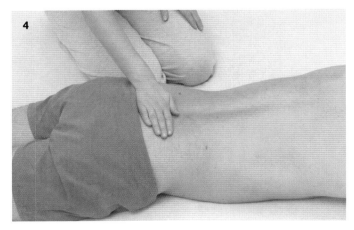

Left: Begin the stroke in the lower back.

Right: Then move your palm toward the buttocks.

Stomach 36—Leg Three Li (Three Lengths to the Foot) (Figures 1 and 2)

How to locate the point: Locate the triangular protrusion of the shinbone below the knee. Stomach 36 is at the level at which the protrusion turns into the front edge of the shinbone, 1 cun toward the outside of the leg.

How to apply pressure to the point: Massage the point using steady pressure and then circling pressure, first clockwise and then counterclockwise, for one to two minutes. Then, using light pressure, rub your palm against the outside of the calf. After two minutes this skin region will have been warmed. Now switch to the other leg and again massage the point before rubbing the skin.

Spleen 6—Three Yin Intersection (Figures 3 and 4)

The sixth point of the Spleen meridian is probably one of the most effective points for the treatment of gynecological problems.

How to locate the point: This point is located one hand-width above the highest point of the inside of the ankle on the back edge of the shin.

How to apply pressure to the point: First warm the area by rubbing it strongly using both hands. Then massage the point using your thumb or the palm of your hand, applying first steady and then circling pressure for one to two minutes each. Then massage the point on the other leg in the same way.

Caution

Spleen 6 must not be massaged during pregnancy, as it can stimulate contractions.

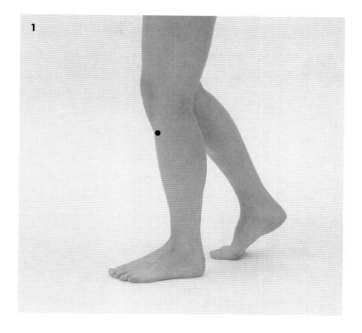

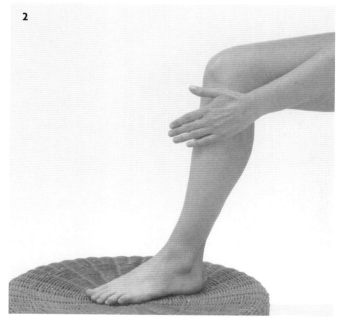

Stomach 36 is located below the knee on the side of the calf.

Use your palm to stroke across Stomach 36.

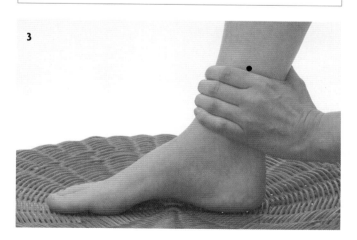

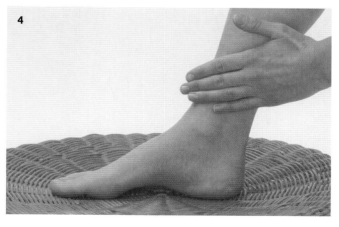

Left: Spleen 6 is located one hand width above the inside of the ankle.

Right: Rub Spleen 6 before applying pressure.

Urinary Tract Infections

Medically speaking, the urinary tract includes the kidneys, ureter, bladder, and urethra. One of the most frequent ailments in this area is the bladder infection, also known as cystitis. It is characterized by a frequent need to urinate, a low volume of urine, and often very strong pain during urination. This ailment is usually caused by an infection of the mucous membranes of the bladder by bacteria that have moved in from the intestines or from the anus. Since the urethra is shorter in women than in men, bacteria can travel more quickly from the anus to the bladder; this is one reason why women suffer much more frequently from bladder infections than men. Bladder infections are especially frequent among people who don't drink enough liquids and whose bladders as a result are not well rinsed.

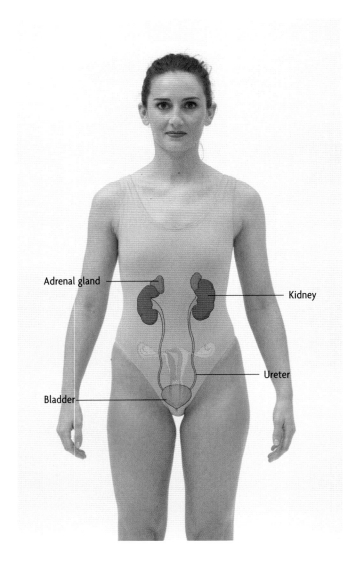

Adrenal gland

Kidney

Ureter

Bladder

The kidneys, ureter, bladder, and urethra are all part of the urinary tract.

What You Can Do

Urinary tract infections must be taken seriously and treated by a physician, since infections in this area can also affect the kidneys. Support medical treatment by drinking at least two to three liters of liquids each day. Teas made from stinging nettle herb, juniper berries, bearberry leaves, and horsetail leaves are especially helpful. During a bladder infection, avoid spicy food, alcohol, and caffeinated drinks, since these can irritate the bladder. To prevent bladder infections, make sure to keep your lower body warm by wearing clothes appropriate for outside temperatures. Take off wet bathing suits immediately after swimming.

It should be noted that people who frequently suffer from bladder infections also tend to have cold feet. Traditional Chinese medicine has an explanation for this: the Urinary Bladder meridian runs along the outside of the feet and the Kidney meridian along the inside of the feet. Acupressure of the points on these meridians has a harmonizing effect on the urinary tract and thus is an effective complementary measure to medical treatment.

How Can Acupressure Help?

Bladder infections are at times accompanied by strong, pulling pain in the abdomen. Acupressure of the points described below relieves pain and resolves tension in the abdomen, while also promoting blood circulation in this part of the body. Whether you carry out the massage on yourself or a partner, the recipient of the massage should have warm hands and feet; you can warm the feet in a footbath before the massage if necessary.

> **Caution**
> Do not carry out this massage during pregnancy!

Massaging the Middle Axis of the Lower Abdomen (Figure 1)

Using your fingertips, massage the body's middle axis on the lower abdomen, at a spot just below the navel, for about ten seconds. Then stroke your palm several times along the skin toward the pubic bone. Bring your hands to a point slightly below the previous one and repeat the massage, again ending with strokes toward the pubic bone. Massage down the middle axis of the lower abdomen point by point in this manner until you reach the edge of the pubic bone.

Rubbing the Sacrum (Figure 2)

Rubbing the sacrum affects the Urinary Bladder meridian, which has several points located there. Taken together, these points affect the lower abdomen and can positively influence ailments such as bladder infections and menstrual problems. These points can be massaged all at once by strongly rubbing the skin above the sacrum. The rubbing causes a pleasurable warming of the skin that will extend all the way to the pelvis minor. Use your whole palm to rub the sacrum back and forth across the body for three to five minutes, until you feel an intense warmth.

Stomach 36—Leg Three Li (Three Lengths to the Foot) (Figures 3–5)

How to locate the point: Locate the triangular protrusion of the shinbone below the knee. Stomach 36 is at the level at which the protrusion turns into the front edge of the shinbone, 1 cun toward the outside of the leg.

How to apply pressure to the point: Begin by applying steady pressure on the point using the tip of your thumb. Then apply circling pressure, first clockwise and then counterclockwise. Altogether the treatment of this point should take two to three minutes. Then switch to the point on the other leg. If you wish, you can also apply a moxibustion warmth treatment to this point, using one of the aids of moxibustion, for two to three minutes on each point.

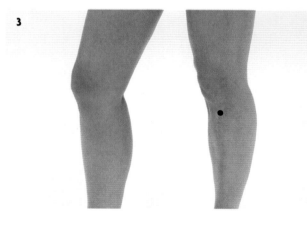

Press the points in the middle of the abdomen.

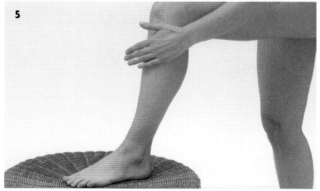

Rub your palm across the sacral bone.

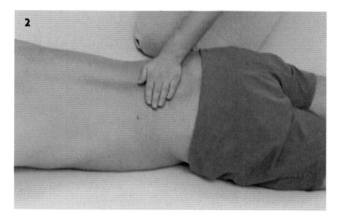

Stomach 36 is located below the knee on the side of the leg.

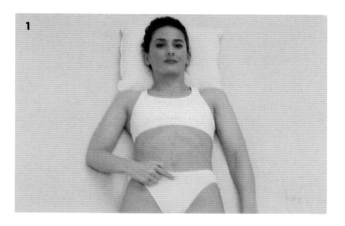

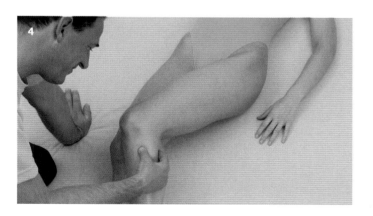

Left: Massage Stomach 36 with the tip of your thumb, applying steady and circling pressure.

Right: Then rub the point using your palm.

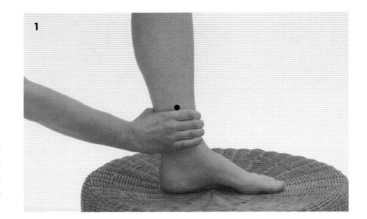

Spleen 6 is located one hand width above the inside of the ankle.

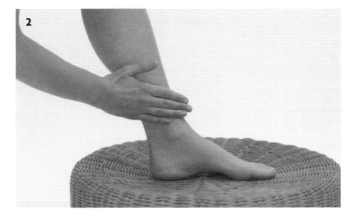

Rub Spleen 6 with your palm before applying pressure.

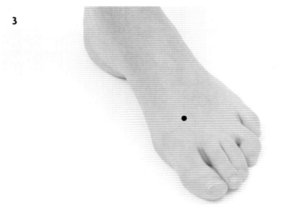

Liver 3 is located on the top of the foot between the first and second metatarsals.

Left: Massage this point using steady and circling pressure.

Right: Then rub your palm across the top of the foot.

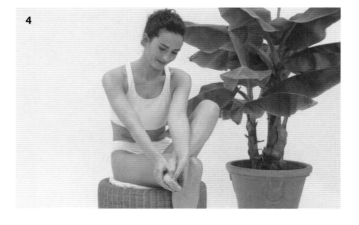

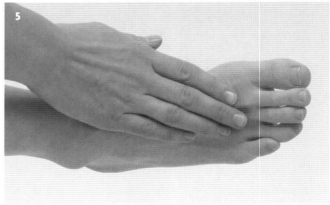

Spleen 6—Three Yin Intersection (Figures 1 and 2)

How to locate the point: Three Yin Intersection is located one hand width above the highest point of the inside of the ankle, on the back edge of the shinbone.

How to apply pressure to the point: First warm the foot by rubbing it vigorously. Then massage the point with steady pressure and then circular pressure, first clockwise and then counterclockwise, for one to two minutes each. You can also rub your palm over the point. Then massage the point on the other leg in the same way.

> **Caution**
>
> Please note that stimulation of Spleen 6 can cause the onset of contractions. It must not be massaged during pregnancy!

Liver 3—Great Surge (Figures 3–5)

How to locate the point: The third point of the Liver meridian is located on the top of the foot between the first and second metatarsals.

How to apply pressure to the point: First warm the top of the foot and the calf by gently rubbing the skin. Then press Liver 3 with the tip of your thumb or index finger as strongly as your partner can bear. Maintain pressure for one to two minutes, then release. Then massage the point using less pressure in circling movements, first clockwise and then counterclockwise, for a minute. Do the same for the point on the other foot.

Acupressure to Treat Menstruation Problems and Urinary Tract Infections

Menstruation Problems/Premenstrual Syndrome

Place your fingertips next to each other on the middle axis of the abdomen at the base of the rib cage. Apply pressure in synchrony with your partner's breathing: apply pressure while she exhales and release it when she inhales. Move downward point by point.

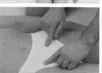

Now massage the points Stomach 28 to 30. These points are arranged in pairs on the abdomen, 2 cun to either side of the body's middle axis. Press the pairs of points one after the other, applying steady and circling pressure.

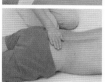

Now have your partner lie on her stomach. Rub the sacral bone for four to five minutes with your palm. Make sure that your palm always remains in touch with your partner's skin to create a pleasant warm sensation in this region of the body.

Stomach 36 is located 3 cun below the indentation of the knee on the outside of the shinbone. Massage it on one leg using steady and then circling pressure, first clockwise and then counterclockwise. Then rub the point using your palm and applying light pressure. Repeat this massage on the other leg.

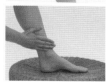

Spleen 6 is one hand width above the highest part of the inside of the ankle, on the back edge of the shinbone. Warm one of the feet by rubbing your palms over it, and then massage the point using steady and then circling pressure, first clockwise and then counterclockwise. Repeat for this point on the other leg.

Urinary Tract Infections

Massage the lower abdomen just below the navel directly on the body's middle axis. Then stroke your palm several times toward the pubic bone. Repeat this sequence, moving from point to point down the abdomen, until you reach the lower edge of the pubic bone.

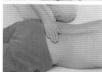

Now have your partner lie on his or her stomach. Rub the sacral bone crosswise for four to five minutes, using your palm. Make sure to maintain contact with your partner's skin at all times to create a pleasantly warm sensation on this part of the body.

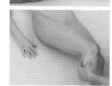

Stomach 36 is 3 cun below the indentation of the knee, on the outside of the shinbone. Massage it with steady and then circling pressure, first clockwise and then counterclockwise. Then use your palm to loosely rub the outside of the calf until you feel a pleasant warmth sensation. Massage both legs in this manner.

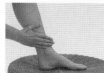

Spleen 6 is one hand width above the highest part of the inside of the ankle, on the back edge of the shinbone. Warm one of the feet by rubbing your palms over it, and then massage this point with your thumb or palm using circling pressure, first clockwise and then counterclockwise. Repeat for the point on the other leg.

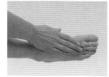

Liver 3 is on the top of the foot between the first and second metatarsals. Warm the foot and calf by gently rubbing the skin, then massage the point with steady pressure. Adjust your pressure to make it tolerable for your partner. Then apply circling pressure, reducing the pressure. Repeat for the other foot.

Problems in the Digestive Tract

Problems in the digestive tract such as chronic constipation or recurring gastrointestinal problems (which are frequently linked to stress) can be positively influenced using targeted acupressure massage. Of course, the application of acupressure can be only one component of a successful treatment, and self-treatment should always be preceded by a professional medical evaluation.

Digestive Problems

Chronic constipation is very common in modern society. In this context it is important to define constipation, since the frequency of bowel movements can vary among people and depends on diet and habits. In the

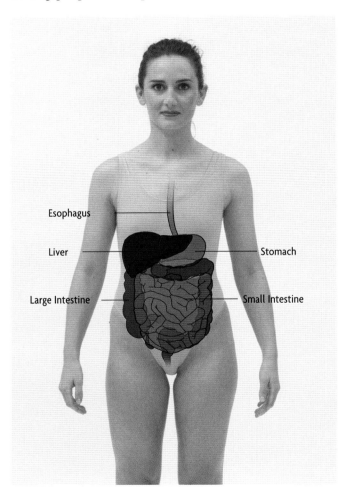

medical sense, constipation is characterized by fewer than three bowel movements a week and stool that is very hard. Chronic constipation can have many causes; lack of exercise and an unbalanced diet are among the most frequent causes of this condition.

The regular use of laxatives in the long run encourages inactivity of the intestines. On the one hand laxatives encourage the excretion that is important for proper digestion; on the other hand, however, the regular ingestion of laxatives can make the intestines dependent on them, leaving the digestive system less able to function on its own.

What You Can Do

Proper digestion and bowel activity rely on a diet containing plenty of fiber, sufficient intake of liquid, and regular physical exercise. Sports that increase stamina such as walking, jogging, and swimming have particularly positive effects. You should not take laxatives unless instructed to do so by your physician. If your intestines have already grown dependent on laxatives, you should begin to gradually reduce your use of them, while at the same time adjusting your diet and activity level according to the guidelines above.

How Can Acupressure Help?

Acupressure massages can complement changes in your diet and exercise activities to help you break free from digestive problems. Acupressure to treat digestion is best done by a partner to ensure that the recipient's abdomen is relaxed.

Begin acupressure for problems in the digestive system by massaging the abdominal skin, followed by the abdominal muscles. Then massage the points Stomach 25, 28, and 36. This acupressure massage can positively influence digestive problems as well as complement any medical treatment that may be necessary. Avoid massaging Stomach 25 and 28 in the case of pregnancy, since both points may cause the onset of contractions.

Esophagus

Liver

Stomach

Large Intestine

Small Intestine

Digestive troubles can indicate a functional problem in the gastrointestinal tract.

Abdominal Massage (Figures 1–3)

Have your partner lie on his or her back on a comfortable surface. Place a small pillow or rolled-up blanket under his or her knees to make sure that the abdomen is completely relaxed. Massage oil can be useful for this massage, since it will help your hands glide more easily across the abdomen. Place your hands on the sides of your partner's abdomen. With a stroking movement, press the skin from both sides toward the middle of the abdomen. From there, use the balls of your thumbs to very slowly stroke the skin toward the feet; at the level of the pubic bone, stroke the skin back toward the sides. Repeat these strokes for three to five minutes. Follow up by gently circling the balls of your hands slowly and steadily clockwise around the navel for two to three minutes.

Lifting the Abdominal Muscles (Figure 4)

Using the index fingers and thumbs of both hands, grasp the skin and muscles of the abdomen first to the right and then to the left of the body's middle axis. Try to move the abdominal muscles in synchrony with your partner's breathing: gently lift the muscles as your partner exhales, and lower them as he or she inhales. Begin by lifting the muscles under the arch of the rib cage, and move point by point toward the feet. Once you have reached the lower abdomen, begin again from the top. Repeat the massage altogether four or five times on each side.

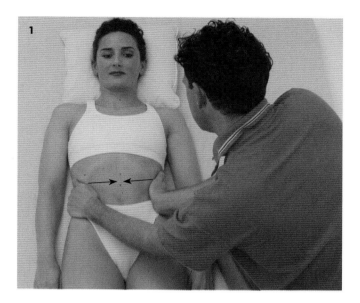

To begin the abdominal massage, press the skin from the sides to the middle.

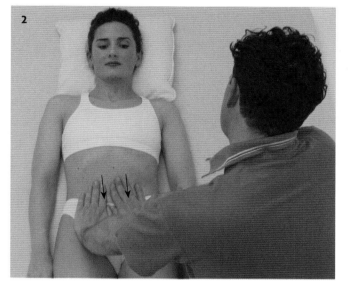

Stroke down from the middle of the abdomen toward the pubic bone.

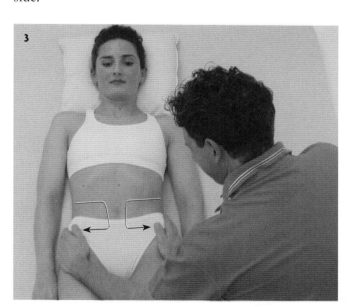

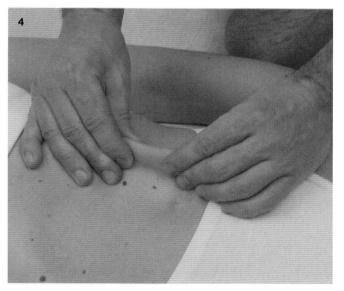

Left: When you reach the level of the pubic bone, glide your hands back toward the sides.

Right: Lift the skin using your thumb and index finger first on one side and then on the other side of the abdomen.

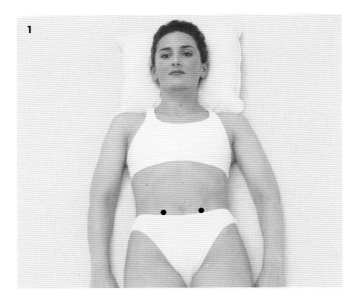

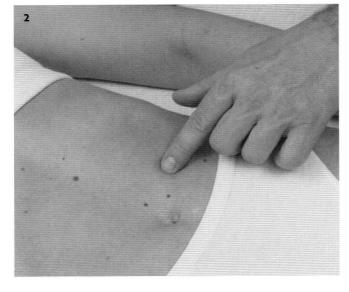

Stomach 25 is located 2 cun to the side of the navel.

Massage Stomach 25 applying steady and circling pressure with the tip of your index finger.

Stomach 25—Celestial Pivot (Figures 1 and 2)

How to locate the point: The twenty-fifth point of the Stomach meridian is located at the level of the navel, 2 cun to the side of the middle axis.

How to apply pressure to the point: Place your fingertips on both points of Stomach 25, one on each side of the abdomen. Apply steady pressure, adjusting your touch based on the reaction of your partner, since this area is often very sensitive. Then apply circling pressure, first clockwise and then counterclockwise for about one minute in each direction.

Stomach 28—Waterway (Figures 3 and 4)

How to locate the point: Locate the navel, and move 2 cun outward. From here, move 3 cun down toward the feet. Here you will find the two points of Stomach 28.

How to apply pressure to the point: Apply only light pressure, since the abdomen in this region is usually very sensitive. Massage the two points of Stomach 28 at the same time, beginning with steady pressure and changing to circling pressure, first clockwise and then counterclockwise for about one minute in each direc-

> **Caution**
>
> Do not massage Stomach 25 and 28 during pregnancy, as they can stimulate contractions.

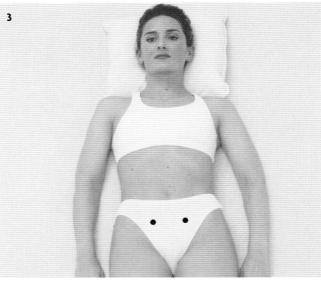

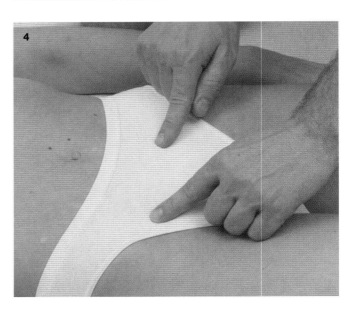

Left: Stomach 28 is located 3 cun below Stomach 25.

Right: Massage the two points of Stomach 28 simultaneously.

tion. If you want to massage the points Stomach 25 to 28 in a sequence, make sure that your fingertips maintain contact with the skin as they glide from one point to the next.

Stomach 36—Leg Three Li (Three Lengths to the Foot) (Figures 1–4)

How to locate the point: Locate the triangular protrusion of the shinbone below the knee. Stomach 36 is at the level at which the protrusion turns into the front edge of the shinbone, 1 cun toward the outside of the leg.

How to apply pressure to the point: To begin your massage of this point, rub the skin above Stomach 36 with your palm, making sure that your hand maintains contact with the skin of the leg. Then apply steady pressure to Stomach 36 using the tip of either your thumb or your index finger, increasing and decreasing the pressure in sync with your partner's breathing. Next apply circling pressure, first clockwise and then counterclockwise. Altogether the massage of this point should take about two to three minutes. When you have finished, massage this point on the other leg in the same way. If you wish, you can also apply traditional warmth treatment to this point (see page 65). Use one of the aids for moxibustion for this purpose: the moxa cigar, the moxa pin, or the loose mugwort in a moxa box. The duration of moxibustion should be two to three minutes for each point.

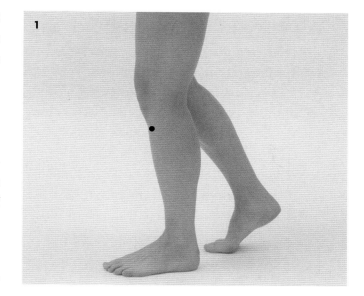

Stomach 36 is located below the knee on the side of the leg.

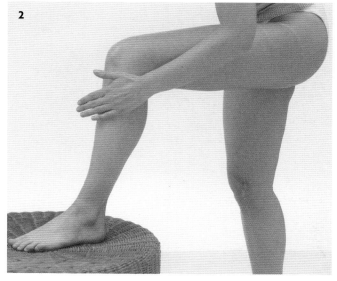

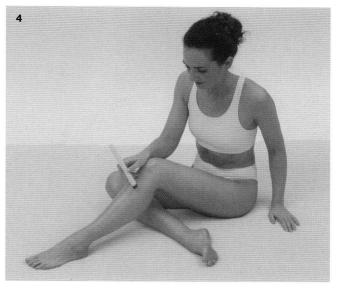

Rub the point before applying pressure.

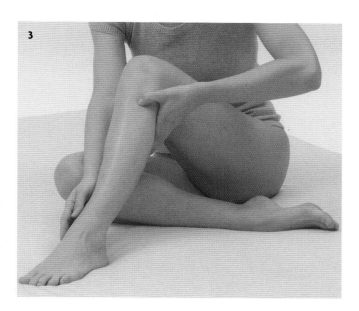

Left: Use the tip of your thumb to massage this point.

Right: You can carry out moxibustion using a moxa cigar.

Gastrointestinal Problems

Many people have had the experience of their belly "rebelling" during times of stress, tension, anger, or worry, characterized by frequently recurring bloating, nausea, burning sensations, and at times even strong, cramping pain. Taken together, these symptoms typify a "nervous stomach" or "sensitive stomach." Typically these symptoms increase in the case of psychological stress. The causes for such discomfort lie in part in an increased production of gastric acid, which is used to break up food into its smallest components. The increased activity of the stomach can also occur as cramping pains. Some medications as well as an excess of alcohol or nicotine can also cause gastrointestinal distress.

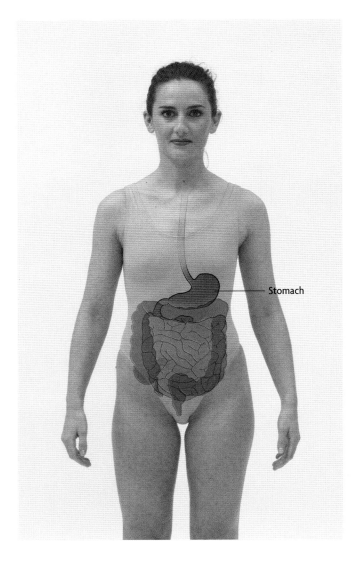

Stomach

Increased production of gastric acid causes stomachaches for many people.

What You Can Do

If you experience recurring episodes of the symptoms listed above, it is important to discuss them with a physician. He or she may prescribe medication to neutralize your gastric acid. While medication can be helpful initially in reducing symptoms, it is not an effective way to address the root causes of the problem. It is thus important to support medical treatment of gastrointestinal symptoms with the following measures.

Unhealthy eating habits often contribute to gastrointestinal problems. Instead, eat a balanced diet containing healthy, fresh, low-fat, high-fiber foods such as fresh fruits and vegetables, steamed foods, and whole grains. Avoid very hot and very cold foods, fatty foods, and late-night meals. Get into the habit of eating slowly, and try to have about five small meals rather than two or three large ones every day. Reduce your consumption of alcohol, caffeine, and strongly spiced foods, since they increase the production of gastric acid and thus place great stress on the stomach's mucous membranes.

Try to avoid stress both at work and at home. Consider practicing special relaxation methods such as progressive muscle relaxation and autogenic training, which can help you overcome stress and prevent pain in the long run. And be sure to get regular physical exercise.

If you experience occasional gastrointestinal pains despite all these preventive measures, you can help yourself with a hot water bottle or a warm wrap against the abdomen. A cup of herbal tea such as chamomile, licorice root, or melissa also will have relaxing and calming effects on the digestive system.

How Can Acupressure Help?

If you suffer from any of the symptoms of gastrointestinal problems described above (bloating, lack of appetite, nausea, and so forth), you can alleviate these ailments greatly through acupressure. While you can carry out the abdominal massage on yourself, it is especially pleasurable when done by a partner.

Massaging the Sternum (Figure 1)

Place the tips of your fingers on the upper edge of the rib cage, on the middle axis of the chest. Apply pressure point by point, moving slowly downward, to the point 1 cun below the lower edge of the sternum. Press this point for about six seconds with moderate pressure. Modulate your pressure in sync with your partner's breathing: increase the pressure when your partner exhales, and reduce the pressure when he or she inhales. The duration of the massage should be two to three minutes.

Stroking the Abdomen (Figure 2)

Now spend four to five minutes stroking the abdomen from side to side with your whole hand. This stimulates the digestion.

Conception Vessel 8—Spirit Gate (Figures 3 and 4)

How to locate the point: This point is located exactly at the navel. Do not use acupressure on this point, however; instead, warm it through moxibustion.

How to perform moxibustion: Pour a little salt into the navel. Then place a fresh, thin slice of ginger on top of the salt. Place a moxa pin on the ginger slice and light it. The pin will burn down after seven to ten minutes, at which point you can carefully remove the ginger slice together with the ashes. The salt should be removed as well. You can carry out moxibustion of the navel once a week. If you wish, you can also use a moxa cigar or loose mugwort in a moxa box for the warmth treatment of this point.

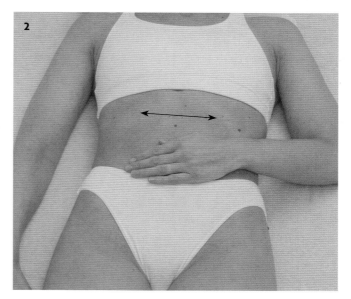

Massage the points on the sternum along the body's middle axis.

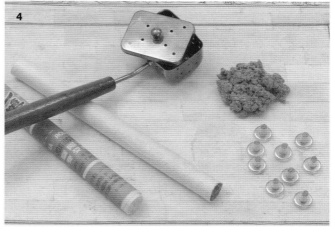

Stimulate digestion by stroking the abdomen from side to side.

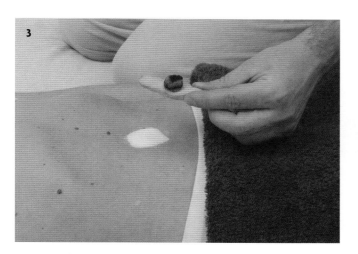

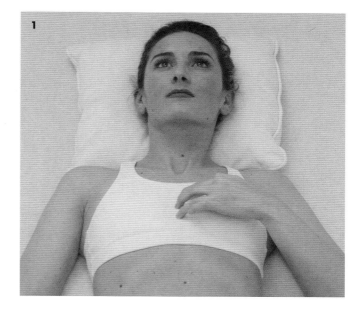

Left: Conception Vessel 8 should not be massaged but rather should be treated with moxibustion.

Right: Use only the specific aids for moxibustion.

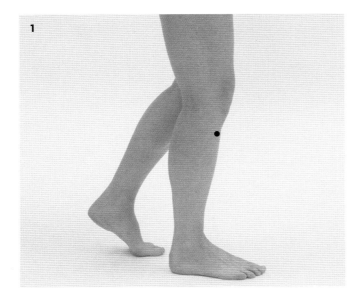

Stomach 36 is located below the knee on the side of the leg . . .

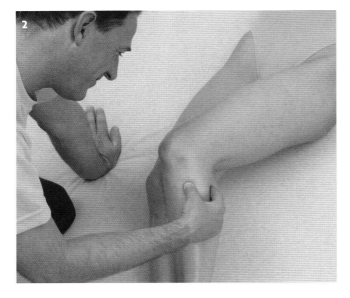

. . . and is massaged with steady and circling pressure using the tip of the thumb.

Stomach 36—Leg Three Li (Three Lengths to the Foot) (Figures 1 and 2)

How to locate the point: Locate the triangular protrusion of the shinbone below the knee. Stomach 36 is at the level at which the protrusion turns into the front edge of the shinbone, 1 cun toward the outside of the leg.

How to apply pressure to the point: Begin by applying steady pressure using the tip of your thumb. Then apply circling pressure, first clockwise and then counterclockwise. Treat the point on both legs in this manner; the treatment of each should take about two to three minutes. If you wish, you can also apply moxibustion to Stomach 36; the duration of this treatment should be two to three minutes for each point.

Liver 3—Great Surge (Figures 3 and 4)

How to locate the point: This point is located on the top of the foot between the first and second metatarsals.

How to apply pressure to the point: First warm the top of the foot by gently rubbing the skin for about two minutes. Then apply steady pressure on the point for about one minute, using the tip of your thumb or index finger. Apply as much pressure as your partner can bear. Then release pressure and carry out small circling movements with less pressure for one minute, moving first clockwise and then counterclockwise.

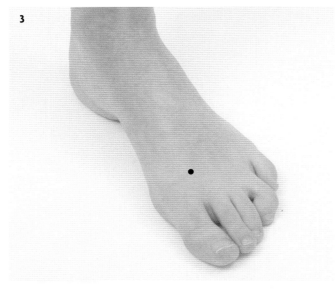

Left: Liver 3 is located on the top of the foot.

Right: Massage Liver 3 using the tip of your thumb.

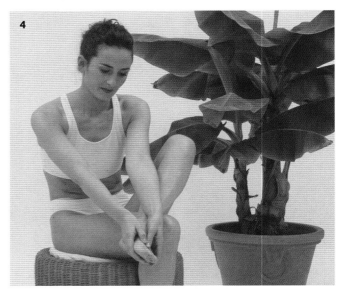

Motion Sickness and Nausea

Dizziness, nausea, and vomiting can make travel by car, plane, or boat a nightmare. These feelings are often caused by sudden and quick movement in different directions, as occurs, for example, on a boat during rough seas, which irritates the balance organ inside the ear. Sometimes these feelings can be countered by concentrating on a nonmoving reference point. Psychological factors also play a role: those who have suffered once from nausea on a certain type of transportation may fear that they will feel the same way the next time around, and these fears by themselves may suffice to cause or amplify the symptoms. This motion illness, called kinetosis in medical terms, has several forms. A mild form is characterized by headache, fatigue, and lack of appetite. A severe form adds nausea and vomiting to the list of symptoms. (If you feel the urge to vomit, you should not fight it.) Very severe forms are characterized by severe vomiting, fatigue, and lack of energy. While the mild form usually ends with the end of the motion, severe forms can persist for several days.

What You Can Do

React at the first indications of sickness. Take a break during car or bus trips, or move to the middle of the vessel on ship and air voyages, since you will experience the fewest movements there. Lying on your back and closing your eyes can sometimes also be helpful. If you suffer from vomiting, counteract the resulting fluid and mineral losses by drinking a lot of fluids such as water or herbal tea.

If you already know that you tend to suffer from motion sickness, it is of course important to take preventive measures. Do not drink alcohol in the twenty-four hours preceding your trip, and eat only easily digestible, low-fat foods before your trip.

How Can Acupressure Help?

Acupressure treatments several days before the beginning of the trip have proven effective in reducing occurrences of motion sickness. Pericardium 6 has long been known for its ability to reduce nausea, which is also helpful during pregnancy. You can massage this point either on yourself or on a partner. It can also be treated on children without any problems. At home, moxibustion of the navel, affecting Conception Vessel 8, is another useful measure.

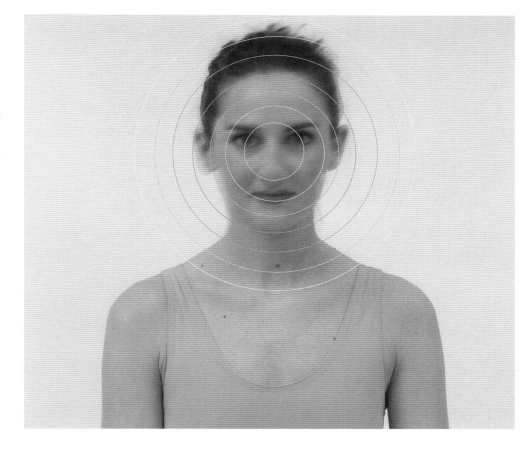

Fatigue, headache, and lack of appetite are among the symptoms of motion sickness.

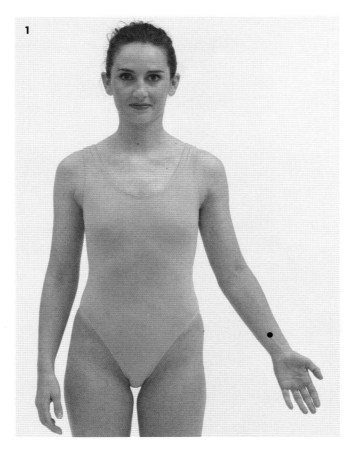

Pericardium 6 is located in the middle of the inside of the arm, 2 cun above the wrist.

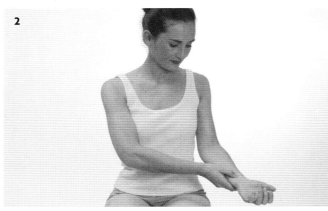

Acupressure Pericardium 6 using steady and circling pressure.

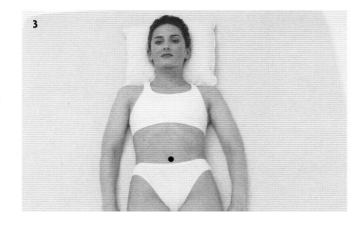

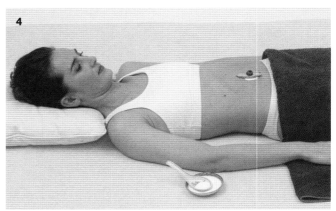

Left: Conception Vessel 8 is located directly on the navel.

Right: Perform moxibustion on Conception Vessel 8.

Pericardium 6—Inner Pass (Figures 1 and 2)

How to locate the point: Pericardium 6 is located exactly in the middle of the inside of the arm between the two tendons, 2 cun above the inside fold of the wrist.

How to apply pressure to the point: First massage the point using steady pressure for one to two minutes. Then apply circling pressure for one to two minutes, first clockwise and then counterclockwise. Massage this point on both arms in this manner.

Conception Vessel 8—Spirit Gate (Figures 3 and 4)

Another possible way to treat nausea is to apply warmth to the eighth point of the Conception Vessel, known as Spirit Gate.

How to locate the point: This point is located exactly at the navel. Do not use acupressure on this point; instead, warm it through moxibustion.

How to carry out moxibustion: Pour a little salt into the navel. Then place a fresh, thin slice of ginger on top of the salt. Place a moxa pin on the ginger slice and light it. The pin will have burned down after seven to ten minutes, at which point you can carefully remove the ginger slice together with the ashes. The salt should be removed as well. If you wish, you can also use a moxa cigar or loose mugwort in a moxa box for the warmth treatment of this point.

Acupressure to Treat Digestive Problems, Gastrointestinal Problems, and Motion Sickness

Digestive Problems

Begin by massaging the stomach. Place both hands on the sides of the stomach and press the skin from the sides to the middle of the stomach. Use the balls of your thumbs to stroke toward the feet and, at the level of the pubic bone, to the sides. Then circle around the navel with your hand.

Working first on the right side and then on the left, grasp the vertical muscles next to the middle axis of the abdomen, below the rib cage, with both hands. Lift the muscles while your partner is exhaling, and release as he or she inhales. Proceed in this manner down to the lower abdomen, then start again below the rib cage, repeating this sequence a total of four or five times on each side.

Stomach 25 is 2 cun to the side of the navel. Press it carefully on both sides of the abdomen with the tip of your index finger, noting that the region around this point is usually very sensitive to pressure. Apply steady and then circling pressure, first clockwise and then counterclockwise.

Stomach 28 is located 3 cun below Stomach 25. Massage it on both sides of the abdomen with steady and circling pressure, applying only light pressure as this region, too, is very sensitive to pressure. Let yourself be guided by your partner.

Stomach 36 is located 3 cun below the indentation of the knee on the outside of the shinbone. Apply steady and circling pressure with the tip of your thumb or index finger, and then loosely rub your palm over this point, creating a feeling of warmth. Massage this point in this manner on both legs.

Gastrointestinal Problems

Apply pressure along the middle axis of the body on the sternum, moving down point by point until you reach about 1 cun below the edge of the sternum. Massage each point with moderately strong pressure for about six seconds, while your partner is exhaling.

Then stroke the abdomen with your palm, using light pressure, from side to side. Make sure that your palm maintains contact with the skin to create a feeling of warmth.

Apply moxibustion to Conception Vessel 8, which is located on the navel. Fill the navel with salt, place a slice of ginger on top of it, and place a glowing moxa pin on the slice. A pleasant warmth will now spread through the abdomen.

Stomach 36 is located 3 cun below the indentation of the knee on the outside of the shinbone. Massage it using steady and then circling pressure, first clockwise and then counterclockwise. Then rub it lightly with your palm. Massage this point on both legs in this manner.

Liver 3 is on the top of the foot, between the first and second metatarsals. Warm the foot and calf through gentle rubbing, and then apply first steady and then circling pressure on the point using the tip of your thumb.

Motion Sickness and Nausea

Locate Pericardium 6 two cun above the wrist, between the tendons on the inside of the arm. Massage it using steady and then circling pressure, first clockwise and counterclockwise. Massage this point on both arms in this manner.

Apply moxibustion to Conception Vessel 8, which is located on the navel. Fill the navel with salt, place a slice of ginger on top of it, and place a glowing moxa pin on the slice. A pleasant warmth will now spread through the abdomen.

Problems in the Musculoskeletal System

Problems in the musculoskeletal system are among the ailments most frequently treated with acupressure. Acute and sudden pain can be effectively alleviated or resolved with just a few massage sessions. For chronic problems, more patience is required, as regular massages over a longer period of time will be necessary.

Neck Pain

Activities that strain one side of the neck over the other, bad posture, stress, and emotional strains can all cause an excess burden on our neck muscles. The affected muscle strings will feel hard and tense and will press on fine nerves and small blood vessels that supply the neck region with nutrients. A vicious cycle ensues that often results in limited range of motion, tense muscles, and bad posture that further exacerbate neck pain.

What You Can Do

For recurring or persistent neck pain you should consult your physician, who may be able to recommend a targeted treatment that will prevent a long period of pain. You should also pay attention to your posture in order to avoid further tensing of the neck muscles as a reaction to bad posture. Carry your head high, and try to keep your spine straight and your shoulder blades held back. To avoid stiffness in the neck, regularly practice relaxation and movement exercises (see page 201). Repeat these as often as you can, ideally hourly, even at the office in the form of small breaks.

If your neck is already tense, a hot, damp wrap or hot water bottle over the tight muscles can ease them, as can acupressure.

How Can Acupressure Help?

Acupressure can help resolve muscle tension, leaving the head and neck freer and more flexible. If you have difficulty reaching the points described here, it is best to have a partner perform the massage. Having a partner give the massage also increases its effectiveness, since the recipient will be more relaxed. Massage the points Large Intestine 4 and Gall Bladder 20, 21, and 39. Also massage the neck area, which will be pleasurable and will help release or prevent tension.

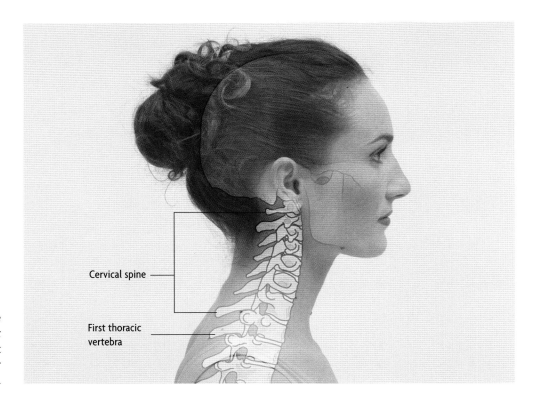

Cervical spine

First thoracic vertebra

One of the most frequent causes of neck pain is improper posture.

Large Intestine 4—Valley of Union (Figures 1–4)

How to locate the point: This point is easiest to locate when you make an O with your thumb and index finger, pressing the tips of the two fingers firmly against each other. This causes a small bulge of muscle to rise just above the web of skin between the index finger and thumb, on the back of the hand; this bulge marks the site of Large Intestine 4.

How to apply pressure to the point: Warm the hand before the massage by rubbing it for two minutes from its base to the tip of the index finger. The rubbing will warm the skin and may redden it slightly.

Grasp the hand in a tweezers grip between your thumb and index finger, with your thumb resting on Large Intestine 4 and the tip of the index finger on the other side of the hand as a balancing point. Apply a pleasant but relatively strong amount of pressure, and maintain this pressure for about two minutes. Then apply circular pressure for two minutes. Massage the other hand in the same way; first rubbing the skin, then applying steady pressure followed by circling pressure.

If you wish, you can also apply a traditional Chinese warmth treatment to Large Intestine 4, using the specific aids of moxibustion, that is, mugwort in a cigar, in a pin, or as loose powder in a moxa box. The duration of moxibustion depends on the sensitivity of the person being treated but generally should last two to three minutes.

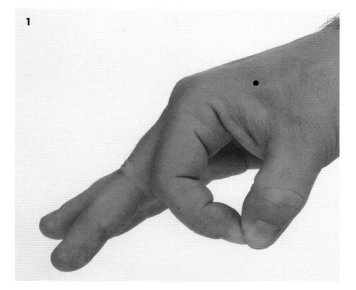

Large Intestine 4 is located on the muscle mass that forms between thumb and index finger when they make an O.

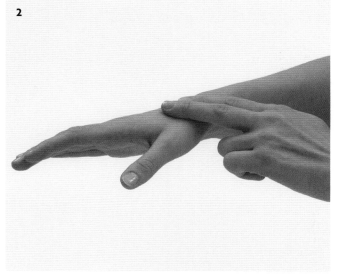

Rub the hand from its base to the tip of the index finger . . .

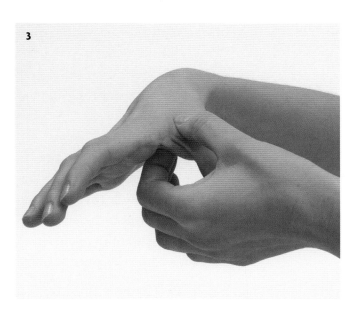

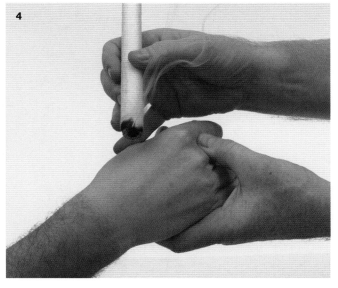

Left: . . . and massage it using steady and circling pressure.

Right: Apply moxibustion with a moxa cigar.

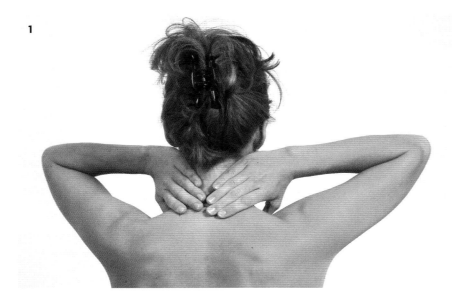

Stroke the neck with both hands, from the middle axis to the sides.

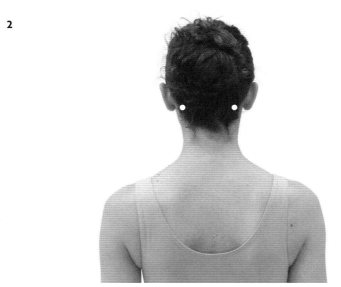

Gall Bladder 20 is located at the sides of the lower edge of the back of the head.

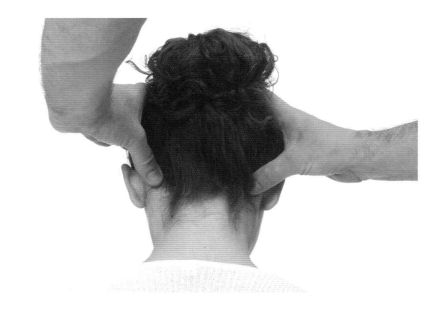

Massage both points of Gall Bladder 20 simultaneously with your thumbs.

Stroking the Neck (Figure 1)

Stroking the neck area is especially helpful in the case of neck pain. For this, place your right hand on the right side of your neck and stroke it five to ten times slowly and steadily to the side. Then use your left hand to massage the other side of the neck in the same way. Or you can massage both sides at the same time. Now place the fingertips of both hands on the sides of the head at the level of the upper edge of the ear, at Gall Bladder 8. Applying pressure, move both hands along the back of the head to the neck, where you will reach Gall Bladder 20. Repeat these strokes for at least three minutes on both sides simultaneously.

Gall Bladder 20—Wind Pool (Figures 2 and 3)

How to locate the point: Wind Pool is located on the lower edge of the back of the head, to either side of the noticeable muscles on the middle axis.

How to apply pressure to the point: Massage the two points of Gall Bladder 20, one on either side of the head, with the tips of your thumbs, using steady pressure and then circling pressure, first clockwise and then counterclockwise, for one to two minutes each. If you are massaging a partner, you can in addition to pressure treatment also apply a traditional Chinese warmth treatment to the points of Gall Bladder 20 using moxibustion.

Gall Bladder 21—Shoulder Well (Figures 1 and 2)

How to locate the point: With your partner leaning his or her head slightly forward, locate the dorsal process of the seventh cervical vertebra. Using your other hand, locate the highest elevation of the shoulder. Shoulder Well is located midway between these two points.

How to apply pressure to the point: Place your hand on the muscle mass above the point, and apply as much pressure as you can without causing pain. Knead and rub the muscles for two to three minutes; this may be slightly uncomfortable. Now apply steady and then circling pressure for two to three minutes. Massage this point on both shoulders.

> **Caution**
> Gall Bladder 21 must not be massaged during pregnancy!

Gall Bladder 39—Suspended Bell (Figures 3 and 4)

How to locate the point: Gall Bladder 39 is located on the outside of the calf, behind the bone and one hand width above the highest point of the outside of the ankle.

How to apply pressure to the point: Massage the point with the tip of your thumb, using first steady and then circling pressure for one to two minutes each. Massage this point on both legs.

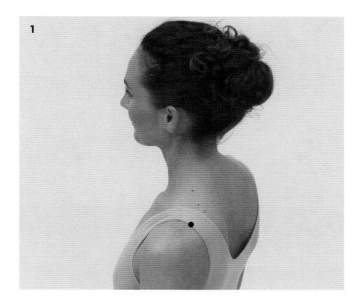

Gall Bladder 21 is on the shoulder muscle.

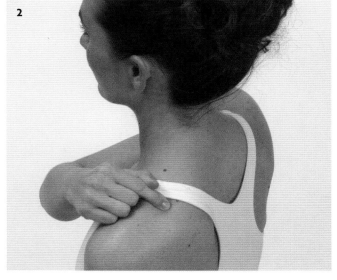

Massage Gall Bladder 21 with steady and circling pressure using your index finger.

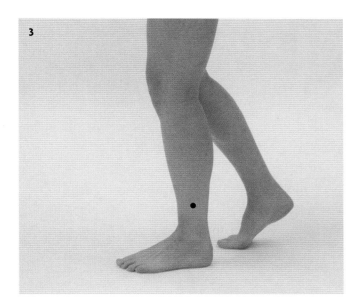

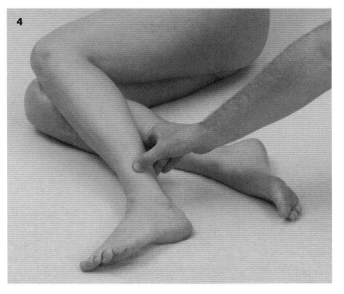

Left: Gall Bladder 39 is one hand-width above the outside of the ankle.

Right: Massage Gall Bladder 39 with steady and circling pressure.

Back Pain/Lumbago

The most common cause of back pain is bad spinal posture. Even in children, damage to the spine from a bend to one side or to the front or back is not rare. The nature of leisure activities has changed, and both children and adults now spend the majority of their day in a sitting position. As a result, the muscles that support the spine are not used sufficiently and begin to atrophy.

> **Caution**
>
> For suddenly occurring back pain, always consult a physician before attempting self-treatment. A slipped disk, in which one of the spinal cartilage disks presses on the nerves of the spine, can have long-term consequences and must be treated by a physician.

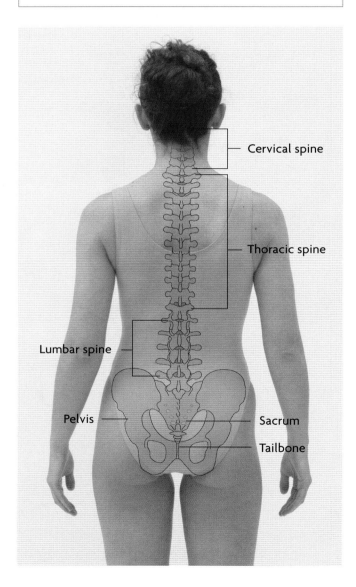

Cervical spine

Thoracic spine

Lumbar spine

Pelvis

Sacrum

Tailbone

Many people today suffer from frequent pain in the lower back.

> **Note**
>
> Have a partner perform acupressure massage of the back for you. This allows you to relax and makes the massage much more effective.

At the same time, the muscles of the buttocks, neck, and shoulders carry an excessive burden that often leads to tension and pain.

Sometimes even small movements initiated from a bad starting position can be enough to cause an unbearable pain in the lower back. This condition, known as lumbago, is characterized by pain in the lumbar spine. In Western medicine, back pain, including lumbago, is frequently categorized as functional, meaning that no organic cause for the symptoms can be detected.

What You Can Do

All activities that strengthen the back help prevent back pain. Learn behavior that is good for your back in everyday life, and make a habit out of it. Many physiotherapists and even community centers offer courses on improving back strength. If you experience lumbago, warm, damp wraps and a hot bath can help alleviate the acute pain. (And be sure to consult a physician as soon as possible.)

How Can Acupressure Help?

In contrast to our Western experience, traditional Chinese medicine sees wind and cold as the most frequent causes of back pain. These two factors are the focus of acupressure treatment, especially in the case of sudden-onset pain. Massage of the points described below (Governor Vessel 3 and 14 and Gall Bladder 30) is helpful in alleviating back pain. A successful course of treatment also includes rubbing the lumbar spine and warming the sacrum region through rubbing. Please note that Governor Vessel 3 must not be massaged in the case of pregnancy.

Governor Vessel 3—Lumbar Yang Pass (Figures 1 and 2)

How to locate the point: This point is located over the lower spine, below the fourth lumbar vertebra. Feel for the upper edge of the pelvic bone and locate this point at that level on the spine.

How to apply pressure to the point: Massage the point with the tips of your thumbs, applying steady and then circling pressure, first clockwise and then counterclockwise, for one minute each. Afterward, rub the skin with your palm for about three minutes.

> **Caution**
> Governor Vessel 3 must not be massaged during pregnancy.

Governor Vessel 14—Great Hammer (Figures 3 and 4)

How to locate the point: Great Hammer is located on the spine between the lowest cervical vertebra and the top thoracic vertebra. It is easiest to locate by bending the head slightly forward, which causes the dorsal process of the lowest cervical vertebra to protrude slightly; Governor Vessel 14 is just below it.

How to apply pressure to the point: Massage the point with the tips of your index and middle fingers, using steady and then circling pressure, first clockwise and then counterclockwise, for one minute each. Then firmly rub the point and the skin around it with your palms for about three minutes.

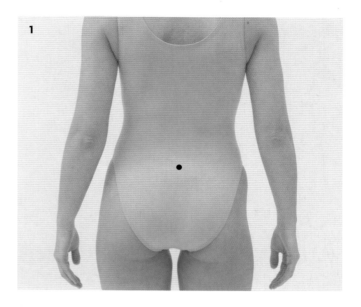

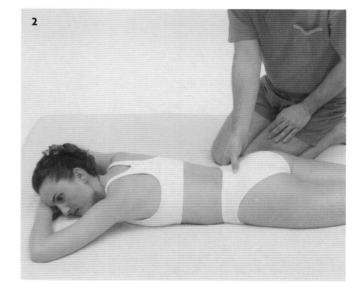

Governor Vessel 3 is located below the fourth vertebra of the lumbar spine.

Massage Governor Vessel 3 using steady and circling pressure.

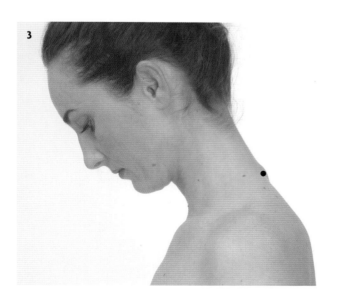

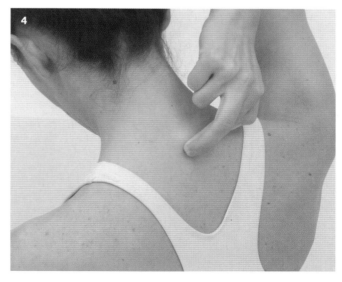

Left: Governor Vessel 14 is between the lowest cervical vertebra and the first thoracic vertebra.

Right: Massage Governor Vessel 14 using the tips of your index and middle fingers.

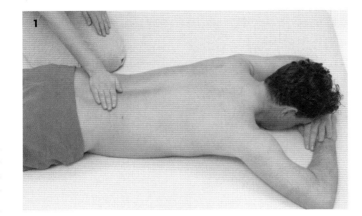

Rub the area above the lumbar spine with your flat hand.

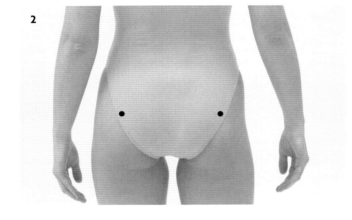

Gall Bladder 30 is located on the rounded top of the buttocks.

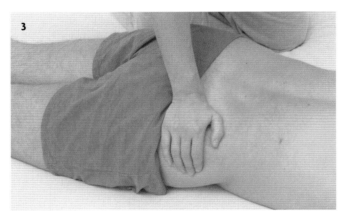

First apply steady pressure to Gall Bladder 30 . . .

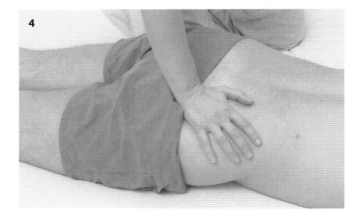

Left: . . . and then circling pressure with the ball of the hand.

Right: Rub the sacral bone with your hands placed on top of each other.

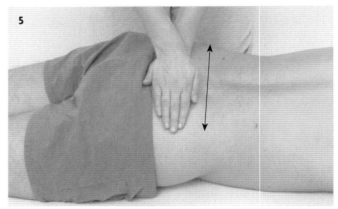

Rubbing above the Lumbar Spine (Figure 1)

At the level of the upper edge of the pelvic bone, rub from side to side across the back with the palm of your hand. Apply slightly stronger pressure when you are moving your hand away from yourself. Rub the skin in this way for three to four minutes, creating a pleasant warmth on the skin.

Gall Bladder 30—Jumping Round (Figures 2–4)

How to locate the point: It is easiest to locate this point with your partner on his or her side and his or her hip joint bent. Imagine a line running from the bottom of the sacrum (at the top of the seam between the buttocks) to the greater trochanter (a prominence at the top of the femur). If you divide the line into three equal parts, Gall Bladder 30 is located at the spot that divides the middle from the outer third.

How to apply pressure to the point: Have your partner lie on his or her stomach. Rub the buttocks muscles for two to three minutes with the balls of your hands, moving your hands from the middle of the body across the large muscles to the outside and then, with less pressure, back to the middle. Then massage Gall Bladder 30 for two to three minutes, using steady and then strong circling pressure, first clockwise and then counterclockwise. Apply as much pressure as your partner can tolerate, and use the ball of your hand.

Warming the Sacrum (Figure 5)

The points Urinary Bladder 27 to 35 (see page 92) are located on the sacrum. Rubbing the area activates these points. This massage is best done by a partner.

Have your partner lie comfortably on either his or her side or stomach. Rub from side to side across the sacrum with the palms of your hands. Make sure that your palms remain in steady contact with the skin, which is necessary to create a pleasurable warmth sensation. Massage the sacral bone in this way for four to five minutes.

Tennis Elbow

Some of the muscles that are responsible for moving the fingers and wrist are fixed to their tendons on a small bone protrusion located on the outside of the elbow. If these muscles are used a lot over an extended period of time, the tendons and the fixed point may become overly exerted. The result is pain in the elbow area that can radiate to the wrist and the shoulder. Since these symptoms are frequently observed among tennis players, the ailment has become known as tennis elbow or tennis arm.

The pain itself is caused by small tears in the tendons. The continued overexertion finally leads to an infection of the involved tissue. Any tension of the lower arm muscles then causes stabbing pain in the muscle roots in the elbow area.

Especially unpleasant is the fact that the pain is difficult to control with ordinary treatment. Therapy is often long, and symptoms have a tendency to recur. Moreover, tennis elbow is caused not only by sport but also by certain professional activities such as working with hammers or other tools.

If you have noticed the symptoms described above on yourself, you should see a physician to determine whether a nerve has been pinched or whether there is any other damage in the elbow joint.

What You Can Do

Sudden-onset pain can be alleviated by applying ice. With a towel between the ice and your skin, ice the area for twenty to thirty minutes. Then take a break of one hour before icing the area again. Persistent elbow pain is best treated with the help of a physiotherapist.

He or she will carry out a movement analysis and give advice as to which muscle areas have to be strengthened through targeted training, and how to avoid overexertion of the elbow in the future.

How Can Acupressure Help?

Acupressure is a good complementary treatment to medical and physical therapy, but one that requires patience: success can be attained only with regular massages over an extended period of time. The goal of acupressure here is to loosen the tense muscle and to alleviate the pain. In the case of chronic pain, massage the points described below once or twice a week on the affected arm. Treat acute pain of the elbow area not on the affected arm but rather on the healthy arm. Acute problems should be massaged by a partner. After an introductory arm massage, treat the points Large Intestine 4, 11, and 15 as well as Triple Heater 10 and Stomach 36.

> **Note**
> In the case of acute pain, massage not the affected arm but rather the healthy arm. For chronic ailments, massage the affected arm.

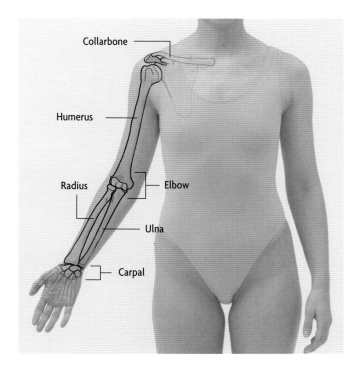

Collarbone

Humerus

Radius

Elbow

Ulna

Carpal

Frequent excessive strain in the arm can cause tennis elbow—and not just among tennis players.

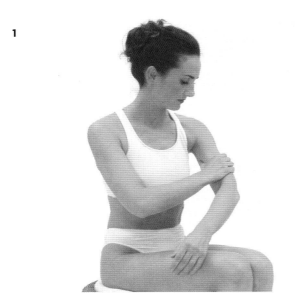

Massage the arm from the shoulder down the upper arm . . .

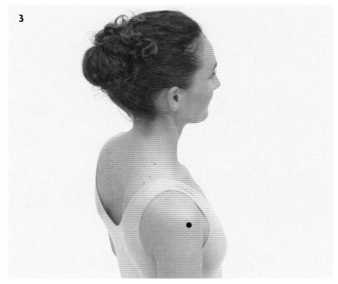

. . . and along the lower arm down to the fingertips.

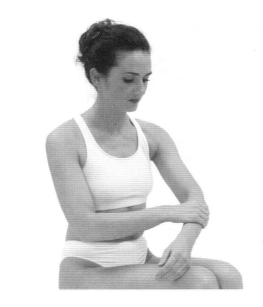

Left: Large Intestine 15 is located at the outside edge of the shoulder.

Right: Massage Large Intestine 15 using steady and circling pressure.

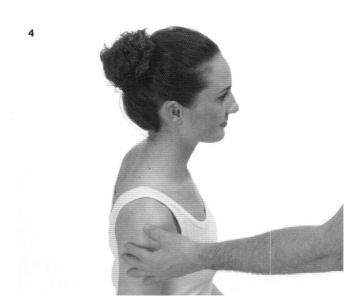

Massaging the Arm (Figures 1 and 2)

If you suffer from problems in the arm such as tennis elbow, it is useful to begin with acupressure of the whole arm. For this, massage one arm from the shoulder joint to the fingertips with strong strokes. Begin on the outside of the shoulder and stroke along the arm to the fingertips. This treatment takes about three minutes. Then switch to the other arm and massage it in the same way. After this, massage the points Large Intestine 15, 11, and 4 one after the other.

Large Intestine 15—Shoulder Bone (Figures 3 and 4)

How to locate the point: When the arm is extended to the side, this point is on the outermost end of the shoulder, just below a bone protrusion between the front and middle parts of the deltoid muscle that begins here.

How to apply pressure to the point: Apply steady pressure to Large Intestine 15 with the tip of your thumb for one to two minutes. Then apply circling pressure, first clockwise and then counterclockwise.

Because of its location, this point is well suited for self-massage. You can also apply moxibustion warmth treatment to this point on both arms.

Large Intestine 11—Pool at the Bend (Figures 1 and 2)

How to locate the point: When the arm is bent, Large Intestine 11 is located midway between the outer edge of the elbow fold and the knobby protrusion of the elbow bone.

How to apply pressure to the point: Massage Pool at the Bend with strong steady pressure for about two minutes. Then apply circling pressure on the point for one to two minutes. If you want to increase the pressure, apply pressure with your middle finger on top of your index finger.

Triple Heater 10—Celestial Well (Figures 3 and 4)

How to locate the point: Celestial Well is located on the outside of the arm in a small indentation above the elbow.

How to apply pressure to the point: Begin by stroking with your fingertips from the shoulder down the outside of the upper arm. Then use the tip of your index finger to apply steady pressure to Triple Heater 10 for about one minute, with your thumb on the other side of the arm for balance; the pressure should be as strong as your partner can tolerate. Afterward, massage the point in small circling movements with slightly less pressure, first clockwise and then counterclockwise for one minute in each direction. Massage this point on both arms in this manner.

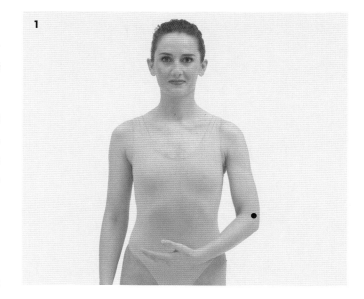

Large Intestine 11 is located on the side of the elbow.

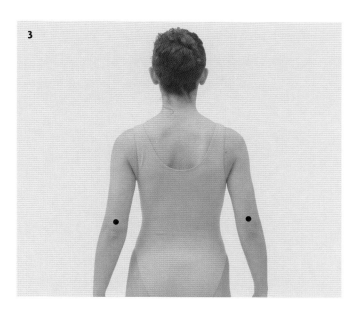

Massage Large Intestine 11 using the tip of your thumb.

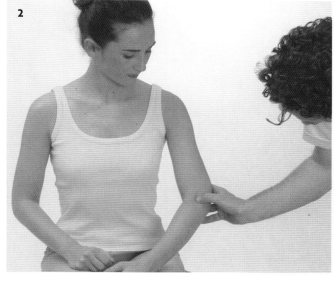

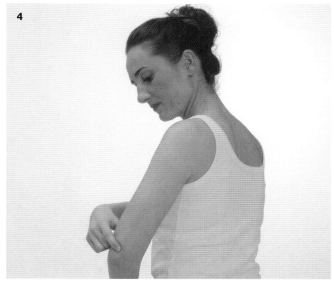

Left: Triple Heater 10 is at the back of the elbow.

Right: Massage this point using the tweezers grip.

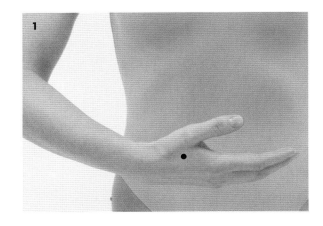

Large Intestine 4 is located on the muscle mass that forms between the thumb and index finger when they make an O.

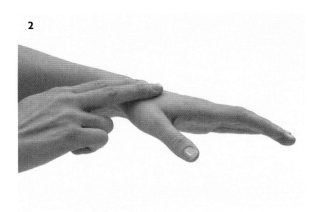

Rub the skin above Large Intestine 4 . . .

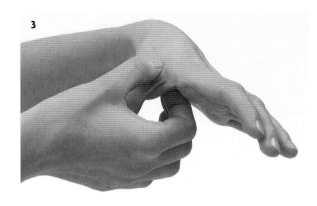

. . . before applying steady and circling pressure.

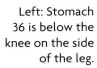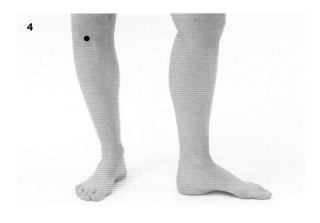

Left: Stomach 36 is below the knee on the side of the leg.

Right: Massage the point with the tip of your thumb, applying steady and circling pressure.

Large Intestine 4—Valley of Union (Figures 1–3)

How to locate the point: This point is easiest to locate when you make an O with your thumb and index finger, pressing the tips of the two fingers firmly against each other. This causes a small bulge of muscle to rise just above the web of skin between the index finger and thumb, on the back of the hand; this bulge marks the site of Large Intestine 4.

How to apply pressure to the point: Rub the thumb side of the hand for one to two minutes, from the base of the hand to the inside of the index finger. This will warm the skin and may cause it to redden slightly. Now place your thumb on Large Intestine 4, and press the point with steady and relatively strong pressure for one to two minutes; adjust the pressure based on the sensitivity of the point. Finally, apply circling pressure to the point. Massage this point on both hands in this manner.

Stomach 36—Leg Three Li (Three Lengths to the Foot) (Figures 4 and 5)

How to locate the point: Locate the triangular protrusion of the shinbone below the knee. Stomach 36 is at the level at which the protrusion turns into the front edge of the shinbone, 1 cun toward the outside of the leg.

How to apply pressure to the point: Massage the point with steady pressure and then circling pressure, first clockwise and then counterclockwise for one minute in each direction. Then lightly rub along the outside of the calf with the palm of your hand for about two minutes. Massage this point on both legs in this manner. You can also carry out moxibustion treatment on this point (see page 65).

> **Caution**
> Large Intestine 4 must not be massaged during pregnancy.

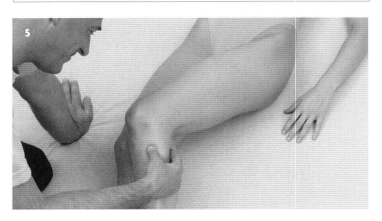

Acupressure to Treat Neck and Back Pain and Tennis Elbow

Neck Pain

Make an O with your thumb and index finger; the point Large Intestine 4 is located on the resulting muscle mass between these fingers. On both hands, rub it with your index and middle fingers, and then massage it with steady and circling pressure.

Stroke the neck toward the front, first with the right and then with the left hand. Use both hands to massage along the base of the back of the head to the neck.

Gall Bladder 20 is located at the base of the back of the head, between the two neck muscles. Massage it on both sides of the middle axis with steady and circling pressure, first clockwise and then counterclockwise.

Gall Bladder 21 is located on the shoulder muscle. Massage it with steady and circling pressure, and then rub it for two to three minutes. Repeat on the other shoulder.

Gall Bladder 39 is located on the outside of the calf, 1 cun above the highest point on the outside of the ankle, behind the bone. Massage it with your thumb, applying steady and circling pressure for one to two minutes each. Repeat on the other leg.

Back Pain

Governor Vessel 3 is located below the fourth lumbar vertebra. Massage it with steady and circling pressure, and then rub over it with your palm.

Governor Vessel 14 is located between the bottommost cervical vertebra and the topmost thoracic vertebra. Massage it with steady and circling pressure, and then rub it strongly with your palm.

Now use your hands to rub across the lumbar spine for three to four minutes. Rubbing with firm pressure creates a pleasant warmth sensation in the pelvis.

Gall Bladder 30 is located on the buttocks. Rub the point with the ball of your hand, and then use your thumb to massage it with steady and strong circling pressure for one to two minutes. Massage both Gall Bladder 30 points in this manner.

Now warm the sacrum by rubbing the balls of your hands over it for two to three minutes with firm pressure. The skin will warm and radiate a pleasant sensation.

Tennis Elbow

Begin by stroking the outside of the arm from the shoulder to the fingertips. The entire massage of the arm should take two to three minutes.

Large Intestine 15 is located on the outside edge of the shoulder, below a bone protrusion and over deltoid muscles. Massage the point with a thumb, applying steady and circling pressure.

Large Intestine 11 is located between the fold of the elbow and the knobby protrusion of the elbow bone. It is easiest to locate when the arm is slightly bent. Massage it with steady and circling pressure.

Triple Heater 10 is located on the outside of the arm, in an indentation above the tip of the elbow. Stroke the upper arm and then massage the point using the tip of your index finger, applying first steady and then circling pressure. Massage this point on both arms in this manner.

Large Intestine 4 is located on the muscle mass that forms between your thumb and index finger when you use them to make an O. Using the tweezers grip, massage it with your thumb, applying steady and circling pressure. Massage this point on both hands in this manner.

Stomach 36 is located on the outside edge of the shinbone, 3 cun below the indentation of the knee. Massage it with steady and circling pressure, first clockwise and then counterclockwise, and then rub it with your palm. Massage this point on both legs in this manner.

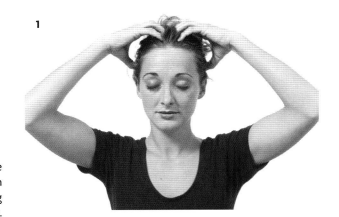

Massage the scalp with small, circling movements.

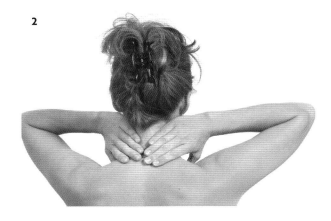

Stroke the neck five to ten times up toward the sides.

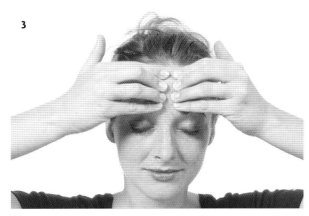

With light pressure, stroke your forehead from the center to the sides.

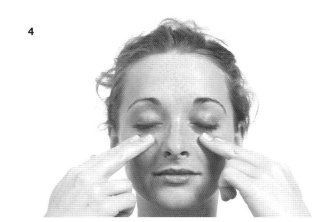

Left: Move from the nose to the hairline stroke by stroke.

Right: Conclude by stroking your chin to the side.

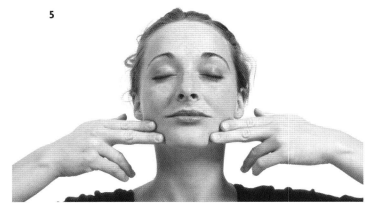

Wellness Massage

Many people consider the face to be a mirror of the soul, since feelings like joy and sadness are first and most prominently reflected in a person's face. Massaging the head and face resolves tension in the face muscles and increases well-being. This massage affects not individual points but zones.

The Head and Neck Massage

You can enjoy a head and neck massage several times a day. You will need about seven to ten minutes for each massage. While you can do this massage on yourself, it is especially pleasurable when carried out by a partner.

Massaging the Scalp (Figure 1)

Place your fingertips along the middle axis of the top of the head, beginning at the hairline. Massage the scalp with your fingertips, using small, circling movements and moving from the middle axis of the head to the sides. Once they have reached the sides, return your fingers to the middle axis, on a point slightly further toward the back of the head. Repeat the massage until you reach the back of the head.

Stroking the Neck (Figure 2)

Place your palms on the neck, with the fingers of each hand facing those of the other. Stroke the neck from the middle axis to the sides five to ten times.

Forehead Massage (Figure 3)

Place your fingers on the middle axis of the forehead, and use them to stroke outward, applying light pressure. After each stroke, move your hands slightly up, so that you massage gradually from the eyebrows up to the hairline.

Cheek Massage (Figure 4)

Stroke from the bridge of the nose to under the eyes using your fingertips. Continue with your fingers across your cheeks and temples to the hairline. Return your fingers to a spot slightly lower on the nose and stroke across the cheeks again. Massage in this way, moving down point by point, until you reach the upper lip.

Chin Massage (Figure 5)

To conclude, stroke your chin several times, from the middle of the chin to the sides of the face.

Relaxation Exercises

After the head and neck massage, you can carry out some relaxation exercises for the head and shoulders. (See figures 6–10.) Slowly turn your head to the left and then to the right; repeat until you have turned your head three times in each direction. Drop your chin to your chest and then slowly raise your head; again, repeat until you have dropped and raised your chin three times.

Make slow and careful circles with your head, circling three times clockwise and three times counterclockwise. With your arms hanging loosely, circle your shoulders five times to the front and five times to the back. Finally, try to pull your shoulders up to your ears, and then let them fall back; repeat this last movement five times too.

6

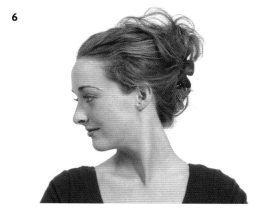

Turn your head to the right and left three times each.

7

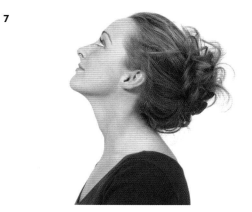

Drop and raise your head three times.

8

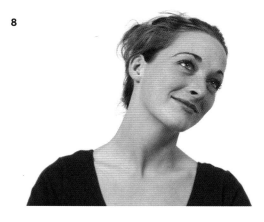

Very carefully circle your head three times in each direction.

9

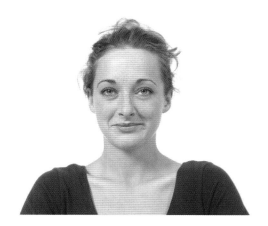

10

Left: Circle your shoulders five times to the front and five times to the back.

Right: Pull your shoulders up and let them drop back down five times.

Whole-Body Massage

The basic acupressure techniques of stroking, kneading, and shaking can also be used to massage the entire body and all the acupressure points on it. It is useful to carry out a whole or partial body massage before acupressure treatment. The whole-body massage illustrated in the following pages is a partner massage, beginning with the front of the body and ending with the back of the body. The complete massage takes about forty-five to sixty minutes.

Massage of the Front of the Body

For this part of the massage, your partner lies on his or her back.

Massaging the Legs (Figure 1)

Place a small pillow or a rolled-up blanket under your partner's knees and neck to support them. Then massage the legs as described below, massaging the left leg first, and then applying the same massage to the right leg.

Introductory Strokes (Figures 2 and 3)

Rub your partner's leg from the foot to the groin. With one hand on each side of your partner's leg, stroke with increasing pressure over the foot, calf, knee, and thigh up to the groin region. Then, applying light pressure and without losing contact with your partner's skin, move your hands back to the original position. From there, carry out another sequence of strokes with increasing pressure. Carry out this stroking sequence a total of ten times.

Left: With your partner lying on his or her back, the massage begins on the front of the body on the left leg and ends on the abdomen and chest. The numbers indicate the work sequence.

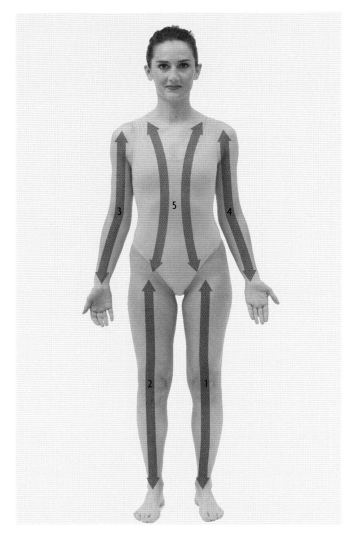

Right: With your partner lying on his or her stomach, the massage begins on the right leg and ends on the back.

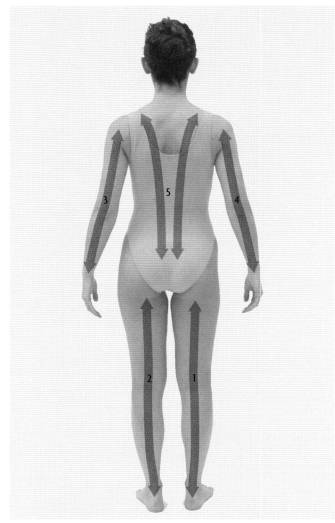

Kneading and Stroking (Figure 4)

Knead the thigh muscles between your thumbs and fingers, making sure to have a lot of skin contact and moving the muscles perpendicular to their fibers. Begin the kneading above the knee and move up to the groin region. Knead for two minutes, and then stroke the leg ten times, as described above.

Shaking (Figure 5)

Prop up your partner's leg, and hold it at the knee with your left hand. Using your right hand, loosen the calf muscles by gently shaking them back and forth.

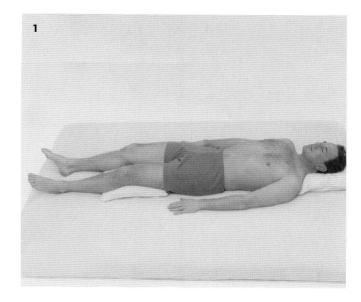

To make your partner comfortable, place small pillows under his or her neck and knees.

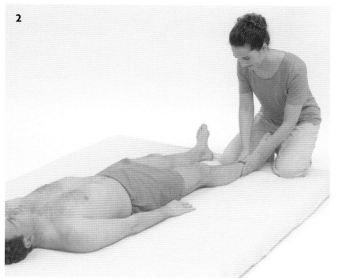

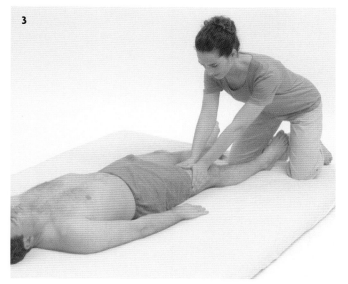

Left: Begin by stroking the ankle . . .

Right: . . . and stroke up the leg to the thigh.

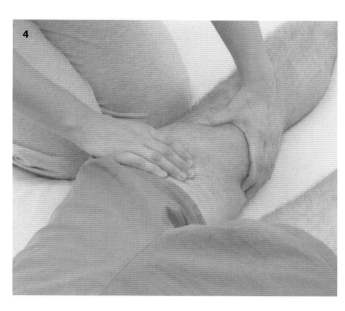

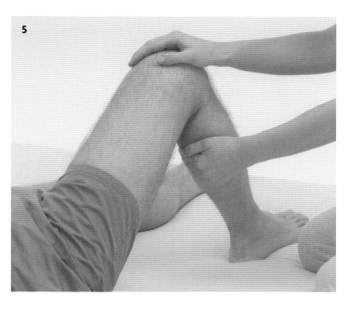

Left: Knead the muscles on the thigh between your thumb and fingers.

Right: Hold the knee while you shake the calf muscles.

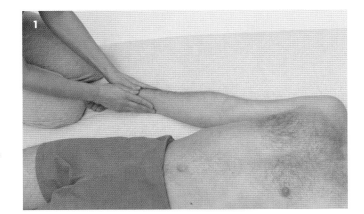

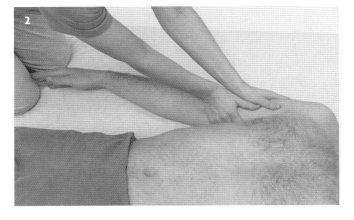

Begin the massage of the arm with strokes from the wrist . . .

. . . up to the shoulder. Make sure to maintain contact with your partner's skin at all times.

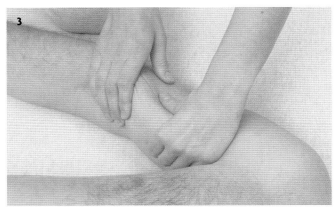

Now knead the muscles of the upper arm between your thumb and fingers.

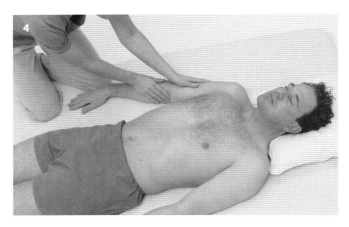

Left: After the kneading, carry out more strokes.

Right: To conclude, shake your partner's arm.

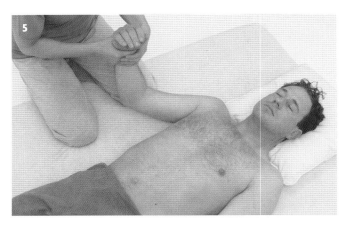

Massaging the Arms

After you have massaged both legs, massage the arms, working first with the right and then the left. Make sure that your partner's arms are loose and relaxed for this part of the massage.

Introductory Strokes (Figures 1 and 2)

Begin the massage on the right arm at the wrist. Take the wrist between your hands, and glide your hands up the arm to the shoulder, gradually increasing your pressure as you move toward the shoulder. Return your hands to their starting position without losing contact with your partner's skin. Perform this stroking a total of ten times.

Kneading and Stroking (Figures 3 and 4)

Now knead the muscles of the lower arm, perpendicular to their fibers. Then knead the biceps on the upper arm. After you have kneaded the lower and upper arm for one to two minutes each, repeat the ten strokes from wrist to shoulder as described above.

Shaking (Figure 5)

Now bend your partner's arm at the elbow and, holding the wrist in both hands, lift the arm a few inches, until the upper arm no longer touches the ground. Shake the arm to the left and right with small movements.

Massaging the Abdomen and Chest

Now turn to your partner's abdomen and chest. Before you begin with this part of the massage, you should warm your hands. Hold your hands in front of your body with your palms facing, but not touching, each other. Focus your attention on your palms, and try to feel the warmth emanating from one hand with the palm of the other. This energetic feeling will transfer to your partner during the ensuing massage. Keep in mind that for this to happen, your hands have to be warm. The more frequently you carry out this exercise (see page 53), the more intensive and fine-tuned will be your perception.

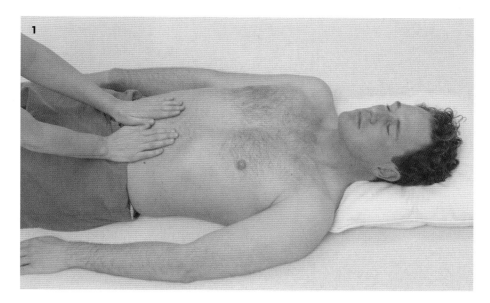

Place your hands on the abdomen . . .

Introductory Strokes (Figures 1 and 2)

Place your hands on both sides of the body's middle axis at the base of the abdomen, with your fingers pointing up the body. Glide your hands up to the outside of the shoulders, gradually increasing the pressure as you move. Return your hands to their starting position without losing contact with your partner's skin. Repeat until you have stroked the arm a total of ten times.

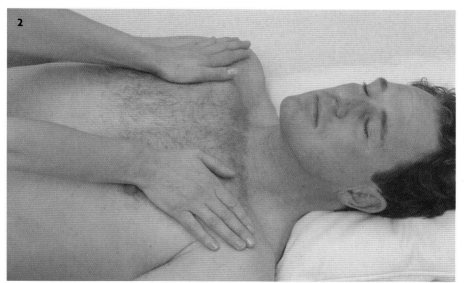

Kneading and Stroking (Figure 3)

Now knead the chest muscles from the armpit to the middle of the chest on both sides for two minutes each. Conclude with ten more strokes from the lower abdomen up to the shoulders, as described above.

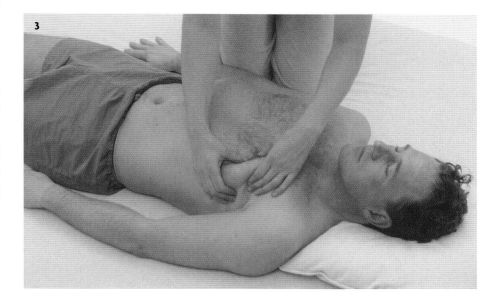

. . . and glide them slowly toward the head.

Knead the chest muscles strongly between thumb and fingers.

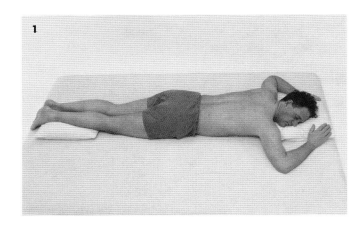

When your partner is lying on his or her stomach, you can relax the spine by placing pillows under his or her head and feet.

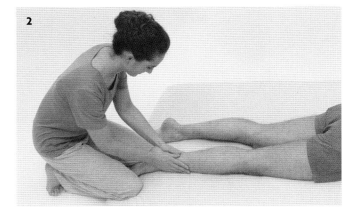

Place your hands on the inside and outside of the foot and stroke the leg up to the buttocks.

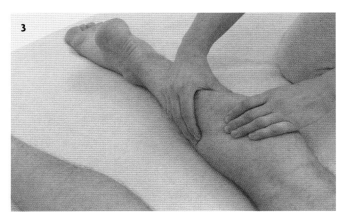

Knead the muscles of the calf . . .

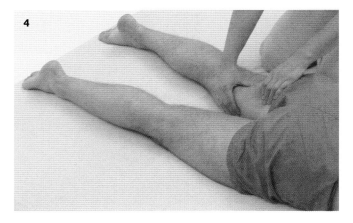

Left: . . . strongly with both hands.

Right: Conclude by kneading the buttocks muscles.

Massage of the Back of the Body

Now ask your partner to lie on his or her stomach. The following techniques will massage their legs and arms again, as well as the back.

Massaging the Legs (Figure 1)

To make this position as comfortable as possible, support the feet and head of your partner with small pillows or a rolled-up blanket. Depending on your partner's preference, his or her arms can be bent or extended along the sides of the body. Begin the massage on the right leg, carrying out the following techniques in their entirety, before switching to the left leg and massaging it in the same way.

Introductory Strokes (Figure 2)

Place your hands on both sides of the foot, that is, on the inside and the outside of the ankle, and stroke the leg from the foot up to the fold of the buttocks, gradually increasing your pressure as you move up. Return your hands to their original position, making sure to remain in contact with your partner's skin as you move, and repeat until you have stroked the leg a total of ten times.

Kneading and Stroking (Figures 3–5)

Now knead the muscles of the calf and the back of the thigh between your fingers and the base of your thumb. Knead the calf and the thigh for two minutes each. Then knead the buttocks muscles for another two minutes. To conclude, carry out another ten strokes as described above from the ankles to the buttocks.

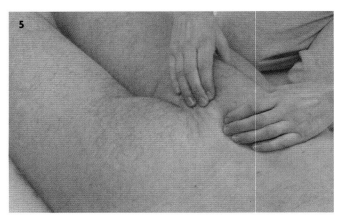

Massaging the Arms

Begin the massage on the left arm. After you have carried out the stroking and kneading, switch to your partner's right arm.

Introductory Strokes (Figures 1 and 2)

Stroke the arm from the wrist to the shoulder ten times.

Kneading and Stroking (Figures 3–5)

Now knead the muscles of the lower arm, the upper arm, and the shoulder. Then stroke the arm ten times again.

Shaking (Figure 6)

Conclude by shaking the arm muscles. To do this, use one hand to hold the arm by the wrist at a right angle away from the body. Place your other hand on the muscles of the upper arm and shake these gently but quickly for at least one minute.

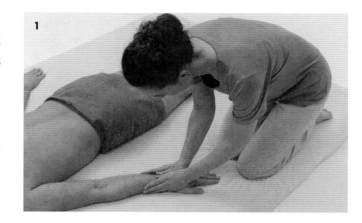

Begin the massage of the arms with strokes starting at the wrist.

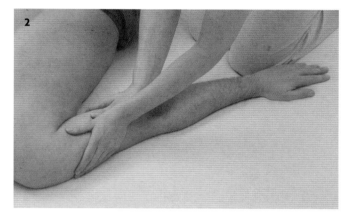

Continue up to the shoulder.

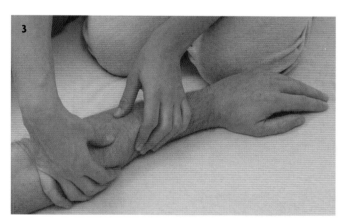

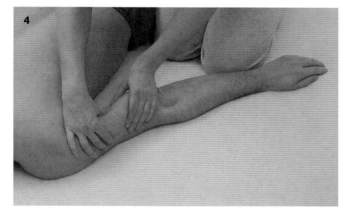

Left: Conclude with kneading the lower arm . . .

Right: . . . and the upper arm.

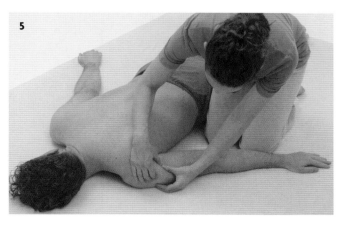

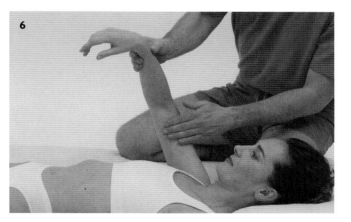

Left: Then knead the area between the upper arm and the shoulder.

Right: After you have finished kneading, shake out the arm muscles.

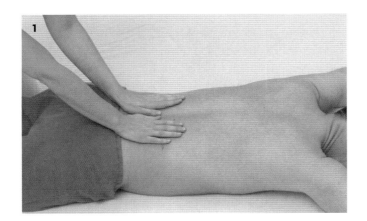

Stroke the back from the sacral bone . . .

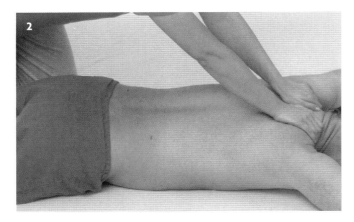

. . . up to the neck.

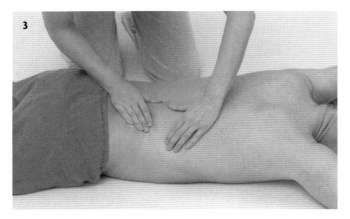

Then knead the muscles next to the spine.

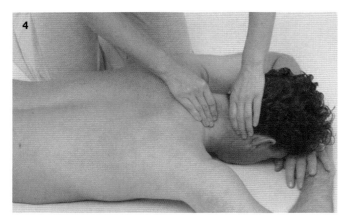

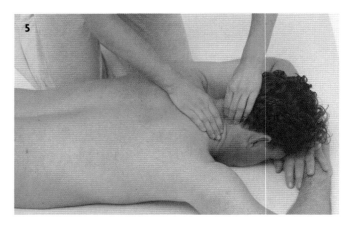

Left and right: Next, knead the neck.

Massaging the Back

Massage the back from the sacrum region up to the neck.

Introductory Strokes (Figures 1 and 2)

Place your hands on both sides of the spine on the lower back. Glide your hands up to the neck, gradually increasing your pressure as you go. Without losing contact with your partner's skin, return your hands to their original position. Carry out ten strokes in this manner.

Kneading (Figures 3–5)

Now knead the back muscles next to the spine. Begin in the sacral area on the side opposite you, and knead in wavelike movements up past the shoulder to the neck. Then massage the other side of the back. Next, massage the neck with both hands, kneading lengthwise in rhythmic wavelike movements for two minutes. Knead the muscles on the sides of the back again, beginning in the sacral area on the side opposite you and moving up to the armpits. Then switch to the side nearest you and repeat.

Circling Pressure (Figures 6 and 7)

Apply circular pressure to the muscles next to the spine from the lower back up to the neck, first on the side opposite you and then on the side nearest you. Make sure that your hands do not glide across the skin (rubbing) but that they are, instead, moving your partner's skin with them. Focus your movements on the depths of the body. Conclude the massage with ten strokes, described above.

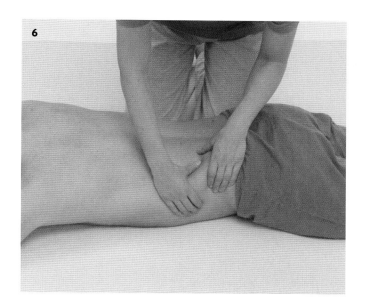

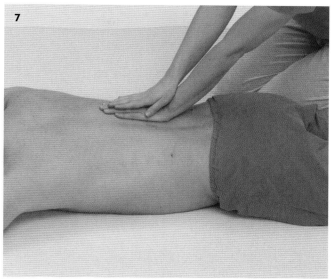

Left: Then knead the muscles on the sides.

Right: Finally, apply circular pressure to the muscles next to the spine from the sacral bone up to the neck.

Wellness Massage at a Glance

Head and Neck Massage

Begin on the head with a scalp massage. Massage the skin with your fingertips using small circling movements, passing several times from the top of the head to the sides.

Now stroke the neck. Place your palms with fingertips toward each other on the neck and stroke to the side five to ten times.

Now turn to the forehead. Stroke with your fingertips from the middle of the forehead outward, applying light pressure. Repeat the stroke a few times, moving from the eyebrows up to the hairline.

Stroke the cheeks outward from the nose to the hairline. Begin on the sides of the nose below the eyes and finish the massage at the upper lip.

Finish the head and neck massage by massaging the chin. Use two fingertips on both sides of the chin and stroke it several times from the middle to the sides.

Relaxation Exercises

The exercises have five steps: Turn your head to both sides, bend it forward and back, and circle it left and right. Then circle and lift the shoulders.

Whole-Body Massage

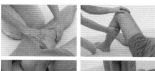

Have your partner lie on his or her back. Massage first the left leg from the foot to the groin. Then switch to the right leg. Make sure to always maintain broad skin contact.

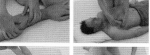

Massage the right arm and then the left one from the hand to the shoulder. Then massage your partner's abdomen and chest.

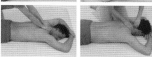

Have your partner lie on his or her stomach. Massage the legs and arms from bottom to top. Then massage the back from the lower back up to the neck.

Appendix

Overview of Acupressure Points

The following pages list all the points mentioned in this book, along with their location and areas of treatment. The exclamation mark (!) in the last column indicates that the point must not be massaged during pregnancy. On later pages you will find illustrations that show the anatomy of the human body and diagrams of the meridians that will help you locate the individual points.

		Name	Location	Indication	!
Lung meridian		Lung 1—Central Treasury	6 cun to the side of the middle axis and 1 cun below the collarbone	Ailments of the respiratory passages; pain in the shoulder or arm	
		Lung 2—Cloud Gate	6 cun to the side of the middle axis, in an indentation below the collarbone	Same as Lung 1	
		Lung 3—Celestial Storehouse	3 cun below the fold of the armpit, on the outside edge of the bicep	Problems in the respiratory passages; nosebleeds	
		Lung 4—Guarding White	4 cun below the fold of the armpit, on the edge of the bicep	Problems in the respiratory passages	
		Lung 5—Cubit Marsh	On the inside of the elbow, on the thumb side next to the tendon of the biceps	Problems in the respiratory passages (bronchitis, bronchial asthma); pain in the elbow	
		Lung 6—Collection Hole	7 cun above the wrist on the thumb side of the inside of the lower arm	Respiratory problems involving coughing and shortness of breath	
		Lung 7—Broken Sequence	1.5 cun above the crease of the wrist on the outside edge of the lower arm	Respiratory problems (coughing, shortness of breath); paralysis in the hand or lower arm	

	Name	Location	Indication	!
Lung meridian	Lung 9—Great Abyss	On the thumb side of the inner crease of the wrist below the ball of the thumb	Same as for Lung 6	
	Lung 10—Fish Border	On the outside edge of the ball of the thumb at the midpoint of the bone	Problems in the respiratory passages	
	Lung 11—Lesser Shang	On the outside lower edge of the thumbnail	Swelling in the mouth and throat; coughing; shortness of breath; loss or impairment of consciousness accompanied by high fever	
Large Intestine meridian	Large Intestine 1—Metal Yang	On the bottom and thumb-facing edge of the nail of the index finger	Acute infections in the mouth and throat area (gum infections, sore throat); unconsciousness	
	Large Intestine 4—Valley of Union	On the small muscle bulge that forms in web of skin between thumb and index finger when they make an O	Problems in the lower arm; colds accompanied by fever; infections in the mouth-throat area; constipation	!
	Large Intestine 5—Yang Ravine	In the indentation that forms on the thumb side of the wrist when the thumb is spread away from the hand	Pain in the joints of the hand; infections of the eyes and ears; ear problems	
	Large Intestine 7—Warm Dwelling	When the elbow is bent, 5 cun up from the wrist on the outside of the lower arm	Infections in the throat-nose-mouth area; nosebleeds	
	Large Intestine 8—Lower Ridge	4 cun from the elbow toward the hand, on the outside of the lower arm	Pain in the elbow joint or the lower arm; headaches; dizziness	
	Large Intestine 11—Pool at the Bend	Between the thumb side of the elbow crease and the knobby protrusion of the elbow bone	Sore throat; pain in the lower arm; psychological and psychosomatic problems; allergies	
	Large Intestine 13—Arm Five Li (Five Lengths of the Hand)	3 cun above Large Intestine 11	Pain in and limitations in the range of movement of the upper arm	

		Name	Location	Indication	!
Large Intestine meridian		Large Intestine 14—Upper Arm	7 cun above Large Intestine 11, on the outside of the upper arm	Pain in the biceps and shoulder; problems with lymph drainage in the neck, throat, or armpit; eye problems	
		Large Intestine 15—Shoulder Bone	With the arm extended to the side, between the front and middle part of the deltoid muscle	Pain in and limitations in the range of motion of the shoulder joint; itchy rashes	
		Large Intestine 16—Great Bone	On the shoulder in an angle formed by the intersection of the collarbone and upper shoulder blade	Pain in the shoulder, back, or arm; problems with the thyroid gland	
		Large Intestine 20—Welcome Fragrance	On the lower side of the nose	Nose problems; facial paralysis	
Stomach meridian		Stomach 9—Man's Prognosis	1.5 cun to the side of the upper edge of the Adam's apple, on the front edge of the sternocleidomastoid muscle	Infection in the throat and mouth; breathing problems	
		Stomach 10—Water Prominence	On the front edge of the sternocleidomastoid muscle, at the height of the lower edge of the Adam's apple	Infections in the mouth (acute tonsil infections); coughing and shortness of breath	
		Stomach 11—Qi Abode	Below the point Stomach 10 and above the collarbone	Acute infections in the mouth; breathing problems (bronchial asthma, bronchitis)	
		Stomach 22—Pass Gate	3 cun above the navel and 2 cun to the side of the middle axis on the front of the body	Acute and chronic gastrointestinal problems	
		Stomach 23—Supreme Unity	2 cun above the navel and 2 cun to the side of the middle axis	Stomachaches; psychosomatic problems	
		Stomach 24—Slippery Flesh Gate	1 cun above the navel and 2 cun to the side of the middle axis on the front of the body	Stomachaches; psychosomatic problems	

Stomach meridian

	Name	Location	Indication	!
	Stomach 25—Celestial Pivot	2 cun to the side of the navel	Menstruation problems; stomachaches; digestive problems (flatulence, constipation)	!
	Stomach 26—Outer Mound	1 cun below the navel and 2 cun to the side of the middle axis	Stomachaches; painful menstruation	!
	Stomach 27—Great Gigantic	2 cun below the navel and 2 cun to the side of the middle axis on the front of the body	Flatulence; stimulates urination	!
	Stomach 28—Waterway	3 cun below the navel and 2 cun to the side of the middle axis on the front of the body	Constipation; painful menstruation; stimulates urination	!
	Stomach 34—Beam Hill	When the knee is bent , 2 cun above the upper and outer edge of the knee	Stomachaches; swelling and pain in the knee area	
	Stomach 36—Leg Three Li (Three Lengths of the Foot)	At the transition from the knee to the front side of the shinbone, 1 cun toward the outside of the leg	Digestive problems; pain and range of motion and sensory problems, such as numbness, in the legs	
	Stomach 38—Ribbon Opening	8 cun below the outside indentation of the knee, on the front edge of the shinbone	Pain in the calf; pain limiting range of motion in the shoulder	
	Stomach 40—Beautiful Bulge	On the same level as Stomach 38, 1 cun farther outward	Respiratory problems; psychological and psychosomatic problems; illnesses with heavy phlegm production	
	Stomach 41—Ravine Divide	In the indentation in the middle of the front fold of the ankle	Constipation; headaches with dizziness; loss or impairment of consciousness; high fever	
	Stomach 44—Inner Court	On the edge of the skin between the second and third toes	Infections in the nose and throat; toothaches; headaches	

		Name	Location	Indication	!
Spleen meridian		Spleen 3—Supreme White (Venus)	On the edge of the foot, just below the base joint of the toe	Acute and chronic gastrointestinal infections; digestive problems	
		Spleen 6—Three Yin Intersection	3 cun above the highest rise on the inside of the ankle, on the back edge of the shinbone	Problems in the reproductive tract; problems with sexual functions; range of motion problems in the leg	!
		Spleen 9—Yin Mound Spring	On the back edge of the shinbone, just below the bulging part of the tibia	Pain in the knee; problems in bladder function; intestinal infections; tendency toward edema	
		Spleen 10—Sea of Blood	With the knee bent, 2 cun above the upper inner edge of the kneecap	Pain on the inside of the thigh; gynecological problems; allergies (eczema)	
		Spleen 13—Bowel Abode	4 cun to the side of the middle axis, slightly above the pubic bone	Tension and bloating in the stomach or intestines; flatulence	!
		Spleen 17—Food Hole	At the level of the gap between the fifth and sixth ribs, 6 cun to the side of the middle axis	Pain in the chest (intercostal neuralgia); difficulty swallowing	
		Spleen 18—Celestial Ravine	At the level of the gap between the fourth and fifth ribs, 6 cun to the side of the middle axis	Pain in the chest; stimulates milk production after childbirth	
		Spleen 19—Chest Village	At the level of the gap between the third and fourth ribs, 6 cun to the side of the middle axis	Pain in the chest	
		Spleen 20—All-Round Flourishing	At the level of the gap between the second and third ribs, 6 cun to the side of the middle axis	Lung problems (coughing, shortness of breath); pain in the chest	
Heart meridian		Heart 1—Highest Spring	In the middle of the armpit	Functional heart problems; paralysis and circulation problems in the arms	
		Heart 2—Cyan Spirit	3 cun up from the elbow, on the inside of the upper arm	Tension in the muscles and tendons; pain in the upper arm	

		Name	Location	Indication	!
Heart meridian		Heart 3—Lesser Sea (Yin Pathway)	Midway between the inside of the elbow and the protrusion of the upper arm bone	Problems in the arms; illnesses of the coronary vessels; sleeping problems; psychological problems	
		Heart 7—Spirit Gate	At the edge of the inside of the wrist, on the pinkie side, 0.5 cun toward the thumb	Illnesses of the coronary vessels; functional heart problems; anxiety	
Small Intestine meridian		Small Intestine 3—Back Ravine	With hand folded loosely into a fist, at the edge of the hand on the outside edge of the fifth base joint, at the end of the large crease	Eye infections; pain in the cervical spine; psychosomatic and psychological problems	
		Small Intestine 5—Yang Valley	On the pinkie side of the wrist	Pain in the wrist; illnesses accompanied by fever; headaches	
		Small Intestine 7—Branch of the Main Pathway	5 cun up from the wrist, on the outside of the lower arm	Psychological and psychosomatic problems; pain in the lower arm	
		Small Intestine 8—Small Sea	Between the tip of the elbow and the protrusion of the ulna	Pain in the shoulder; psychosomatic and psychological problems; colds accompanied by fever	
		Small Intestine 9—True Shoulder	When arms hang loosely to the side of the body, 1 cun above the back of the armpit fold	Pain in the shoulder and upper arm; lymph drainage problems in the neck, throat, or armpit area	
		Small Intestine 10—Upper Arm Shu	In line with Small Intestine 9, below the upper edge of the shoulder blade	Pain in the shoulder and upper arm; lymph drainage problems in the neck or throat area	
		Small Intestine 11—Celestial Gathering	At the transition from the top third to the bottom two-thirds of the shoulder blade	Pain in the neck, elbow, shoulder, or upper arm; lung problems	
		Small Intestine 12—Grasping the Wind	In line with Small Intestine 11, in a small indentation above the spire of the shoulder blade	Pain in the neck, shoulder, or upper arm	
		Small Intestine 13—Crooked Wall	At the inside end of the upper shoulder blade	Pain in the shoulder or neck; muscle and tendon tension	

		Name	Location	Indication	!
Small Intestine meridian		Small Intestine 14—Outer Shoulder Shu	At the height of the space between the first and second thoracic vertebrae, 3 cun to the side of the middle axis	Pain in the neck or shoulder; muscle tension	
		Small Intestine 15—Central Shoulder Shu	At the height of the space between the seventh cervical and first thoracic vertebrae, 2 cun to the side of the middle axis	Pain in the neck; problems in the respiratory passages (cough, infections with fever)	
		Small Intestine 18—Cheek Bone Hole	Below the outside edge of the eye, in an indentation below the zygomatic bone	Pain in the face; facial paralysis; trigeminal neuralgia; tics; illnesses caused by drafts	
		Small Intestine 19—Auditory Palace	With the mouth slightly open, in an indentation in front of the ear	Ear problems; trigeminal nerve pain; toothaches	
Urinary Bladder meridian		Urinary Bladder 2—Bamboo Gathering	In an indentation on the inside edge of the eyebrows	Headaches; sinus infections; eye problems	
		Urinary Bladder 6—Light Guard	On the line that runs 1.5 cun parallel to the middle axis, 2.5 cun from the hairline	Headaches	
		Urinary Bladder 7—Celestial Connection	On the line that runs 1.5 cun parallel to the middle axis, 4 cun from the hairline, toward the back of the head	Headaches under the roof of the skull	
		Urinary Bladder 8—Declining Connection	On the line that runs 1.5 cun parallel to the middle axis, 1.5 cun behind Urinary Bladder 7	High blood pressure; psychosomatic problems	
		Urinary Bladder 10—Celestial Pillar	1.5 cun to the side the middle axis, in an indentation just under the bony edge of the back of the head	Headaches; sleeping problems; pain in the cervical spine	
		Urinary Bladder 11—Great Shuttle	On the line that runs 1.5 cun parallel to the middle axis, at the level of the gap between the fist and second thoracic vertebrae	Problems in the upper respiratory passages; pain in the cervical spine	
		Urinary Bladder 12—Wind Gate	On the same line as point Urinary Bladder 11, at the level of the gap between the second and third thoracic vertebrae	Infections of the upper respiratory passages (acute and chronic bronchitis)	

Urinary Bladder meridian

	Name	Location	Indication	!
	Urinary Bladder 13— Lung Shu	On the line that runs 1.5 cun parallel to the middle axis, at the level of the gap between the third and fourth thoracic vertebrae	Illnesess of the respiratory passages (bronchial asthma); lung problems	
	Urinary Bladder 14— Pericardium Shu	On the line that runs 1.5 cun parallel to the middle axis, at the level of the gap between the fourth and fifth thoracic vertebrae	Cardiovascular problems; cough	
	Urinary Bladder 15— Heart Shu	On the line that runs 1.5 cun parallel to the middle axis, at the level of the gap between the fifth and sixth thoracic vertebrae	Cardiovascular problems; psychological and psychosomatic problems	
	Urinary Bladder 16— Governing Shu	On the line that runs 1.5 cun parallel to the middle axis, at the level of the gap between the sixth and seventh thoracic vertebrae	Stomachaches; abdominal pain; cardiovascular problems	
	Urinary Bladder 17— Diaphragm Shu	At the level of the gap between the seventh and eighth thoracic vertebrae	Asthma; nosebleeds; hiccups; anemia	
	Urinary Bladder 18— Liver Shu	At the level of the gap between the ninth and tenth thoracic vertebrae	Ailments of the liver and gallbladder; eye problems; psychological and psychosomatic problems	
	Urinary Bladder 19— Gall Bladder Shu	At the level of the gap between the tenth and eleventh thoracic vertebrae	Ailments of the gallbladder	
	Urinary Bladder 20— Spleen Shu	At the level of the gap between the eleventh and twelfth thoracic vertebrae	Chronic infections of the stomach's mucous membranes; digestive problems (diarrhea)	
	Urinary Bladder 21— Stomach Shu	At the level of the gap between the twelfth thoracic vertebra and the first lumbar vertebra	Acute and chronic infections of the stomach lining; stomachaches	
	Urinary Bladder 22— Triple Heater Shu	At the level of the gap between the first and second lumbar vertebrae	Acute and chronic gastrointestinal infections; digestive problems	
	Urinary Bladder 23— Kidney Shu	At the level of the gap between the second and third lumbar vertebrae	Sexual dysfunctions; menstruation problems; lower back pain	

		Name	Location	Indication	!
Urinary Bladder meridian		Urinary Bladder 24—Sea of Qi Shu	At the level of the gap between the third and fourth lumbar vertebrae	Lower back pain; painful menstruation	!
		Urinary Bladder 25—Large Intestine Shu	At the level of the gap between the fourth and fifth lumbar vertebrae	Lower back pain; disruptions of intestinal functions	!
		Urinary Bladder 31—Upper Bone Hole	On the sacral bone at the level of the first sacral foramen	Sexual dysfunctions; gynecological problems (menstrual anomalies)	!
		Urinary Bladder 32—Second Bone Hole	Below Urinary Bladder 31, at the level of the second sacral foramen	Gynecological problems (menstrual anomalies, infections of the pelvis minor); paralysis of the legs	!
		Urinary Bladder 33—Central Bone Hole	At the level of the third sacral foramen, below Urinary Bladder 32	Pain in the sacral bone region; gynecological problems (infections of the uterus)	!
		Urinary Bladder 34—Lower Bone Hole	At the level of the fourth sacral foramen, below Urinary Bladder 33	Acute and chronic intestinal infections; inability to urinate	!
		Urinary Bladder 37—Gate of Abundance	On the back of the thigh, 6 cun below the buttocks	Pain in the back and groin area	
		Urinary Bladder 40—Bend Middle	On the back of the knee	Range of motion problems and cramps in the legs; pain in the lower back area; stomachaches	
		Urinary Bladder 41—Attached Branch	3 cun to the side of the dorsal process of the second thoracic vertebra, at the level of Urinary Bladder 12	Pain in the shoulder, neck, or back	
		Urinary Bladder 42—Po Door	3 cun to side of the middle axis on the back, between the third and fourth thoracic vertebrae, at the level of Urinary Bladder 13	Lung problems (asthma, bronchitis); pain in the shoulders, neck, or back	

Urinary Bladder meridian

	Name	Location	Indication	!
	Urinary Bladder 43—Gao Huang Shu	Below Urinary Bladder 42, at the level of the gap between the fourth and fifth thoracic vertebrae	Pain in the shoulder, neck, or back; chronic bronchitis	
	Urinary Bladder 44—Spirit Hall	At the level of the gap between the fifth and sixth thoracic vertebrae	Chronic and acute bronchitis; bronchial asthma	
	Urinary Bladder 45—Yi Xi (Ow, That Hurts!)	At the level of the gap between the sixth and seventh thoracic vertebrae	Same as Urinary Bladder 44	
	Urinary Bladder 46—Diaphragm Pass	At the level of the gap between the seventh and eighth thoracic vertebrae	Chronic stomachaches	
	Urinary Bladder 47—Hun Gate	At the level of the gap between the ninth and tenth thoracic vertebrae	Chronic and acute gastrointestinal infections	
	Urinary Bladder 48—Yang Headrope	At the level of the gap between the tenth and eleventh thoracic vertebrae	Acute and chronic gastrointestinal infections; infections of the gallbladder	
	Urinary Bladder 49—Reflection Abode	At the level of the gap between the eleventh and twelfth thoracic vertebrae	Acute and chronic gastrointestinal infections	
	Urinary Bladder 50—Stomach Granary	At the level of the gap between the twelfth thoracic vertebra and the first lumbar vertebra	Acute and chronic gastrointestinal ailments; digestive problems in children	
	Urinary Bladder 51—Huang Gate	At the level of the gap between the first and second lumbar vertebrae	Chronic constipation; swelling of the liver or spleen	
	Urinary Bladder 52—Will Chamber	At the level of the gap between the second and third lumbar vertebrae	Problems of the male sexual functions; urinary tract infections; pain in the lower back area	

		Name	Location	Indication	!
Urinary Bladder meridian		Urinary Bladder 54—Sequential Limit	3 cun to the side of the middle axis on the back of the body, at the level of Urinary Bladder 34	Pain along the course of the sciatic nerve; prostate ailments; hemorrhoids	
		Urinary Bladder 56—Sinew Support	5 cun below the knee, between the two heads of the calf muscle	Calf cramps and pain; hemorrhoids	
		Urinary Bladder 60—Kunlun Mountains	Midway between the highest rise of the outside of the ankle and the Achilles tendon	Pain in the heel, lower back, or neck	!
		Urinary Bladder 67—Reaching Yin	Next to the outside edge of the nail of the small toe	Malposition of the fetus; weak contractions	!
Kidney meridian		Kidney 3—Great Ravine	In the indentation between the highest rise of the inside of the ankle and the Achilles tendon	Problems of sexual functions; illnesses in the throat and mouth	
		Kidney 6—Shining Sea	In the indentation below the lower edge of the inside ankle	Gynecological problems; chronic mouth infections; fatigue	
		Kidney 7—Recover Flow	2 cun above the highest rise of the inside ankle, in front of the Achilles tendon	Lack of or excessive sweat secretion; edema	
		Kidney 15—Central Flow	1 cun below the navel and 0.5 cun to the side of the middle axis	Constipation; menstruation anomalies	!
		Kidney 16—Huang Shu	0.5 cun to the side of the navel	Bloating; stomachaches; constipation	!
		Kidney 17—Shang Bend	2 cun above the navel and 0.5 cun to the side of the middle axis	Stomachaches; digestive problems	

Kidney meridian

	Name	Location	Indication	!
	Kidney 18—Stone Pass	3 cun above the navel and 0.5 cun to the side of the middle axis	Pain in the upper abdomen; acute stomachaches	
	Kidney 19—Yin Metropolis	4 cun above the navel and 0.5 cun to the side of the middle axis	Pain in the upper abdomen; acute stomachaches	
	Kidney 20—Open Valley	5 cun above the navel and 0.5 cun to the side of the middle axis	Acute and chronic infections of the stomach lining	
	Kidney 21—Dark Gate (Pylorus)	6 cun above the navel and 0.5 cun to the side of the middle axis	Acute and chronic infections of the stomach lining; infections of the esophagus; hiccups	
	Kidney 22—Corridor Walk	At the level of the gap between the fifth and sixth ribs, 2 cun to the side of the middle axis	Chest pains; acute and chronic infections of the respiratory passages	
	Kidney 23—Spirit Seal	At the level of the gap between the fourth and fifth ribs, 2 cun to the side of the middle axis	Problems in the respiratory passages; acute infections of the mammary glands	
	Kidney 24—Spirit Ruins	At the level of the gap between the third and fourth ribs, 2 cun to the side of the middle axis	Acute and chronic infections (bronchial asthma, chronic bronchitis)	
	Kidney 25—Spirit Storehouse	At the level of the gap between the second and third ribs, 2 cun to the side of the middle axis	Chest pains; acute and chronic infections of the respiratory passages	
	Kidney 26—Lively Center	At the level of the gap between the first and second ribs, 2 cun to the side of the middle axis	Acute and chronic infections of the respiratory passages (coughing, shortness of breath)	
	Kidney 27—Shu Mansion	On the lower edge of the collarbone, 2 cun to the side of the middle axis	Chest pains; acute and chronic infections of the respiratory passages	

		Name	Location	Indication	!
Pericardium meridian		Pericardium 1—Celestial Pool	At the level of the gap between the fourth and fifth ribs, 5 cun to the side of the middle axis	Lung and bronchial problems (cough, bronchial asthma); cardiovascular problems	
		Pericardium 2—Celestial Spring	2 cun below the upper end of the armpit on the front	Acute and chronic bronchitis; pains in the chest	
		Pericardium 3—Marsh at the Bend	In the middle of the elbow, on the side of the tendon of the bicep muscle	Cardiovascular problems caused by constricted coronary vessels; acute infections of the stomach lining; restlessness	
		Pericardium 6—Inner Pass	2 cun up from the wrist, on the line between the points Pericardium 3 and 7	Nausea and vomiting; pain in the lower arm; stomachaches; pain or constriction of the chest	
		Pericardium 7—Great Mound	With the wrist bent, in the middle of the fold	Psychological and psychosomatic problems; pain caused by constricted coronary vessels	
		Pericardium 8—Palace of Toil	On the palm at the spot where the tip of the middle finger touches the palm when making a fist	Psychological and psychosomatic problems; infections in the mouth; nosebleeds	
Triple Heater meridian		Triple Heater 4—Yang Pool	On the back of the wrist, in the center of the crease	Pain in the wrist, shoulder, or back	
		Triple Heater 5—Outer Pass	2 cun up from the wrist, in the space between the radius bone and ulna bone	Pain in the back or arm; headaches; problems in the respiratory passages, eyes, or ears	
		Triple Heater 10—Celestial Well	With the elbow bent, in the indentation behind the elbow	Pain in the upper arm; swellings of the lymph passages in the neck, throat, or armpit area	
		Triple Heater 13—Upper Arm Convergence	On the back of the upper arm, directly below the shoulder	Thyroid ailments; infections of the lymph passages in the neck, throat, or armpit area	

	Name	Location	Indication	!
Triple Heater meridian	Triple Heater 14—Shoulder Bone Hole	With the arm extended to the side, in the indentation of the deltoid muscle	Range of motion problems in the shoulder	
	Triple Heater 15—Celestial Bone Hole	At the end of the upper shoulder blade, about 1 cun up towards the spine	Pain in the shoulder; range of motion problems in the neck	
	Triple Heater 16—Celestial Window	Slightly below the mastoid process, on the back edge of the sternocleidomastoid muscle	Pain in the neck or throat area; hearing problems (hearing loss)	
	Triple Heater 17—Wind Screen	Behind the earlobe, in an indentation between the mastoid process and the lower jaw	Hearing problems (deafness, sounds in the ears); facial paralysis	
	Triple Heater 21—Ear Gate	At the front of the ear at the point where the upper edge of the zygomatic bone meets the ear	Ear problems (sounds, infections); infections of the trigeminal nerve	
	Triple Heater 23—Silk Bamboo Hole	On the side of the eyebrow, next to the edge of the eye socket	Headache; eye problems (cornea infections, muscle problems)	
Gall Bladder meridian	Gall Bladder 2—Auditory Convergence	In an indentation in front of the ear, on a line between the lower edge of the zygomatic bone and the ear	Headaches on one side; pain in the jaw; toothaches; hearing problems	
	Gall Bladder 3—Upper Gate	At the upper edge of the zygomatic bone, above the point Gall Bladder 2 and slightly toward the nose	Hearing problems; toothaches in the upper jaw	
	Gall Bladder 4—Forehead Fullness	On the temples	Headache on one side; high blood pressure	
	Gall Bladder 7—Temporal Hairline Curve	On the side of the head above the ear	Headache on one side; infections of the large parotid gland	

Gall Bladder meridian

	Name	Location	Indication	!
	Gall Bladder 8—Valley Lead	1.5 cun above the highest point of the ear	Headache on one side; balance problems; high blood pressure	
	Gall Bladder 12—Completion Bone	On the back area of the mastoid process in a small indentation	Headaches; pain in the cervical spine; circulation problems in the vessels that supply the brain	
	Gall Bladder 14—Yang White	When looking straight ahead, straight above the pupil and 1 cun above the eyebrows	Headache; sinus infections; eye problems	
	Gall Bladder 20—Wind Pool	Behind the ear, at the same level as and to the side of the point Gall Bladder 12	Migraine; tension in the neck; circulation problems in the vessels that supply the brain	
	Gall Bladder 21—Shoulder Well	Midway between the seventh cervical vertebra and the upper end of the shoulder blade	Shoulder and back pain; infections of the mammary glands	!
	Gall Bladder 25—Capital Gate	On the lower edge of the free end of the twelfth rib	Pain in the lower back; ailments of the urinary tract system; gastrointestinal problems	
	Gall Bladder 28—Linking Path	Slightly below the front iliac crest	Menstruation anomalies	!
	Gall Bladder 30—Jumping Round	At the transition from the middle to the outer third on an imaginary line between the buttocks fold and top of the buttocks	Problems in the lower extremities; pain in the sciatic nerve and the lower back	
	Gall Bladder 31—Wind Market	7 cun above the knee on the outside of the thigh	Pain and paralysis in the leg area	
	Gall Bladder 34—Mound Spring	In front of and slightly below the head of the calf	Pain in the knee; ailments of the gallbladder and biliary tract; one-sided paralysis	

		Name	Location	Indication	!
Gall Bladder meridian		Gall Bladder 39—Suspended Bell	3 cun above the highest rise of the outside of the ankle, on the side of the calf	Problems in the neck; pain; lack of strength	
		Gall Bladder 41—Foot Overlooking Tears	On the top of the foot between the fourth and fifth metatarsals	Pain in the foot, groin, or abdomen; one-sided paralysis; one-sided headache	
Liver meridian		Liver 3—Great Surge	On the top of the foot in the indentation between the first and second metatarsals	Menstruation problems; incontinence; difficulty urinating; range of motion problems in the legs and feet	
		Liver 8—Spring at the Bend	On the inside of the thigh, at the side of the knee in an indentation between the two tendons	Limited range of motion in the knee; problems in male sexual function; gynecological conditions	
		Liver 10—Foot Five Li (Five Lengths to the Foot)	3 cun below the upper edge of the pubic bone	Problems urinating; prostate infections	
		Liver 11—Yin Corner	2 cun below the upper edge of the pubic bone	Menstrual problems; fertility problems	
		Liver 13—Camphorwood Gate	On the lower edge of the eleventh rib	Gastrointestinal infections; diarrhea; acute and chronic ailments of the liver and gallbladder	
Governor Vessel		Governor Vessel 3—Lumbar Yang Pass	Below the fourth lumbar vertebra, at the level of the upper edge of the pelvis	Pain in the groin or leg	!
		Governor Vessel 14—Great Hammer	On the middle axis, in an indentation below the dorsal process of the seventh cervical vertebra	Pain in the neck or shoulders; fever; colds and flus	
		Governor Vessel 16—Wind Mansion	1 cun above the hairline on the back, exactly on the middle axis	Migraine; infections accompanied by fever; sinus and throat infections	

		Name	Location	Indication	!
Governor Vessel		Governor Vessel 19—Behind the Vertex	On the middle axis, 5.5 cun from the front hairline toward the back of the head	Psychological and psychosomatic problems accompanied by high blood pressure	
		Governor Vessel 20—Hundred Convergences	0.5 cun toward the nose from Governor Vessel 19, on the middle axis	Headache; dizziness	
		Governor Vessel 21—Before the Vertex	From the front hairline, 3.5 cun toward the back of the head on the middle axis	High blood pressure; depression	
		Governor Vessel 22—Fontanel Meeting	From the hairline, 2 cun toward the back of the head on the middle axis	Headaches under the roof of the skull	
		Governor Vessel 26—Water Trough	On the middle axis of the face, exactly between the nose and upper lip	Unconsciousness; psychological and psychosomatic problems	
Conception Vessel		Conception Vessel 8—Spirit Gate	On the navel	Pain in the navel area; acute and chronic intestinal infections	!
		Conception Vessel 17—Chest Center	On the sternum between the nipples	Asthma; stimulates milk production after childbirth	
		Conception Vessel 22—Celestial Chimney	On the middle axis above the bony edge of the sternum	Problems in the respiratory passages (bronchial asthma, hoarseness, loss of voice)	
Extra point		Yintang—Hall of Seal	On the middle axis between the eyebrows at the top of the nose	Headaches; dizziness; eye and nose problems	

The Skeletal and Meridian Systems: Illustrations

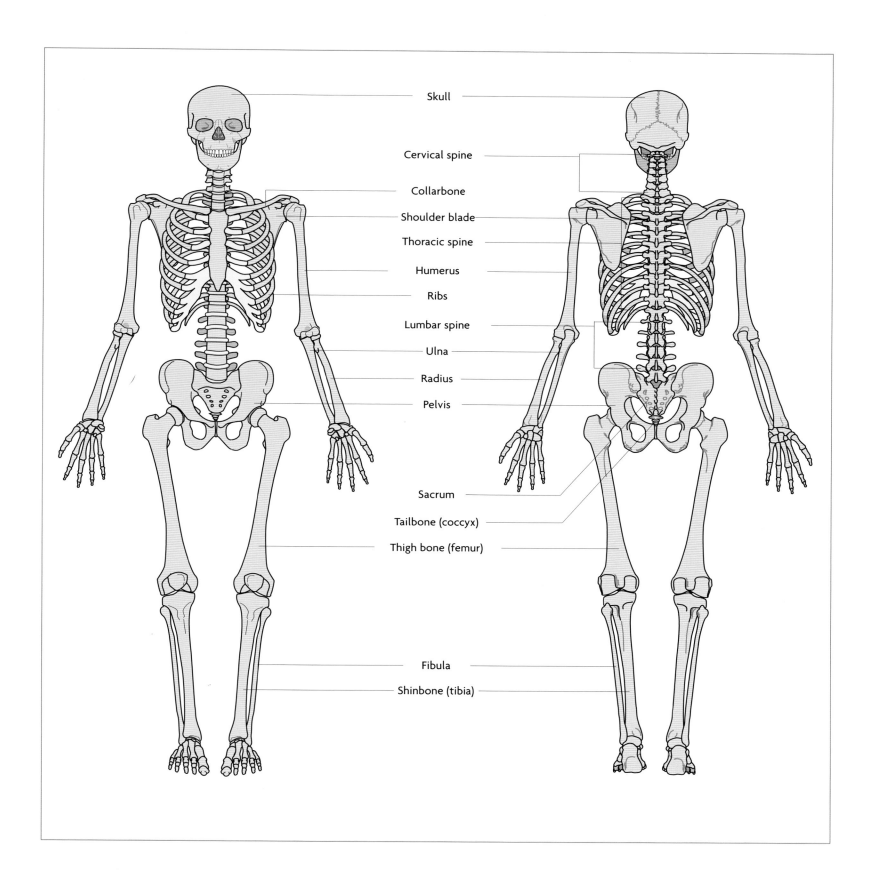

Skull

Cervical spine

Collarbone

Shoulder blade

Thoracic spine

Humerus

Ribs

Lumbar spine

Ulna

Radius

Pelvis

Sacrum

Tailbone (coccyx)

Thigh bone (femur)

Fibula

Shinbone (tibia)

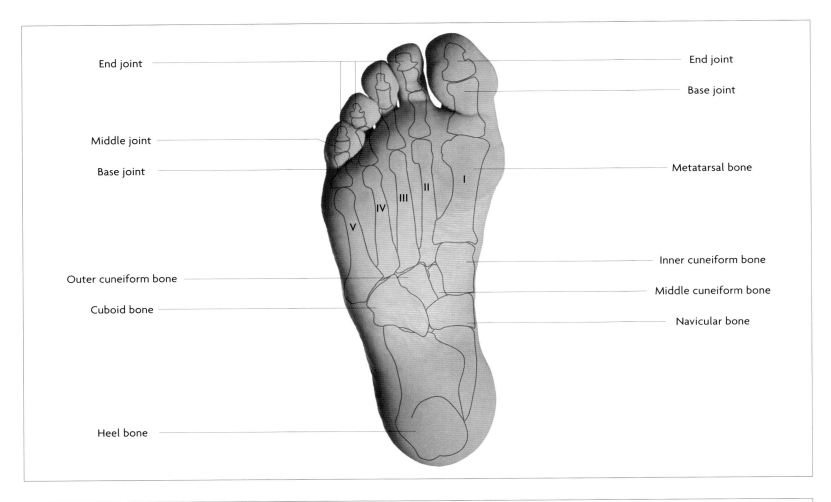

End joint —
Middle joint —
Base joint —

Outer cuneiform bone —
Cuboid bone —

Heel bone —

— End joint
— Base joint

— Metatarsal bone

— Inner cuneiform bone
— Middle cuneiform bone
— Navicular bone

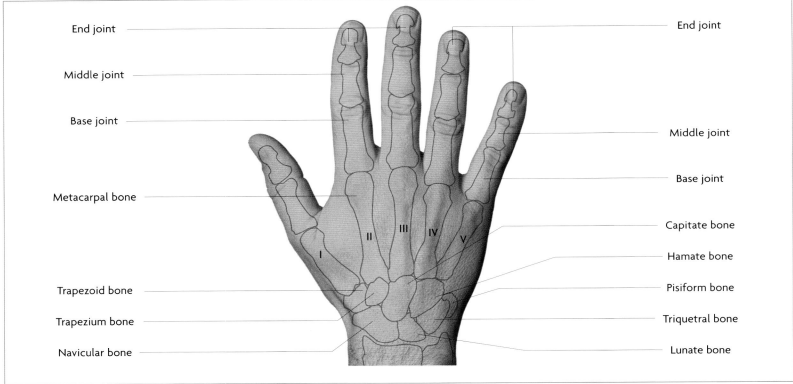

End joint —
Middle joint —
Base joint —

Metacarpal bone —

Trapezoid bone —
Trapezium bone —
Navicular bone —

— End joint

— Middle joint

— Base joint

— Capitate bone
— Hamate bone
— Pisiform bone
— Triquetral bone
— Lunate bone

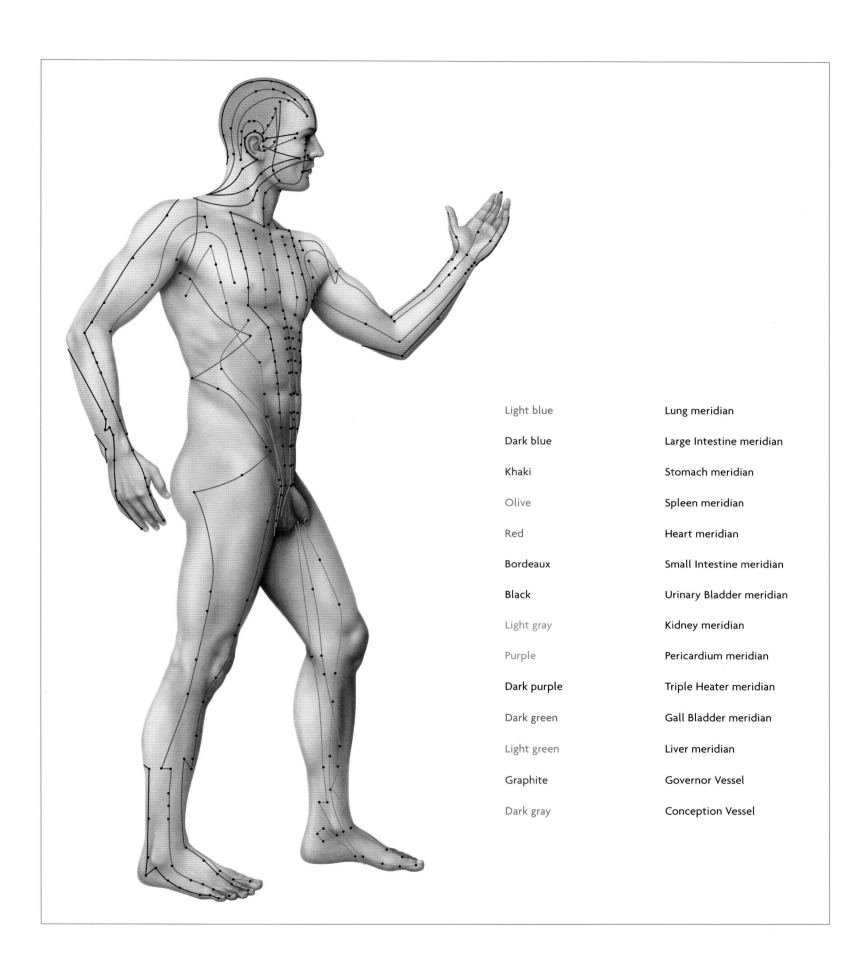

Light blue	Lung meridian
Dark blue	Large Intestine meridian
Khaki	Stomach meridian
Olive	Spleen meridian
Red	Heart meridian
Bordeaux	Small Intestine meridian
Black	Urinary Bladder meridian
Light gray	Kidney meridian
Purple	Pericardium meridian
Dark purple	Triple Heater meridian
Dark green	Gall Bladder meridian
Light green	Liver meridian
Graphite	Governor Vessel
Dark gray	Conception Vessel

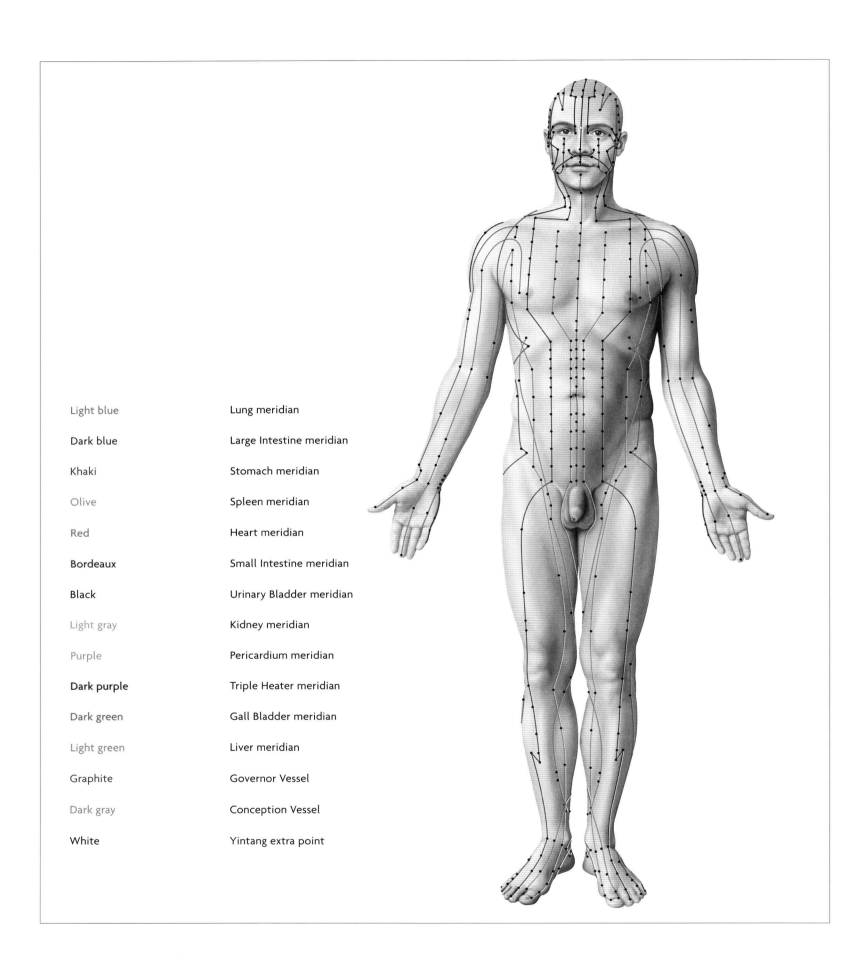

Light blue	Lung meridian
Dark blue	Large Intestine meridian
Khaki	Stomach meridian
Olive	Spleen meridian
Red	Heart meridian
Bordeaux	Small Intestine meridian
Black	Urinary Bladder meridian
Light gray	Kidney meridian
Purple	Pericardium meridian
Dark purple	Triple Heater meridian
Dark green	Gall Bladder meridian
Light green	Liver meridian
Graphite	Governor Vessel
Dark gray	Conception Vessel
White	Yintang extra point

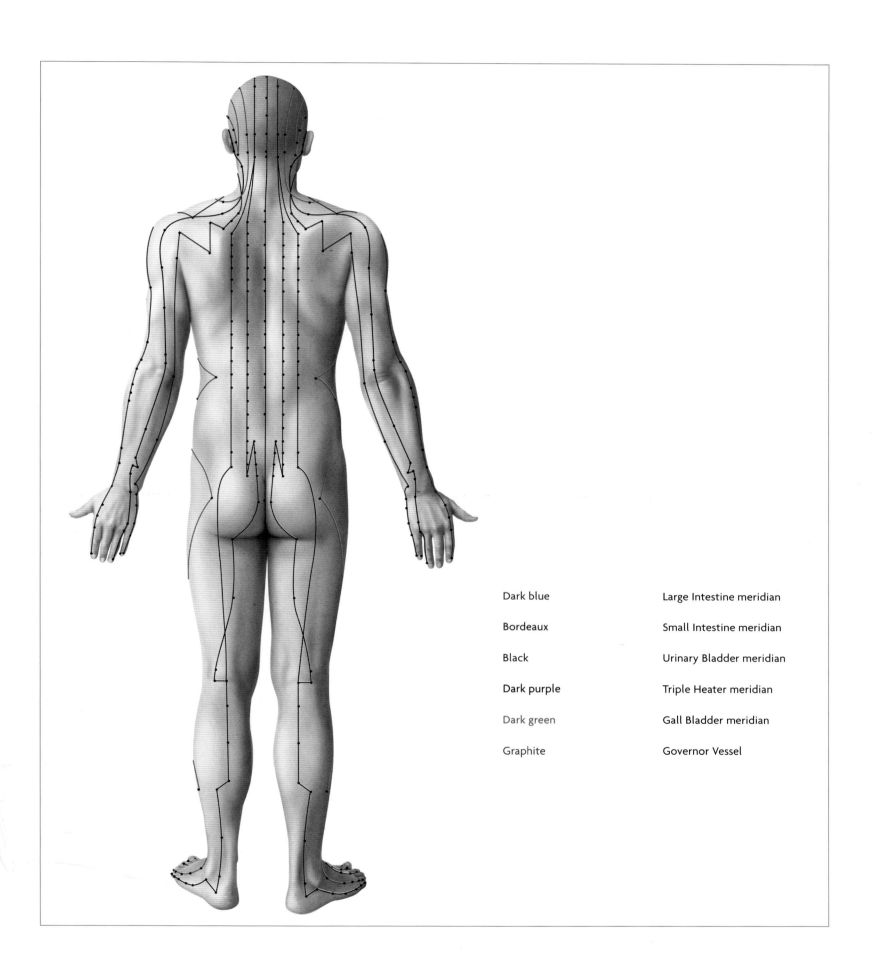

Dark blue	Large Intestine meridian
Bordeaux	Small Intestine meridian
Black	Urinary Bladder meridian
Dark purple	Triple Heater meridian
Dark green	Gall Bladder meridian
Graphite	Governor Vessel

Glossary

AMENORRHEA
Absence of menstruation.

ANEMIA
Deficiency of the number of red blood cells or of iron-based hemoglobin.

AUTOGENIC TRAINING
An easily learned stress management technique developed by German psychiatrist Johannes Schultz. Practitioners use repetition of a set of visualizations that induce relaxation.

AUTONOMIC NERVOUS SYSTEM
Autonomous, compared to the central nervous system. Regulates muscles of intestines, sensory organs, glands, blood vessels, heart, and genitals.

BRONCHIAL ASTHMA
Shortness of breath due to a sporadic contraction of the bronchi caused by an oversensitivity of the respiratory passages, for example during an allergic reaction.

CENTRAL NERVOUS SYSTEM
The part of the nervous system composed of the brain and spinal cord.

CONSTITUTIONAL TYPE
Refers to the entirety of the physical, mental, and psychological characteristics that a person is born with. A constitutional type also includes susceptibility to certain types of illnesses.

CYSTITIS
Bladder infection, meaning infection of the bladder's mucous membranes and in severe cases of the entire bladder wall.

DORSAL PROCESS
The back part of a vertebra that forms the visible relief of the spine on a person's back.

EDEMA
Painless, colorless swelling caused by a collection of watery fluids in the folds of tissue, for example in the skin and mucous membranes.

ENDORPHINS
Endogenous substances formed in the central nervous system that have relaxing and pain-inhibiting effects.

FACIAL PARALYSIS
Paralysis of the facial muscles due to nerve damage. Generally affects only half of the face. On the affected side, among other things the mouth can no longer be moved and the eye no longer closed.

FUNCTIONAL DISEASE
Disruptions in the function of an organ without recognizable damage. Clinical examinations cannot detect changes to the organ.

INTERCOSTAL NEURALGIA
Pain between the ribs caused by irritation of the nerves between the ribs.

LUMBAGO
Suddenly occurring pain in the lower back.

MOXIBUSTION
Chinese warmth treatment. Warming of certain acupressure points using specific preparations based on mugwort.

NEUROVEGETATIVE
Something linked to the autonomic nervous system, which regulates body processes essential to life such as breathing, digestion, and blood circulation.

PARASOMNIA
Term for abnormal sleep patterns or disruption of the quality of sleep.

PSYCHOPHARMACEUTICALS

Synthetic psychotropic substances, medicines that influence especially the central nervous system and have effects on psychological functions. They influence mood, affect, and emotions.

QIGONG

Breathing and meditation exercises of traditional Chinese medicine. In carrying out certain movements, practitioners focus the mind, reach internal calm, and guide the breath through the meridians.

SCIATICA

Pain caused by irritation of the sciatic nerve. Pain goes from the buttock region down the back or side of the leg to the outside edge of the foot.

SINUSES

Maxillary sinus, frontal sinus, ethmoidal sinus, and sphenoidal sinus: air-filled cavities surrounded by mucous membranes that are connected to the nose.

SINUSITIS

Acute or chronic inflammation of the sinuses

STERNOCLEIDOMASTOID MUSCLE

Muscle in the neck that moves the head. It is most noticeable when the head is bent forward.

TAI CHI

Traditional Chinese physical training to strengthen the body and prevent illnesses, and also as self-defense. Facilitates the harmonious connection of consciousness and imagination with breathing and the continuous, slow, and steady body movements. Similar to qigong.

TAOISM

"Tao" = way. Law of nature. Chinese philosophy according to which the world and all living things inside it are in a continuous cycle.

TRIGEMINAL (NERVE)

Name for a three-part nerve in the brain.

TRIGEMINAL NEURALGIA

Term for the occurrence of severe pain attacks in the area of one or several of the branches of the trigeminal nerve.

TROCHANTER

Bone protrusion on the upper end of the thigh. Differentiates into the greater trochanter, to which most hip muscles are attached, and the lesser trochanter, to which the groin muscle is attached.

TUI NA

A form of massage of traditional Chinese medicine consisting of about thirty-five techniques. Initially pressure-sensitive points on the body surface were pressed and rubbed; later, hard and sharp objects were used to increase the pressure. The main effect is stimulation of blood circulation and mobilization of stiff joints.

TWEEZERS GRIP

A grip used in acupressure in which the tips of the thumb and index finger join to form an O and pressure is applied between the tips.

YANG

The male principle in traditional Chinese medicine. Embodies the positive charge, activity, heat, light, strength, and summer.

YIN

The female principle in traditional Chinese medicine. Embodies the negative charge, passivity, coldness, darkness, inactivity, night, and winter.

ZHEN JIU

Chinese term for the combined application of acupressure and moxibustion.

Resources

Acupressure

AcuGuide—A Beginner's Guide to Acupressure

www.geocities.com/jrh_iii/acupressure/

Online guide by James Roy Holliday III that offers good illustrations of acupoints to massage for allergies, anxiety, fear control, memory, migraines, smoking control, vertigo, flatulence, heart attack, vomiting, and more.

Acupressure Massage Articles & Self-Care

www.acupressure.com/articles.htm

Hosted by the Acupressure Institute's main site, this collection of articles offers introductory information on acupressure as well as self-care practices for colds and flus and immune-system boosting. The Acupressure Institute offers acupressure training and certification classes.

Acupuncture/Acupressure Internet Resources Database

www.holisticmed.com/www/acupuncture.html

This website offers extensive acupuncture/acupressure links to articles, national and international organizations, practitioner databases, discussion forums, education and training information, and journal websites.

ACUXO—Interactive Acu Database

www.acuxo.com/index.asp

This acupuncture database allows users to follow the points and paths of each meridian using excellent illustrations. It also offers a library of conditions and acupuncture protocols.

Unihealth—Comprehensive Alternative Health Solutions

www.unihealth.ca/online_community/do.cfm

This commercial (pay-for-access) site offers information regarding acupressure and reflexology self-help for a variety of problems.

Shiatsu

American Organization for Bodywork Therapies of Asia (AOBTA)

AOBTA National Headquarters
1010 Haddonfield-Berlin Road
Suite 408
Voorhees, NJ 08043-3514
Phone: 856-782-1616
Fax: 856-782-1653
Web site: www.aobta.org
E-mail: office@aobta.org

The American Organization for Bodywork Therapies of Asia is a professional membership organization that promotes Asian bodywork and its practitioners. Its website defines several different forms of shiatsu and includes a state-by-state search page for locating certified member practitioners. It also lists schools with shiatsu training programs and provides links to other shiatsu-related sites.

Bibliography

Bahr, Frank R. *Akupressur: Erfolgreiche Selbstbehandlung bei Schmerzen und Beschwerden.* München: Mosaik-Verlag, 1991.

Beresford-Cooke, Carola. *Praktische Einführung in die Akupressur: Punkte, Praktiken und therapeutische Anwendung.* München: Hugendubel-Verlag, 1996.

Bihlmaier, Susanne. *Die Akupunktur: Lehrbuch, Bildatlas, Repetitorium.* Berlin, Heidelberg: Springer-Verlag, 2003.

Chaling, Han. *Leitfaden Tuina: Die manuellen Techniken in der TCM.* München, Jena: Urban & Fischer-Verlag, 2002.

Chmelik, Stefan. *Chinesische Heilkräuter.* Köln: Benedikt Taschen-Verlag, 2000.

Frohn, Birgit. *Akupressur und Shiatsu: Alltagsbeschwerden, Schmerzen und Krankheiten selbst behandeln.* München: Cormoran-Verlag, 1999.

Gach, Michael Reed. *Heilende Punkte: Akupressur zur Selbstbehandlung von Krankheiten.* München: Droemersche Verlagsanstalt Th. Knaur Nachf, 1992.

Gleditsch, Jochen M. *Reflexzonen und Somatotopien als Schlüssel zu einer Gesamtschau des Menschen.* Schorndorf: WBV, Biologisch-Medizinische Verlags-Gesellschaft, 1985.

Hin, Kuan. *Chinesische Massage und Akupressur.* Reinbek: Rowohlt-Verlag, 1997.

Kaptchuk, Ted J. *Das groß Buch der Chinesischen Medizin.* München: Heyne-Verlag, 2001.

———. *The Web That Has No Weaver: Understanding Chinese Medicine.* New York: McGraw-Hill, 2000.

Kolster, Bernard C. *Akupressur: Heilsame Selbstbehandlung mit sanfter Druckmassage.* Marburg: KVM-Verlag, 1999.

———. *Partner Massage: Gentle Treatment for Body and Soul.* Trans. Sandra Harper. Koeln: Konemann, 1999.

Kolster, Bernard C., and Astrid Frank. *Look After Your Back.* Trans. Phil Greenhead. Koeln: Konemann, 1999.

Kolster, Bernard C., and Astrid Waskowiak. *The Reflexology Atlas.* Rochester, Vt.: Healing Arts Press, 2005.

Kolster, Bernard C., and Gisela Ebelt-Paprotny (Hrsg.). *Leitfaden Physiotherapie.* Neckarsulm: Jungjohann-Verlag, 1996.

Lawson-Wood, Denis und Joyce. *Akupunktur und chinesische Massage: Theorie und Praxis.* Freiburg/Brsg.: Aurum-Verlag, 1977.

Lian, Yu-Lin, Chun-Yan Chen, Michael Hammes, Bernard C. Kolster. *Seirin-Bildatlas der Akupunktur: Darstellung der Akupunkturpunkte.* Marburg KVM-Verlag, 1999.

Ogal, Hans P. "Schädelakupressur." In Bernard C. Kolster and Gisela Ebelt-Paprotny (Hrsg.), *Leitfaden Physiotherapie.* Neckarsulm: Jungjohann-Verlag, 1996.

Pschyrembel, Willibald. *Pschyrembel: Klinisches Wörterbuch.* Berlin, New York: Walter de Gruyter-Verlag, 1994.

Schwegler, Johann S. *Der Mensch—Anatomie und Physiologie: Schritt für Schritt Zusammenhänge verstehen.* Stuttgart, New York: Thieme-Verlag, 1998.

Wagner, Franz. *Akupressur: Heilung auf den Punkt gebracht.* München: Gräfe & Unzer-Verlag, 1998.

———. *Reflexzonentherapie.* München: Gräfe & Unzer-Verlag, 1999.

Weinmann, Marlene. *Schmerzfrei durch Fingerdruck: 200-Akupressurpunkte gegen die häufigsten Beschwerden.* Augsburg: Midena-Verlag, 2001.

Xinnong, Cheng. *Chinese Acupuncture and Moxibustion.* Beijing: Foreign Languages Press, 1987.

Index